The International Behavioural and Social Sciences Library

COLLECTED PAPERS:
THROUGH PAEDIATRICS TO
PSYCHO-ANALYSIS

TAVISTOCK

CHILD DEVELOPMENT
In 9 Volumes

I	Delinquent and Neurotic Children
	Ivy Bennett
II	A Study of Children's Thinking
	Margaret Donaldson
III	Studies of Troublesome Children
	D H Stott
IV	Discussions on Child Development: Volume 1
	Edited by J M Tanner and Bärbel Inhelder
V	Discussions on Child Development: Volume 2
	Edited by J M Tanner and Bärbel Inhelder
VI	Discussions on Child Development: Volume 3
	Edited by J M Tanner and Bärbel Inhelder
VII	Discussions on Child Development: Volume 4
	Edited by J M Tanner and Bärbel Inhelder
VIII	Collected Papers: Through Paediatrics to Psycho-Analysis
	D W Winnicott
IX	The Child and the Outside World
	D W Winnicott

COLLECTED PAPERS

Through Paediatrics
to Psycho-Analysis

D W WINNICOTT

First published in 1958 by
Tavistock Publications Limited

Reprinted in 2001 by
Routledge
11 New Fetter Lane, London EC4P 4EE

Routledge is an imprint of the Taylor & Francis Group

Transferred to Digital Printing 2003

Printed and Bound in Great Britain

British Library Cataloguing in Publication Data
A CIP catalogue record for this book
is available from the British Library

Collected Papers: Through Paediatrics to Psycho-Analysis
ISBN 0-415-26405-7
Child Development: 9 Volumes
ISBN 0-415-26506-1
The International Behavioural and Social Sciences Library
112 Volumes
ISBN 0-415-25670-4

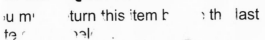

D. W. Winnicott

F.R.C.P.(LOND.)

Collected Papers

THROUGH PAEDIATRICS
TO PSYCHO-ANALYSIS

TAVISTOCK PUBLICATIONS

First published in 1958
by Tavistock Publications Limited
2 Beaumont Street, London, W.1

Printed in Great Britain
in 10 pt. Times Roman
by Simson Shand Ltd, The Shenval Press,
London, Hertford, and Harlow

Contents

PREFACE   *page* ix

ACKNOWLEDGEMENTS   x

PART 1

| I | A Note on Normality and Anxiety | 1931 | 3 |
| II | Fidgetiness | 1931 | 22 |

PART 2

III	Appetite and Emotional Disorder	1936	33
IV	The Observation of Infants in a Set Situation	1941	52
V	Child Department Consultations	1942	70
VI	Ocular Psychoneuroses of Childhood	1944	85
VII	Reparation in Respect of Mother's Organized Defence against Depression	1948	91
VIII	Anxiety Associated with Insecurity	1952	97
IX	Symptom Tolerance in Paediatrics: a Case History	1953	101
X	A Case Managed at Home	1955	118

PART 3

XI	The Manic Defence	1935	129
XII	Primitive Emotional Development	1945	145
XIII	Paediatrics and Psychiatry	1948	157
XIV	Birth Memories, Birth Trauma, and Anxiety	1949	174
XV	Hate in the Countertransference	1947	194
XVI	Aggression in Relation to Emotional Development	1950	204
XVII	Psychoses and Child Care	1952	219
XVIII	Transitional Objects and Transitional Phenomena	1951	229
XIX	Mind and its Relation to the Psyche-Soma	1949	243
XX	Withdrawal and Regression	1954	255
XXI	The Depressive Position in Normal Emotional Development	1954	262
XXII	Metapsychological and Clinical Aspects of Regression within the Psycho-Analytical Set-Up	1954	278

CONTENTS

XXIII Clinical Varieties of Transference   1955   295
XXIV   Primary Maternal Preoccupation   1956   300
 XXV   The Antisocial Tendency   1956   306
XXVI   Paediatrics and Childhood Neurosis   1956   316

BIBLIOGRAPHY   322

INDEX   326

Figures

1	*page*	109
2		109
3		109
4		110
5		110
6		113
7		114
8		114
9		223
10		223
11		223
12		223
13		224
14		224
15		224
16		226
17		226
18		227
19		240
20		240

Preface

THIS BOOK collects together various contributions that I have addressed to scientific audiences.

The student will not turn to these pages for instruction in basic psycho-analytic concepts and techniques. A knowledge of these I was able to take for granted since my audience was composed chiefly of analysts. I have been concerned with putting forward my own point of view and testing out my own ideas as they came to me in the course of my clinical work.

My clinical experience has been varied. I have never cut loose from paediatric practice which was my starting point. It has been valuable to me to keep in touch with social pressure, which I have had to meet as physician at a children's hospital. Also I have enjoyed the constant challenge of private practice and the therapeutic consultation. These interests have provided me with an opportunity for applying in a general way what I have at the same time been learning through the practice of psycho-analysis proper.

My hope is that this book will show that paediatrics is one of the legitimate ways into psycho-analysis, and indeed a good one.

*   *   *

It has been found convenient to group the papers into three sections. In the first section are reprinted two chapters from an earlier book (Winnicott, 1931), now out of print, and in these chapters is represented my attitude as a paediatrician prior to my training in psycho-analysis. I wrote as a paediatrician to paediatricians.

The papers in the second section can be recognized as coming from a paediatrician—one, however, who has become psycho-analytically orientated.

The third section is my personal contribution to current psycho-analytic theory and practice.

1957

D. W. WINNICOTT, F.R.C.P. (Lond.)
Physician, Paddington Green Children's Hospital, London W.2
Physician-in-Charge, Child Department, London Clinic of Psycho-Analysis,
London W.1

ACKNOWLEDGEMENTS

I wish to acknowledge my debt to my secretary, Mrs Joyce Coles.

I am grateful to Mr M. Masud R. Khan for compiling the index and for many helpful criticisms and suggestions.

Thanks are recorded to the following individuals, publishers, and organizations for permission to publish material that has already appeared in print: the Editor of the *British Journal of Medical Psychology*; the Editor of *Case Conference*; Mrs W. M. Davies and Jonathan Cape Limited for the poem 'Infancy', from *The Collected Poems of W. H. Davies*, which appears on p. 166; William Heinemann Limited; the Editor of the *International Journal of Psycho-Analysis*; the Ophthalmological Society; the Editor of *Psyche*; the Editor of the *Revue française de Psychanalyse*; the Royal Society of Medicine.

PART 1

Chapter I

A Note on Normality and Anxiety[1]
[1931]

BY TAKING the weights of a large number of children it is easy to work out what is the average weight for any given age. In the same way an average can be found for every other measurement of development, and a test of normality is to compare the measurements of a child with the average.

Such comparison may give very interesting information, but there is a complication that can arise and spoil the calculation — a complication not usually mentioned in the paediatric literature.

Although from the purely physical standpoint any deviation from health may be taken to be abnormal, it does not follow that physical lowering of health due to emotional strain and stress is necessarily abnormal. This rather startling point of view requires elucidation.

To take a rather crude example, it is very common for a child of two to three years old to be very upset at the birth of a baby brother or sister. As the mother's pregnancy proceeds, or when the new baby arrives, a child that has hitherto been robust and has known no cause for distress may become unhappy and temporarily thin and pale, and develop other symptoms, such as enuresis, temper, sickness, constipation, nasal congestion. If physical illness should occur at this time — e.g., an attack of pneumonia, whooping cough, gastro-enteritis — then it is possible that convalescence will be unduly prolonged.

Joan, aged two years five months, was an only child till thirteen months ago, when a brother was born.

Joan had been in perfect health till this event. She then became very jealous. She lost her appetite, and consequently got thin. When left for a week without being forced to eat, she ate practically nothing and lost

[1] From *Clinical Notes on Disorders of Childhood*. London, Heinemann, 1931.

weight. She has remained like this, is very irritable, and her mother cannot leave her without producing in her an anxiety attack. She will not speak to anyone, and in the night she wakes screaming, even four times in a night — the actual dream material not being clear (wants pussy, etc.).

She pinches and even bites the baby, and will not allow him things to play with. She will not allow anyone to speak about the baby, but frowns and ultimately intervenes. When she was put in a welfare centre she worried a great deal, and, having no one to bite, bit herself, so that she had to be taken home again after three days.

She is scared of animals.

'If she sees the boy on the chamber she heaves until she is sick'. If given chocolate she puts it in her mouth and keeps it there till she gets home, then she spits it all out again.

She constantly prefers men to women.

The parents are exceptionally nice people, and the child is a perfectly healthy and lovable child.

Now, had the new baby not arrived, with all that this implies to a child, Joan would have remained in robust health, but the value of her personality would have been to some extent diminished owing to her having missed a real experience at the proper age. Such an occurrence justifies the statement that it can be more normal for a child to be ill than to be well.

A doctor who does not understand the processes underlying such unwellness will think out a diagnosis and treat the illness as determined by physical causes. A doctor who understands a little about psychology will guess the underlying cause of the illness and take active measures to help the patient; for instance, he will instruct the parents not to make a difference in their treatment of the child after the baby's arrival, or will send the child away to stay with an aunt, or advise the parents to allow the child animal pets. As a prophylactic measure he will advise parents to answer fearlessly their children's questions about where babies come from, and generally to act without anxiety.

It is possible to go further and to say that a doctor who knows still more about psychology will be content to hold a watching brief, and do nothing at all, except be a friend. For he realizes that the experiencing of frustrations, disappointments, loss of what is loved, with the realization of personal unimportance and weakness, forms a significant part of the child's upbringing, and, surely, a most important aim of education should be to enable the child to manage life unaided. Moreover, the forces at work in determining the behaviour both of the parents and of the child are so hidden, with foundations so deep in the unconscious, that intellectual attempts to modify events resemble the scratching of initials on the pillars of a cathedral — they do little more than reflect the conceit of the artist.

To illustrate this 'normal unwellness' an obvious example has been taken, one that can be observed in any practice that includes the care of children from birth to school age. But this particular emotional situation has only a certain frequency, whereas every child experiences similar, or even more disturbing, internal and external emotional situations which he or she must live through, and discover means of facing and altering or tolerating. When actual situations are absent, imagined ones are ever present — indeed these are often the more powerful — and it is not necessarily the normal child that passes through the first few years of life without showing in delayed physical development and impaired physical health the existence of emotional conflict.

This aspect of symptom formation is one which enables the observer to catch a glimpse of the cause of an enormous number of childish ailments, and in any work on clinical paediatrics the part played by anxiety must be frequently discussed. Such an explanation of deviations from the normal has the advantage that it violates no biological principle. If enuresis is explained as a disturbance of the pituitary or thyroid gland, the question remains, how is it that these glands are so very commonly affected in this way? If cyclical vomiting is explained along biochemical lines the question must be asked: Why is the biochemical balance so easily upset, when everything points to the stability of the animal tissues? The same applies to the toxaemic theory of tiredness, the glycopoenic theory of nervousness and the theory that stuttering is due to lack of breathing control. All these theories lead to blind alleys.

The theory which explains these symptoms by giving to emotional conflict the respect due to it is not only capable of proof in individual cases, but is also satisfactory biologically. These symptoms are typically human and the great difference between the human being and other mammals is, perhaps, the much more complicated attempt on the part of the former to make the instincts serve instead of govern. And in this attempt is naturally to be sought the cause of the illnesses which are common in man and practically absent in animals.

If normal development leads often to disturbance of physical health it is clear that abnormal quantities of unconscious conflict may cause even more severe physical disturbances.

In spite of the recognition that ill-health may be normal, it is legitimate, from another point of view, to use disturbance in physical health as one criterion of psychological ill-health, and to say that a child's difficulties have become pathologically intense if physical health is so disturbed that, directly or indirectly, health is more than temporarily impaired, or even life itself is threatened.

At the same time it is necessary to remind a doctor who has under his care a child whose ill-health is due to difficult emotional development that he must keep a constant look-out for physical disease, not only because physical disease, e.g., encephalitis, chorea, etc., may co-exist with, and even bring out, anxiety, but also because continued debility due to emotional causes undoubtedly predisposes to certain diseases, such as, for instance, tuberculosis and pneumonia, by lowering general resistance. For this reason clinical medicine is complicated, but in early childhood complications can be unravelled which in adult life would be hopelessly complex.

ANXIETY

Anxiety is normal in childhood. The story of almost any child might be cited as illustrating some phase or other of anxiety.

Case

A mother came into my room at hospital carrying a baby boy of two months and leading a little girl of two years. The little girl appeared frightened, and said very loudly: 'He's not going to cut his throat, is he?' She was afraid I would cut the baby's throat.

The baby boy had an ulcer of the soft palate, and on a previous occasion I had told the mother he must not be allowed a dummy, as the constant rubbing of the rubber against the soft palate was obviously keeping up the ulceration. It happened that the mother had already tried to break the little girl's love of a dummy, and had once threatened, 'I'll cut your throat if you don't stop it!' and the little girl formed a logical conclusion, that I must be longing to cut the baby's throat.

It must be understood that this was a healthy little girl, and the parents, though poor and uncultured, were kind, ordinary people.

For a while my attitude of obvious well-wishing succeeded in reassuring her, but eventually the fears broke out again: 'He won't cut his throat, will he?' 'No, but he'll cut yours if you don't stop fidgeting,' answered the exasperated parent.

This new light on the emotional situation did not appear to affect the child, but in a half a minute she said, 'I want to wee-wee', and had to be taken post-haste to the lavatory.

This episode may be used to illustrate everyday anxiety in childhood.

Superficially there appears the love of the baby brother, the hope that he will not be hurt, and a request for reassurance from the mother. Deeper seated is the wish to hurt, due to unconscious jealousy, which is accompanied by a fear of being hurt in a similar way, represented in consciousness by anxiety. The mother's last remark produced deeper anxiety. This showed in no immediate obvious mental change, but in a physical symptom, namely, the urgent desire to micturate.

The following case, which is representative of innumerable others, illustrates the onset of anxiety without obvious cause:

Lilian, aged two years six months, is brought to see me because a month ago she woke screaming, and has since then been very nervous. She is the only child.

She was born normally and naturally. She was at the breast till four months, when she was put on to a bottle because the mother had a breast abscess. After this she was even more healthy, having been a little cross when on the breast.

She has developed normally and has been very contented; she slept so soundly in her cot beside the parents' bed that the parents congratulated one another. She had always been on the best of terms with both parents.

Then suddenly, without any ascertainable change in environment, the child woke up at 6 a.m. terrified, and said: 'There's no bikes in this room', and since then she has been a different child. In the night she has to have the side of the cot down so as to be close to her mother; in fact, several times she has had to be taken into the parental bed because of being terrified. In the day she is all the time scared, won't leave her mother, but follows her round, even when she goes downstairs to get water. Instead of being her own contented self, she now gets quickly tired of things, losing interest in one toy after another. Her appetite, now again good, was for some days very poor. She is always picking herself, and is fidgety and unmanageable. There are no physical signs of disease. Defaecation and micturition remain normal.

It is in the years between one and five that the foundations of mental health are laid, and here, too, is to be found the nucleus of psychoneurosis.

The importance of the feelings of early years can be proved in the case of any one individual in the course of a psycho-analysis, and is illustrated (as Freud and others have shown) in all forms of art, in folk-lore and in religions.

The knowledge of these details of underlying unconscious wishes and conflicts is of little or no direct clinical use, except in actual treatment by psychoanalysis. But it is often important to realize the intensity of the emotional strains and stresses even in normal emotional development, so that due allowance can be made for the anxiety basis of physical ill-health and abnormal behaviour.

When the child becomes four or five years old the wishes and fears associated with the position of the child in relation to the two parents or their surrogates become less intense, to be rekindled at puberty.

At ten or eleven years the child begins a new emotional development, according to the pattern of emotional development worked out in early childhood, but this time with physical development of the genital organs, and also with the power that comes with years to perform in reality what the child can only do in fantasy and in play.

The paediatrician, and the teacher and the parson, have great opportunities for observing the success or failure of children in this great early struggle, and without the desire to recognize the strength of the forces at work each must fail to understand the manifestations of failure to reach the ideal, whether it be in health, learning, or morals.

The following illustrates a common type of case where symptoms are apparently the result of alterations in the surroundings:

Veronica was a normal healthy infant until, when she was one year and five months old, her mother went into hospital and stayed there a month. The mother has now been home a month, and she brings the baby for advice because she is unwell, eats very little, vomits after food, and is nervous.

Whilst the mother was in hospital an unmarried friend, aged forty-three, looked after the infant. She seemed an ordinary sort of woman, but her treatment of the infant seems to have been tinged with cruelty. For instance, she kept a strap on the table as a constant threat to the child. The strap was to be used if she did not eat. Neighbours report how the child used to squeal, refusing food as a reaction to the apparent loss of her mother. But the woman was also fond of the child.

While Veronica was with this woman she grew nervous. For instance, it was noted by her father that she seemed afraid to go to him, though she had never shown fear before. When the mother came home and tried to undo the harm that had been done she only partially succeeded. It was some time before the child would go to her father without fear, and play again in a contented way by herself (she is an only child, another having died some years ago).

But besides the lack of appetite, for which the child is brought to me, there are also micturition and defaecation difficulties. Whereas formerly micturition was normal, now she has increased urgency and frequency by day, and enuresis, especially at night; also constipation has become obstinate.

At the second visit the mother tells me the child has pain with micturition, and for three days she has refused to defaecate. The urine is not infected and is normal.

The mother also explains that an attempt even to wash the perineal region gives rise to terror on account of the fact that the woman used to put her finger up the child's anus in order to produce a motion. 'You dare not let the child see a pot of vaseline.'

Formerly sleep was normal. Now the child wakes frequently and cries out for her mother.

Actual trauma, however, need have no ill-effect, as shown by the following case; what produces the ill-effect is the trauma that corresponds with a punishment already fantasied.

Helen, aged one year three months, is brought to me because of a cough. I notice a scar in the front of the neck and am told the following history:

When she was just over a year old, her brother, aged two, took advantage of his mother's momentary relaxation of vigilance to heat a poker and stick it in the baby's neck, just below the thyroid cartilage. He just did it for spite. He is rather a jolly and intelligent child, though apt to reply to his mother's threats with 'O shut up!'

The baby did not cry much. She was taken to the infirmary, where she was kept for six weeks.

The child seems to have been very little affected by these experiences. There is no symptom referable to the incident. She looks happy and well and does not show undue anxiety when the same brother snatches away a toy from her hand, and in other ways tries to provoke her while I am speaking to her mother.

In this case it happened that having a hot poker put against her neck corresponded with nothing already in the infant's mind. As a result little ill-effect can so far be noted. Nevertheless, when the child reaches a more advanced level of emotional development, anxiety will quite possibly be referred back to the incident, which may then come to represent to her the cruel assault that it was.

An obvious example of trauma that only caused illness because it touched on a sore point is the case of Peggy.

Peggy, aged ten, was a highly intelligent and vivacious child. She came to me because of the change that took place in her when a child shouted at her in the street words to the effect that she was not the child of her parents.

This remark of a friend made a great alteration in her, so that, instead of being clever at school and good at acting comic music-hall turns (dressed as a boy, with top hat and cane), she now became nervous, picking her fingers, etc. She lost her memory for facts, and had become unwilling, and indeed unable, to act. She started night terrors, and would get out and put her head through the bedstead bars and call for mum and dad.

From the same time she had increased urgency and frequency of micturition, and lost her appetite.

In ordinary conversation she showed big and obvious memory gaps. She could not even give the outlines of her life before she was six. Actually she was an adopted child; but it was useless to speak of this for she was quite incapable of taking in what was said. The facts were only elicited with difficulty from the 'mother' (Mrs B.), who said she had always avoided speaking of this subject with the child.

Mr and Mrs B. had had one child that had died many years ago. Peggy knows of the child. Peggy is by birth the only child of Mrs B's. sister; her father died soon after her birth and her mother neglected her. Mrs B. looked after Peggy till she was two, after which the child was taken over by Dr Barnardo's till she was four. Then Mrs B. legally adopted the child, so that for six years Peggy has lived with Mr and Mrs B. as their only child, calling them father and mother. The intention was that she should never have reason to question the truth of this satisfactory fiction. However, at odd times, and once when Peggy was five, a woman (the real mother) turned up like a bolt from the blue. Confusion had followed. Once the front window was pushed in, and the woman was arrested.

Peggy had, till the friend jeered at her, successfully avoided dealing with these facts in consciousness. She came to me one hour twice a week for about six weeks. In this short investigation I was able to learn something about her unconscious fears.

Very few people really believe in the unconscious. The majority of people would tell me to treat this girl by getting her confidence and then telling her the whole truth. However, this would have been futile because (1) she would not accept the facts, and (2) she was already in possession of them.

Actually the material that came forward during the superficial investigation had to do with the origin of babies, and with the facts of conception and of coitus. I can imagine two critics here, one saying that a healthy-minded girl of ten does not think of these things, the other that any girl of ten would have already found out for herself at least the rough outlines of the answer to these questions. The truth was that, although when she first came to see me she was most abysmally ignorant of such matters, as distrust gradually broke down she enlightened herself, practically without my intervention. Her observations of animals had provided her with all the information she wished for, but she would not accept it, preferring to believe in the origin of babies from pear trees, and so on.

As she grew able to accept the truth, so she became able to remember facts she had observed, and at the same time the symptoms arising from the friend's remark disappeared. Once more she held her own in invective, she did well at school, and could act comic turns again, and the facts of her own home complications became so unimportant that she took no more trouble over them.

It seems possible that the parents' taboo of sexual matters had been an important factor in her illness, more important than the unusually complicated nature of the home life she had experienced. Through meeting my attitude towards sexual matters, which was relatively free from anxiety, she was enabled to deal with the material that was already present in her mind. In other words, what the child needed, and got, was sexual enlightenment; but I did not directly enlighten her, I only provided a blackboard on which she chalked up her own observations. This could not have been successful in so short a time if she had been a markedly neurotic individual.

Physical Symptoms of Anxiety

It has been observed that anxiety often produces or is accompanied by some physical symptom. Frequently the parent brings the child for advice because of such a symptom, for instance, on account of frequency of micturition, or increased urgency of micturition or defaecation, symptoms that occur several times in these case histories. If the emotional situation is not inquired into, these children are liable to be diagnosed as suffering from urinary tract infection, worms, etc.

As a further introduction to the study of these physical symptoms and signs of anxiety the following case of anxiety hysteria is instructive:

Rosina is thirteen years old. She is tall and thin and has long fair curls. She is fully intelligent. Her father will 'only allow medicinal treatment', a fact which partly explains her unchanged condition over a period of five years.

Her mother is healthy and fairly sensible. Her father suffers from severe anxiety hysteria, and has been three times in a mental home. Probably in his case there is an underlying psychosis. There have been no other children.

Rosina was born one month prematurely after the mother had been in labour three days. The mother states labour was brought on by the daylight air raid over London in 1917. She puts down Rosina's anxiety directly to this trauma of birth.

Half an hour after birth Rosina cried, and she cried a great deal from this time onwards. She was nervous from the start, as soon as she could show signs of nervousness. From three to eighteen months she had minor convulsions asleep or awake, also attacks in which she went blue. At this time her father was at the war.

She was fed at the breast (supplemented) till nine months old. In infancy she was extremely constipated, receiving for this frequent injections till she was nine months old. Even in infancy she had 'breakdowns', in which she simply lay in her cot, and the doctor said she was exhausted on account of nervousness. At two years old she started to have frequent night terrors.

At five years, in spite of nervousness, she went to school and did fairly well. She was liked at school, and as she grew older, owing to her love of acting, was in demand for school concerts. However, she gradually gave up acting because excitement always led to illness.

At eight years she was first seen by me, being sent as a case of chorea. The fidgetiness was, however, not new, and was not like that of chorea. It was recognized that the restlessness was an outward sign of inward anxiety.

At this time it was complained of her that she would tip over the ink at school, and drop plates at home. She was always discontented. At night she would sweat excessively and feel very cold. Sleep varied; at times she would talk and sing in her sleep, at times she would wake frightened. There were no physical signs of disease.

In the course of the next few years she suffered in turn from innumerable symptoms, some obviously psychological and some simulating one or other physical disease. Never has any physical disease developed, and her heart has remained healthy.

Pains in the legs and across the instep on walking led to her being sent to me as rheumatic. There was no joint swelling. With this she had times at which she became extremely irritable and liable to fly into passions, after which she would cry, being very sorry, and have a headache. Rheumatism could not be diagnosed.

Soon she was sent to me as a case of cyclical vomiting, excitement always leading to bilious attacks and prostration. The father refused to allow her to go away on a holiday that had been arranged with a view to estimating the part played in her illness by her surroundings. She did well in an examination, in spite of missing much schooling, and was moved up two classes in consequence. At the same time she started habit spasms of two varieties.

At ten years she had joint pains again, and was kept in bed for some time. She was tired, discontented, fretful. Lying in bed made her nervousness worse. She became oversensitive to noise. A knock at the door terrified her. She could not bear to be left alone.

All the time a careful watch was kept on her heart. At ten years there was a heart irregularity which was shown to be due to premature ventricular beats. A shower of these would occur immediately the stethoscope was placed on the chest, after which they would occur very infrequently. This condition persisted for years. The possibility of subacute rheumatism at this time necessitated her being treated by rest, though it is possible now to say that she was not rheumatic (that is, liable to rheumatic heart disease). Wassermann negative.

She was next brought to me because of sharp pains all over, a generalized hyperaesthesia. She developed cramps in the hands, was very excitable, showed a tendency to lean up against everything. She was liable to sickness after eating fats. At times she had an excessive appetite, and had to be restrained from eating.

When eleven years old she often fainted. She suffered from recurring sharp 'pains in the heart', pseudo-angina, that made her cry. She would come over very hot and sweat profusely; or she would suddenly feel ill at 2 a.m., and be found to be cold and trembling, these turns being closely associated with nightmares. In the day she was incessantly blinking. Her skin became sensitive at this time, and she would easily get erythema patches that were very irritating.

When about twelve years old she came because of headaches, and continual nervousness. She must bite. She had a habit cough. If left alone she got what she called 'dreadful dreads'.

School became too much for her. She broke down, lay prostrate for days, and was so sensitive to noise that the 'rattling of tissue paper was too much for her'. She frequently woke up in extreme anxiety, seeing snakes everywhere.

At this time she still slept in her parents' room, and all attempts to alter this failed, partly because of the parents' unwillingness to give up the pleasure of having someone to make jealous, and partly owing to the child's own fear of being alone.

By day she dreaded bus, tram, and train. Any journey made her vomit. She vomited one Wednesday, and afterwards dreaded Wednesdays, simply because they reminded her of vomiting.

She became excessively anxious at seeing insects so that she could not go into the garden. She often fell down; if she carried an umbrella she would be constantly dropping it. She would hate to be asked anything, preferring to tell on her own if she made a mistake or did anything she should not have done.

This description of Rosina's symptoms rouses in the reader a feeling of nausea; it seems that the child must be so ill as to be uninteresting. But actually, in spite of unfortunate internal conflicts that absorb more and more of her energy, Rosina seems to be trying hard to be normal, and is not unattractive. She also has ambitions, and writes short stories that indicate a natural aptitude, though terribly inhibited.

Enough has been said to show that physical health is often disturbed in childhood as a result of non-physical factors. The ways in which nervous and nervy children may suffer from secondary disturbances of physical health will now be described in greater detail.

PHYSICAL CHANGES DUE TO EMOTIONAL CAUSES

One physical effect of anxiety is the tendency to produce thinness. This may be partly due to an increased rate of metabolism, and certainly anxious children may at times overeat enormously and obsessively and yet remain thin. But anxious children often do not enjoy routine meals, and are brought to the doctor because of lack of appetite.

Undoubtedly the ever-present anxiety is the chief cause of the thinness, but when sleep is disturbed by night terrors there is, in addition, increased debility due to lack of good sleep. It must be remembered that manifest anxiety by day need not be present, so that were it not for nightmares, or an excessive reaction to some trivial event — such as a dog jumping up or the passing of a fire engine — there would be little to show the true emotional state. On the other hand, the child may be anxious all day, scared of a knock on the door, or of seeing a spider, worried when the father comes home late from work, or upset by any show of hostility (accidents, quarrels between parents, chastisement of animals or of other members of the family, broken dolls, etc.). In such a case the cause of the debility is obvious to any observer.

Such a combination of thinness, pallor, liability to feverishness, liability to sweating, fainting, migrainous headaches, and bodily aches and pains makes the doctor suspect physical disease. Frequently the difficulty of diagnosis is increased by the fact that such children may have a temperature of 100 deg. F. when brought to the consulting-room.

Whereas a few years ago these children were classed as 'pre-tuberculous', they are now considered 'pre-rheumatic' by those who do not recognize the anxiety factor. They often have 'growing pains' — aches and pains in muscles and ligaments and in the chest and abdominal walls, and this makes subacute rheumatism seem yet more likely. The overacting heart, perhaps dilated during examination, leads to the child's being kept in bed as a rheumatic suspect. But in reality there is no rheumatism, and rest in bed is bad treatment for the condition.

Another common set of symptoms caused by anxiety includes fidgetiness, the compulsion to be always doing something, and inability to sit still at meals. Children so afflicted are a source of worry to parents and school teachers, and the doctor frequently makes the mistake of diagnosing chorea in such cases. The fidgetiness affects the whole child, is not more marked in the arm and leg of one side as in early chorea. Treatment by rest in bed is very bad for a fidgety child that has not chorea (see Chapter II, Fidgetiness). Increased frequency and urgency of micturition are common in fidgety children. Underlying the condition is anxiety associated with the battle over masturbation.

The anxiety state is always present or latent in such children, but symptoms do not necessarily appear all the time. Symptoms tend to appear in *attacks*, recurring at more or less regular times, with intervals of health. In this way the recurrence of colic or 'collywobbles' in these children may produce a picture closely simulating that of smouldering appendicitis, and has led to the removal of a large number of innocent appendices. Or, the intestinal hurry of these patients leads to a false diagnosis of colitis, and colon wash-outs can convert such innocent colon irritability into serious colon disease. If the proper diagnosis were known, such a colon would be left without local treatment.

Celia, nine years old, belongs to a healthy family. She has three sisters, all younger. Her mother stutters.

At times she gets attacks in which she has a severe headache, and vomits a great deal. She is at first flushed, and then goes deathly white. With the vomiting she yawns again and again. She also gets pain across the chest. The vomit is green and watery and seldom contains food; during the attack the urine is reported to contain a white deposit; sometimes there is associated increased frequency and urgency of micturition. After the sickness she is well again, almost suddenly. Sometimes during the attacks she becomes 'hysterical', laughing and crying and then lying prostrate. The attacks are not frequent; ten months have separated one group of attacks from another.

She is always a fidget — especially is this noticed at meal-times. 'There's no sitting in her.' Although a happy sort she is liable to be nervous. Knowing she was to see the doctor, she was so anxious that 'she wouldn't let her mother move, even to go and wash herself'. She goes to bed early, but lies awake for hours; she complains of headache, 'creeping pains'. 'I feel as if someone is chopping the back of my head.' There are no physical signs of disease.

If the intervals between the attacks of vomiting are regular and the vomiting is severe, the name 'cyclical vomiting' is applied; indeed this name has led to the mistaken view that recurrent vomiting can be a disease in itself. Really it is one symptom of underlying anxiety — except where a definite physical cause is present (such as some form of intestinal obstruction, subacute appendicitis, pyelitis).

Headaches, often worthy of the name 'migrainous', may recur in anxious children. In some of these cases the headaches are fairly clearly the result of frontal or ethmoid sinus congestion; in other cases no such mechanism seems to be operative. There may be associated convulsive attacks.

Periodic nasal and paranasal congestion is also a way in which the excitement of anxious children appears. It is as if they need to show rage, but being unable to let themselves do so (owing to the intensity of the feeling) they become congested in various places. Congestion of the nose leads to dryness of the mucous membranes, which not only leads to discomfort, the formation of crusts and nose-picking, but it is also a harmful condition. Mucous membrane in its natural state is moist, and it is probable that when dry it is a less efficient barrier against infection. In this way a hint can be thrown out as to a possible explanation of the recurring colds of over-excitable and nervous children and of children who are pampered, or are constantly being physically stimulated by someone.

Along with nasal congestion goes the tendency to epistaxis.

Children liable to asthma usually to some extent develop attacks in relation to anxiety — that is to excess of excitement over capacity for discharge. In some cases this is the important factor. Anxious children are liable to attacks of difficult or heavy breathing associated with night anxiety attacks, which are not infrequently mistaken for asthma.

Many children are brought to a doctor because they show a tendency to faint, especially at school during morning prayers or when standing is necessary in a hot room or along with a crowd of other children. This may lead to, or seem to confirm, a suspicion of heart disease, and may lead a doctor to keep in bed for long periods a child that is really healthy.

A boy was brought to me because he fainted in school. 'Anaemia, possible rheumatic heart disease' had been diagnosed. Actually he had fainted because, during the reading lesson, the word 'blood' had occurred, and he could not think of blood without experiencing extreme anxiety because of its meaning to him. He was physically quite healthy.

Similarly, the tendency to have fits is not always independent of the emotional state of the patient. Children liable to epilepsy may, especially in the very early stages, throw a fit where another child would be angry or terrified. In some cases the fits are only brought on in situations of emotional tension, and in the extreme case may only occur at the height of a bad night terror. Also, an anxiety attack may occur so suddenly, apropos of nothing, that a fit is suspected, though no tendency to true convulsive attacks is really present. Recognition of this is important, for treatment over a long period by bromide, which is of doubtful benefit to an epileptic, is certainly very bad for a child who is only anxious, and therefore not necessarily abnormal.

It is appropriate here to try to trace the mechanisms, in so far as they are understood, by which physical disease is simulated, or actually produced, by causes that lie in the emotional life of the child. It will be at once recognized that much depends on the child's ability to tolerate the amount of anxiety present. The ability to tolerate anxiety varies as well as the degree and content of the anxiety.

Any physical alteration that can be produced by hypnotism can also be met with in the medical clinic. The power of the unconscious over the body is only just being appreciated, but it seems true that metabolism can be reduced almost to a standstill, that the cutting of teeth can be delayed, that wounds can be kept from healing, and that hair can fall out, simply as a result of a deep-seated wish. It also seems that sores sometimes do not heal simply as a result of a general lack of interest on the part of the child, and of the tissues, in living. A new interest may revive both the child and the healing power of the tissues. Tissues other than the skin also show variations in healing power associated with the child's desire to live (e.g. recovery from pneumonia). It is fairly certain that lack of satisfactory oral gratification can delay infantile development, and produce late walking, clumsiness of movements, late talking, absence of ability to play and to establish contact with people. The mechanism involved here is not clear.

Better understood are the organ changes due to excitement. Erotic fantasies are normally accompanied by erection and sensitization of the glans penis (or clitoris) throughout childhood as at adolescence, and the complete orgasm with heightened pleasure, vasomotor changes, and rhythmic body movements, followed by prostration and sweating and desire for sleep, occur in normal children, including the very young.

One of the effects of anxiety over the fantasy material is to bring about a lingering at the early stages of the act and simultaneously there is likely to be an obsessive attempt to masturbate in order to compensate for the lack of self-confidence that results from the inhibition.

The effects of this prolonged excitation may be divided into hyperaemia, hyperaesthesia, and vasomotor instability.

A boy's penis may be observed to be always flabby and the skin of the scrotum not contracted. This lack of support of the testicles, combined with a general hyperaemia of the soft tissues, causes the neuralgia or dragging sensation of these regions of which boys sometimes complain. The continued hyperaesthesia of the glans may make games difficult because the friction of the trousers becomes intolerable. Balanitis and tender lymph-glands in the groin are associated with these events, and the corresponding disorder among girls probably includes the common vaginal discharge.

But more remote effects follow unsatisfactory forms of masturbation, and these have as their pattern the associated hyperaemia of the anus and hyperaesthesia of the urinary tract, muscles and ligaments, which accompany regression to fantasies of pregenital stages of emotion development.

The main tendency of a body that is altered by prolonged excitement is towards local hyperaemia. Stuffy nose is the common example, but almost any tissue can undergo a change that corresponds to erection of the erectile tissue.

Another tendency is towards sensitization of the skin resulting in anal irritation, a general urticarial reaction to irritation, or spontaneous urticaria.

Vasomotor skin changes show in the mottling of the skin of dependent parts, in oedema of the ankles, in 'poor circulation', and in certain modifications of the normal tendency to bleed from skin wounds.

In illustration of these tentative suggestions as to the mechanisms at work in the production of some physical disorders, the eye, the nose, the throat will be taken in turn.

The Eyes

Hysterical not seeing, symbolizing blindness (punishment for looking). No physical changes.

Anxiety over good sight (unconscious sense of guilt), constant self-testing leading to tiredness of ocular muscles; wearing of glasses for minute defects (resulting in destruction of good looks, neutralization of sense of guilt, better general health; also, on the other hand, glasses are felt to be 'swanky').

A child in a state of partial excitement looking at forbidden objects in order to derive excitement with tired eyes due, probably, in part to hyperaemia, and in part to the extra work involved in moving the eyes because of conflict—('I want to see' *plus* 'I do not want to see').

Obsessional blinking, another method of dealing with the sense of guilt over seeing.

Chronic blepharitis kept up by secret rubbing (masturbation equivalent).

The Nose

The main disturbance is congestion of continual excitement directly associated with anal congestion and excitement, and with fantasies of a certain nature. Such fantasies are cruel and are associated with extremely destructive wishes of which the child is not aware.

The hyperaemia results in

A sensation of stuffiness, habit sniffing, tendency to epistaxis.

Obstruction to flow of air, mouth breathing.

Dryness of the mucous membranes, with the formation of crusts and possibly a heightened liability to infection; and

Obstruction to flow of secretion from the sinuses with increased tension and resulting headache, and liability to sinusitis; moreover infected sinuses in such individuals do not recover easily, or tend to recur.

Usually associated with congestion is increased sensitivity of the nasal mucous membrane, and nose-picking. The destruction of mucous membrane, even leading to haemorrhage, reflects the cruelty that is in the associated fantasy material, of which, however, the child is chiefly unconscious. The parents' tendency to ascribe nose-picking to worms is an intuitive understanding on their part that the nose-picking really stands for anal masturbation.

The Throat

Hysterical mutism and aphonia (no physical change); these have direct symbolic value to the subject.

Anxiety dryness, sensation of sore throat, hoarseness with sticky mucus (desire to drink water to relieve dryness).

Anxiety may have associated with it the tendency to follow with the throat all talking and music, and even noise; this leads to tiredness and exaggerates the dryness and hoarseness. Many people, when they read, must follow what they read with vocal chord movements, as if they were reading aloud. This leads to tired voice and accounts for the advice frequently given to singers that they should not read before a recital. An anxious situation increases this tiresome throat, and it seems clear that much unconscious hostility is dealt with by the symptom.

This condition may be used as a hysterical symptom (punishment by loss of beautiful voice, relief of sense of guilt over good voice) in a patient who would not develop hysterical aphonia.

Alone or added to these disorders may be an obsessional hawking. In so far as this tends to make the voice worse, this will also be a self-destruction.

Sometimes a boy at puberty cannot make use of the new power of manly speech, but either must speak falsetto, or else unconsciously imitate the voice of a girl or woman he has known. This may lead to throat tiredness, and is quite likely to be associated with anxious throat. A girl may, in a similar way, speak at a low pitch and imitate manly speech, or the speech of a man she has known, but this is less likely to be associated with secondary physical change.

Most of these symptom-formations, like physical disease, can be used by a child (unconsciously) for the gratification of unconscious wishes and the neutralization of a sense of guilt (also unconscious); or a child may, so to speak, specialize in one or other morbid tendency according to the interest taken in the disorder (as when the doctor calls it by a name, or orders some interesting form of treatment); also the inconvenience resulting from the symptom with its treatment is often particularly well suited to the neutralization of guilt, as when tachycardia prevents (as it should not) indulgence in sports of which a boy is very fond, but about which he feels guilty when he is successful, or when recurring headaches (not due to vision defect) prevent a girl from reading books which she is reading in the hope or fear that they may give sexual enlightenment.

It is because of the tendency to make a hysterical mountain out of an anxiety molehill that it is essential that doctors should get a clear knowledge of the common anxiety picture; for it is important that such physically healthy but emotionally unstable children should not be labelled as suffering from rheumatism, chronic appendicitis, colitis, etc., and be kept in bed — perhaps for months — or possibly be subjected to an operation.

Moreover, by understanding management of an anxious child, which usually means inactive observation *without anxiety on the part of the doctor*, return to health can in many cases be hastened.

PHYSICAL CAUSES OF NERVOUSNESS

In this study of the common causes of nervousness emphasis has been laid on its non-physical basis. It is the non-physical basis that tends to be ignored, owing to unwillingness on the part of doctors and others to recognize the unconscious, and to admit the importance and intensity of childish erotism and hostility.

But physical disease itself may profoundly alter a patient's psychological state. An everyday example of this truth is provided by the feverish patient who temporarily speaks nonsense, gets over-excited by the visit of a relative, or may even become maniacal. Sometimes the only clinical manifestation of pneumonia is acute mania, or delirium.

Disease of the brain is capable of producing alteration of temperament to any degree, and can affect the happiness, reliability, intelligence, or mental speed of the patient attacked. A common example is chorea, which causes emotional instability, exaggerated reactions, and fluctuating control.

Encephalitis lethargica, as a result of its epidemic nature, may at any time become a common cause of altered personality due to brain disease. Immoral, unsocial, neurotic, or psychotic behaviour may appear in a previously normal individual as a result of encephalitis, chiefly by modification of the forces that lead normal human beings to become more or less civilized. The brain disease has upset the nice balance.

Apart from chorea, an increase of nervousness accompanies rheumatic fever, whether acute or smouldering. This suggests an interesting problem which can be stated as follows:

Does active rheumatic fever cause emotional instability? Does nervousness predispose to rheumatic fever? Are there nervous children whose nervousness is caused by rheumatic fever that is not at the moment manifesting itself in any other way (absence of arthritis, carditis, chorea, etc.)?

1. The first proposition is undeniably true and is generally accepted.

2. It is not certain whether nervousness predisposes to rheumatic fever.

3. It must be admitted as a possibility that in rare cases emotional instability might be due to rheumatic fever prior to the appearance of arthritis, carditis, etc.; this would then be an unusual mode of onset of rheumatism. Latent rheumatism is not, however, a common cause of nervousness.

ANXIETY MASKING PHYSICAL DISEASE

Real physical illness, occurring in a nervous child, may be masked by the anxiety symptoms. Not only does feverishness increase the liability to emotional disturbance, but also a child may be so alarmed at having a pain, or at feeling ill, that the resulting symptoms of alarm may mask the real disease, such as rheumatic heart disease, influenza, tuberculous disease of the spine or hips, poliomyelitis.

Further, anxiety may lead to incomplete physical examination, as when the struggle against accepting a spatula leads the doctor to miss diphtheria, or when the child's fear of being undressed causes failure to find rheumatic nodules, or heart disease, or an inflamed peritoneum. Lastly, a nervous child can appear to be full of energy and life when he or she is in a physical state that would make a more normal child lie prostrate and exhausted, the idea of illness being symbolical of something so laden with guilt that to be ill has become, for the particular child, impossible.

Chapter II

Fidgetiness[1]
[1931]

THREE KINDS of fidgetiness are commonly met with in general practice: fidgetiness of anxious excitement, tics, and chorea. As the last, which is less common than the other two, carries with it a liability to rheumatic fever and heart disease, the differential diagnosis between one kind of fidgetiness and another is a matter of importance. A mistake may mean either that a child who is not liable to heart disease is kept in bed when he would be better up and about, or else that a child with chorea is punished at school for fidgetiness that is not under voluntary control, and made to do drill and play games just when the heart should be allowed the maximum rest. Either mistake is deplorable.

Fortunately each kind of fidgetiness has its distinguishing features, so that, assuming reasonable care, only seldom need there be any doubt as to diagnosis.

COMMON ANXIOUS RESTLESSNESS

Common fidgetiness has no physical basis, is quite unrelated to chorea, and consequently to rheumatic heart disease, and is usually best left untreated, and as far as possible unnoticed.

Usually this common fidgetiness does not appear as a new thing, but is, so to speak, part of the child's nature, and for this reason can be distinguished from chorea on the history alone.

Sometimes there is a history of onset following some event that was so exciting or so productive of anxiety that the child could not deal with it, the idea behind the event producing feelings that the child found intolerable. Such an event might be too sudden and unexpected, as when a sudden gale blows open the window, and the door bangs, and all is in confusion; or too great fear or

[1] From *Clinical Notes on Disorders of Childhood*. London, Heinemann, 1931.

rage may be evoked by some event such as unwanted sexual enlightenment, the sight of the parents in bed together, or witnessing a quarrel between adults, the birth of a baby brother or sister, the sight of a man with a paralysed leg, or of someone's false teeth, etc., etc. (Chorea can also start after some such anxiety-producing event, or after mental striving, as for an examination.)

These excited, fidgety children must always be doing something or going somewhere. Excitement leads immediately to increased fidgetiness (as also in chorea). Whereas the movements of chorea possess the child, the movements of the anxious child are part of the child's effort to master the anxiety. The child is a 'worry', is restless, is up to mischief if left with a moment unoccupied, and is impossible at table, either eating food as if someone would snatch it away, or else liable to upset tumblers or spill the tea, so that everyone is glad to grant the request 'May I get down?'

All manner of variations are found: one child is unbearable at home but as good as gold at school; another is sent to the doctor by the teacher as a case of chorea, while the parent has noticed no abnormality.

The underlying condition is anxiety, and usually other evidence of anxiety is to be found. The commonest other symptom is increased urgency and frequency of micturition. There may be increased urgency of defaecation with or without colic, or attacks of severe colic alone, causing pallor and prostration, but soon over. Sleep is usually restless. There may also be an apparent lack of need for sleep, so that the child is the last to go to sleep and the first up in the morning. Sleep may be disturbed by night terrors, though this is not as characteristic of these 'nervy' children as it is of the 'nervous' child. For these children are over-excitable or 'nervy' rather than nervous of things, people, the dark, being alone, etc. Of course, the two conditions are frequently blended.

Such a child makes friends, plays wildly all day long, and is often happy, though irritable if restricted in activity. Picturing such a child one remembers countless children of between five and ten years old, thin and wiry, quick in the uptake and eager.

REPEATED MOVEMENTS—TICS

It is also an everyday experience to meet with repeated movements — blinking, head-jerking, shoulder-shrugging — in physically healthy children. Some movement, perhaps originally designed with some purpose, has become an obsessive act. The fact that the same movement is exactly repeated enables chorea and common fidgetiness to be ruled out in the diagnosis. A tic may persist when a child also develops chorea, or tics may occur in excitable children. Obviously, local conditions should be investigated — for instance the eyes tested in a case of blinking — but the abnormality lies in the internal need to perform the repeated act, so that if one movement is cured the likelihood is that some other movement will appear. The best treatment is to leave the movement unnoticed. It may persist, but in that case the various treatments that are usually prescribed would not have affected it.

CHOREA

Nothing is more easy than the diagnosis of a straightforward case of chorea by someone who is familiar with the picture of the disease. The child is kept restless by unintentional movements of odd muscles, no one movement being repeated, no one part of the body being entirely quiet. Speech tumbles over itself and becomes unintelligible; walking becomes dangerous; even lying supine is an exhausting task. Emotional instability is shown in alternate jerky smiling and uncontrolled crying.

The characteristic explosive responses are brought out when the child is told to put out the tongue and then allowed to draw it in again. If, when the child tries to maintain a grip on the doctor's fingers, the doctor forces the child's hand alternately into pronation and supination, the choreic child tends to lose grip and to grip again each time the position is changed and the new position reached; a child that is not suffering from chorea can maintain an even grip continuously during passive movements of the forearm. A child with chorea, unless too jerky to hold a pencil, will draw a line on paper that demonstrates both irregular control and over-compensation. If a choreic child obeys the order to hold out the hands in front of the body with the fingers spread and extended, it is typical for the hands to be flexed at the wrists and the fingers hyper-extended. If the movements are more pronounced on one side it is on that side that this position of the hands and fingers is most marked.

There is also a unique quality about choreic movements that defies description, so that typical chorea becomes one of the diseases that is diagnosed as soon as the child is seen — indeed in hospital the ideal time to diagnose slight chorea is often when another patient is being examined and the choreic child, as yet unselfconscious, is waiting to be seen next.

Chorea is a physical brain-tissue disease intimately associated with rheumatic sore throat, arthritis, carditis. The brain tissue change must be more of the nature of oedema than inflammatory reaction, for no permanent symptom or sign ever results.

Recovery from chorea can be confidently expected, and can sometimes be slightly hastened by aspirin. The only danger is from the associated rheumatic carditis. The majority of chorea attacks are uncomplicated, but they tend to recur, and eventually rheumatic arthritis or carditis appears instead of, or in association with, the chorea. It is a little unusual for carditis to complicate chorea in a child who has not, or has not at some time had, rheumatic joint swelling.

Typically chorea starts on a certain day, with paresis of an arm and leg on one side associated with involuntary movements of the same arm and leg. Either paresis or movements may be present alone at the start. *It is quite rare for the movements to be symmetrical at the start*, though they usually become generalized after a few days. When the movements are localized they never affect the upper limb on one side and the lower limb on the other, and it is very seldom that movements are noticed in one limb and are not demonstrable in the other limb of the same side.

The paresis is made more obvious by incoordination, and also voluntary effort produces a result that is both delayed and explosive. When no voluntary movement is attempted, the whole body or the parts chiefly affected are constantly moving. Whenever possible the child makes the movement into a purposive one as if ashamed of moving without purpose.

'As a rule, the extremities can scarcely be kept still for a moment. They are continually performing sprawling movements and wonderful contortions. The shoulders are sometimes raised, sometimes sunk, the head drawn down to the side, and more or less rotated. The facial muscles also participate, the eyes are alternately shut and opened, the forehead wrinkled and quickly smoothed again, the corners of the mouth are twisted to one side or the other. . . .' (Henoch, 1889, p. 197.)

During chorea the child reacts in an exaggerated way to every emotional event, and this emotional instability persists in many cases for months or years after the chorea has cleared up. The same mental change is found in some cases of rheumatic fever, even without choreic movements.

There are certain other interesting points about chorea, though they do not help in diagnosis. Chorea affects three girls to one boy; there seems to be no reason for this favouritism. On the other hand, common fidgetiness is, if anything, more commonly seen in boys than in girls. Chorea is slightly seasonal, common fidgetiness and the tics are not. Chorea is related to district and social standing, common fidgetiness and the tics are ubiquitous.

In some cases attacks of chorea appear repeatedly and without producing rheumatic arthritis or carditis. In one case the child started chorea on her birthday for several years in succession. It would seem that it will eventually be possible to weed out of any hundred cases of true chorea a percentage not liable to rheumatic manifestations; but at present this is not possible, and all children with chorea must be treated as potential heart cases.

There is no treatment for chorea except rest in bed and prevention of emotional strain. In a ward it may be advisable to screen off the bed, but not if this makes the child feel anxious, as if being punished. In the home a room must be found where the other children cannot bounce in and produce excitement. Much can be done by quiet and sympathetic nursing, and during convalescence occupation for the fingers and food for the mind must be supplied, as in all long illnesses. Some children tolerate rest very badly, for in bed they cannot make use of their ordinary devices for dealing with the anxiety produced by their thoughts. It must be remembered that for such a child the presence of a too-loving parent may indirectly, through stimulation, be a form of torture, in which case the child could be expected to improve more rapidly away from home. But it is just the too-loving parent who cannot tolerate the child's removal from home, even for the child's good.

Treatment by drugs is unsatisfactory, as shown by the number advocated.

Untreated, chorea nearly always clears up. The only serious complication is heart disease, and for this no treatment is known except rest.

DISCUSSION OF DIAGNOSIS

Although chorea can nearly always be easily diagnosed it is not uncommon for fidgetiness of other kinds to be mistaken for chorea, and for this reason it is expedient to summarize the details of differential diagnosis, at risk of repetition.

In a typical case of common fidgetiness the restlessness is part of the child's nature. It is the whole child that is affected. Associated with the movements are usually some increased urgency and frequency of micturition. On the contrary, a careful inquiry into the history of onset of true chorea will usually reveal the fact that a more or less normal child on a fairly definite date became fidgety. The movements at the onset will nearly always be found to have affected the arm and leg of one side more than of the other. There is often an associated paresis, and this paresis is always of the more fidgety arm and leg; that is, the paresis and movements go together. Micturition is usually unaffected.

After a few days, when the child is in bed in a hospital or nursing home, these points may be very much less obvious, and the one-sidedness and the initial paresis may have passed off.

The history of onset of the tics is not important in diagnosis — the movements may have suddenly appeared, may follow a fright, may be associated with change in temperament. Habit spasms are peculiarly annoying to those who must see them.

It is usually possible, then, to diagnose chorea from the history alone. If the movements are typical but the history unusual, the diagnosis of chorea should be questioned. Diagnosis of common fidgetiness is usually easy, but in some cases the fidgetiness so much resembles that of chorea that only by the careful taking of a history of the case can a diagnosis be made. The presence of some heart sign that leads to suspicion of rheumatic carditis, old or new, is often responsible for unnecessary and unfortunate restriction of activity in the case of an anxious child who is not choreic.

It is necessary to emphasize here the fact that the term pre-choreic has no meaning in the present state of knowledge. Common fidgetiness does not directly predispose to chorea, and there is no relation between tics and chorea. It is true that chorea is sometimes related to overstrain (e.g., school examinations) and can be started by a fright; the link between chorea and the child's straining to do well, or reacting to fright, is not understood. But it remains true that chorea is a physical brain disease and appears in normal and excitable and nervous children indiscriminately. In differential diagnosis the tics, common fidgetiness, and chorea must be taken at present to be unrelated.

The athetoid movements associated with certain diseases of the central nervous system are not easily mistaken for chorea. Acute epidemic encephalitis lethargica may, on the other hand, start as generalized chorea, quite indistinguishable clinically from common chorea.

The following case illustrates the unusual sequence: trauma—chorea—rheumatic carditis and arthritis.

Lily was well until at eight years old she experienced two frights in one week: she was knocked down by a bicycle, and on another occasion she was afraid to come home because a man and woman were after her (this was probably her imagination, but none the less productive of anxiety). At about the same time she began to be unsteady, especially in her left arm and leg. She went thin and pale. After a few weeks of this she complained once of pain in her hands.

Since the frights she had been miserable. Also she spoke funnily at times, she could not get her words out right. Sleep was normal except for some kicking and 'twittering of the limbs'. She had never been nervous or subject to night terrors.

Past History. She had had measles, and once had swollen tonsillar glands in the neck. She had had no growing pains. Tonsils had not been removed.

Family History. She was one of eight children, of whom one had had rheumatic fever.

On examination, apart from slight fever (100 deg.), no additional positive facts were noted. The movements were typical of chorea, though slight, and the heart was entirely natural.

Course. The movements quickly improved, but remained more obvious on the left side than on the right. While lying in bed she developed stiff neck, presumably a rheumatic arthritis. The tonsils were very small and healthy; in fact, on first inspection it seemed they must have been removed.

After three months the child was apparently well and the heart remained unaffected.

She was not seen again for four months, but she then returned immediately on being taken ill, apparently as a result of getting a headache in the hot sun. She now had definite movements again, but not joint pains or swellings; her temperature was 100 deg. and she seemed ill. The heart signs were as follows: the impulse was heaving; the apex beat was just within normal limits (half an inch to the left in the fifth space); in a quiet room the continuation of the second sound as a murmur could be heard low down on the left of the sternum. This appearance of a diastolic murmur necessitated a diagnosis of active endocarditis of the aortic cusps, causing aortic regurgitation.

After fifteen weeks' institutional treatment she was well, except that her heart still showed evidence of aortic regurgitation. There was no demonstrable hypertrophy.

In spite of all care the movements returned, and though they remained slight the heart developed a new sign — a mid-diastolic murmur, heard at the apex when the patient was examined lying down. This might have been associated with the aortic regurgitation, but the possibility of early mitral stenosis was noted.

Twenty-one months after the first attack of chorea the child developed smouldering rheumatic fever, with swelling of the ankles. She was treated in institutions for another seven months, at the end of which time she was well.

Thirty-two months after the first attack she developed chorea again. At this time the heart showed evidence of hypertrophy, advanced mitral stenosis and aortic regurgitation, and, in view of the active chorea, active carditis had also to be presumed.

This illustrates the course the disease may follow in spite of all possible care and supervision.

The following case illustrates the common fate of a fidgety child:

Doris was originally sent to me at five years old by a school medical officer on account of 'rheumatism', which is always a sound reason for periodic overhaul and observation of a child.

Past History. Scarlet fever twice, tonsils and adenoids removed at three.

Family History. The mother had rheumatic fever twice, and her heart is said to have been affected at the time.

There is a sister aged eight years and a baby brother of six months.

Case Notes. The child is happy and lively and eats well, but is liable to 'growing pains' in the thighs and legs, and frequent 'colds'. She has never had joint swellings. The fact that the child admits having pains is a sufficient justification for careful investigation.

The mother also complains that the child is fidgety and makes faces. There has been no date of onset of these odd symptoms; they have, so to speak, grown with the child.

Routine questioning of the parent brings out the following facts: the little girl sleeps fairly well, except that she talks in her sleep, but in the day she is very nervous and constantly over-excited. Excitement makes her talk incessantly, and she becomes more and more fidgety. In fact, she is never still, and associated with this, as usual, are increased urgency and frequency of micturition (but no enuresis).

The fidgetiness found on examination of the child corresponds with this anxious restlessness and is not choreic. No physical signs of disease are found and the heart is normal. When asked to lie down the child has to overcome a strong dislike of the idea, and this shows in thumping of the heart.

Further Notes. I learned that the fidgetiness had been diagnosed as chorea at a hospital not long previously, but the fidgetiness that remains after chorea is so characteristic that I felt quite confident in sending the following report: this child is healthy physically; she is anxious, and this can account for the pains and fidgetiness.

At times she was kept from school for going pale, for fainting, and again for an illness with feverishness, pains all over, and pins and needles in a hand. Each time after a few days in bed she was well again. Anxious children commonly get this type of illness without physical signs.

The next I heard of her was that she had been diagnosed as a case of chorea at another hospital, which seemed to go against my diagnosis; but when she came to me again I found there had been no change in her fidgetiness, which was not choreic.

She was next kept in a hospital as a case of erythema nodosum. However, it happens that bruising of the skin over the shins and elsewhere is, in her case, a familial condition, shared by her brother and sister, and the diagnosis 'erythema nodosum' had been a false one. There was actual bleeding under the skin at one time, and the bumps formed by the coagulated blood had been called rheumatic nodules. The heart was found to be dilated, and the case was labelled active rheumatism and carditis. With this diagnosis she was sent back to me, but I found her exactly the same as she had been ever since I first saw her. Her heart had remained normal.

She is, in fact, not a rheumatic subject, nor is she subject to chorea.

Postscript (1957)

Rheumatic fever and chorea have become very much less common since the time when this was written. The incidence of common anxious restlessness and of tics has not altered.

PART 2

Chapter III

Appetite and Emotional Disorder[1]
[1936]

IN THE PSYCHO-ANALYTIC and other psychological literature I find it generally agreed that disturbances of appetite are common in psychiatric illnesses, but perhaps the full importance of eating is not recognized. It is rare, for instance, to meet the word 'greed' in psychological writings, and yet greed is a word with a very definite meaning, joining together the psychical and the physical, love and hate, what is acceptable and what is not acceptable to the ego. The only psycho-analytic discussion I know in which the word greed enters inherently into the theme is *Love, Hate and Reparation* by Melanie Klein and Joan Riviere (lectures 1936, published 1937).

A discussion is overdue on the relationship of appetite to greed. I should like to put forward the suggestion that greed is never met with in the human being, even in an infant, in undisguised form, and that greediness, when it appears as a symptom, is always a secondary phenomenon, implying anxiety. Greed means to me something so primitive that it could not appear in human behaviour except disguised and as part of a symptom complex.

Careful history-taking has had a profound effect on my outlook, for it has made clear to me the clinical continuity of appetite disorders as they present themselves in earliest infancy, in childhood, in adolescence and in adult life. For some years now I have been teaching that history-taking reveals the fact that there is no sharp dividing line between the following conditions: anorexia nervosa of adolescence, the inhibitions of feeding of childhood, the appetite disorders in childhood that are related to certain critical times, and the feeding inhibitions of infancy, even of earliest infancy. Examples of crises would be: birth of new baby, loss of first nurse, removal from first home, first feeding with the two parents, attempts to induce self-feeding, introduction of solids or even simply of thickened feeds, anxious reaction to breast-biting.

[1] Read before the Medical Section, British Psychological Society, 1936.

33

These cases occur in one big grouping; at the one end of the scale are the feeding difficulties of infants, and at the other end are melancholia, drug addiction, hypochondria, and suicide. In other words, in illnesses of all kinds as well as in health we find that eating may be affected.[1]

Through analysis of older children and of adults very clear insight is gained into the many ways in which appetite becomes involved in defence against anxiety and depression. It can only be inferred, then, that the psychology of the small child and of the infant is not so simple as it would at first seem to be, and that a quite complex mental structure[2] may be allowed even to the new-born infant.

First in the appreciation of oral function there comes the recognition of oral instinct. 'I want to suck, eat, bite. I enjoy sucking, eating, biting. I feel satisfied after sucking, eating, biting.'

Next comes oral fantasy. 'When hungry I think of food, when I eat I think of taking food in. I think of what I like to keep inside, and I think of what I want to be rid of and I think of getting rid of it.'

Third comes a more sophisticated linking up of this theme of oral fantasy with the 'inner world'. There is a tremendous elaboration of the two parts of the fantasy I have just briefly outlined, namely ideas of what happens inside oneself and, along with this, ideas of what is the state of the inside of the source of supply, namely the mother's body. 'I also think of what happens at the source of supply. When very hungry I think of robbing and even of destroying the source of supply and I then feel bad about what I have inside me and I think of means of getting it out of me, as quickly as possible and as completely as possible.'

This sort of oral fantasy can be deduced from observations on the infants and little children who play with an object, as I hope to show.

It is this limitless elaboration that constitutes an 'inner world'. The word 'inner' in this term applies primarily to the belly, and secondarily to the head and the limbs and any part of the body. The individual tends to place the happenings of fantasy inside and to identify them with the things going on inside the body.

---

[1] Mothers will often say that their infants who are inhibited in their desire for food will nevertheless crave for medicines. I have been told this more than once of infants under one year old, and very many times of older infants and young children.

[2] At this time it was not usual to look for the cause of psychological illness in the infant. My view was therefore somewhat original, and was disturbing to those analysts who saw only castration anxiety and the Oedipus conflict. In my later papers I have devoted myself to a development of the theme of the infant whose emotional development can be healthy or distorted at any age, even before the time of birth. At the present time (1956) there is a general acceptance among psycho-analysts of the view that there is a psychology of the new-born infant.

Although I was all the time influenced by Melanie Klein, in this particular field I was simply following the lead given me by careful history-taking in innumerable cases.

This inner world is normally a live world of movement and feelings. It may be kept inactive when feared and in illness it may get over-controlled, or some of its elements may take control over the individual.

This part of oral fantasy seems to me to be but little acknowledged as such, and if I do rather press for its recognition the reason is that I do all the time need to understand it as a paediatrician. No case of collywobbles in a child, of vomiting or of diarrhoea, or of anorexia or constipation can be fully explained without reference to the child's conscious and unconscious fantasies about the inside of the body.

Even if we want to confine our attentions to *physical* disease within the body we still have to say that no study of a child's reaction to a physical illness could be complete without reference to the child's fantasies about his inside. It must seem very funny to a child when his doctor obviously knows less about his inside than he knows himself. Most doctors prefer to keep to the simple idea of pain without fantasy content, but the fact remains that children will often give an account of their inner world, when asked about their inner discomforts. One child says that there is a war going on inside between Spaniards and English who fight with swords. Another recounts a fantasy of little people sitting round a table in his stomach, waiting for the food to be passed down. A little boy of four said he could hear little men knocking their plates about after he had eaten. Another said that there was a row of children sitting on a fence inside mother, and a birth occurs when father goes in and knocks one off with a crowbar.

Occasionally an artist who can paint an ordinary picture will give us a set-piece of his inner world in terms of guts[1]. The result is terrible to most people; they see bits and pieces everywhere, from which a butcher's shop is a relief. One can admire such an artist's courage, even if one feels bothered by his flight from fantasy to anatomy.

The following incident seems to me to illustrate the way in which acknowledgement of fantasy about the world inside the belly is made through the exercise of a sense of humour.

Case 1. A mother brought her son to hospital and in trying to tell me that he had a malformation of the penis (hypospadias) she said: 'The doctor said he looked as if he had been circumcised before he was born, and I was that scared, I can tell you.' The boy had an exceptionally dark skin, and I was asking her to tell me whether this darkness had come on recently or whether it was natural to him. Evidently she had always been disturbed by this pigmentation. She parried; it was due to the summer holiday (which was obviously false) and so on. At last she said, 'Oh, I remember, he was

---

[1] I was thinking of certain surrealist pictures, in some of which crude anatomical features appeared.

born like that; the doctor said that he looked quite sunburnt.' So I said, 'Well, he seems to have had quite a time in there, one way and another.'

Fantasies of pregnancy cover crude fantasies about the true inside, and afford relief from fears about destructive elements, so much so that it is sometimes hard for a child to give them up. But the fact is that the womb is not the inside. Boys adopt this defence as commonly as girls do. Mother becomes pregnant and then the swelling goes down and behold a nice little human being emerges. So the idea is adopted.

Case 2. A little boy was brought to hospital for a belly pain. I often get asked to see children who have pains that have not yet been localized. This boy had not yet decided where to have the pain, but it had something to do with his inside. Actually he himself had not yet decided even to have pain, but he had something. This something was to do with mother's having just had a baby. He believed he had a baby inside. It must be a boy baby. He did not want to lose the baby, would prefer to keep it inside. It had something to do with love of daddy.

This kind of nascent fantasy is easily obtainable, but I do not think the child gains much by the fact of one's having reached to it. And of course in certain cases it would be actually harmful for a child to have his or her inner secrets forced. But the material is lying around for anyone to gather.

Here is another case in which I took the trouble to let a child tell me about her fantasies in regard to her body.

Case 3. My assistant asks for my advice about a girl of seven called Heather, who since two has habitually scratched her genitals, so that they are constantly inflamed and sore. Recently she has only scratched at school, but teachers have complained. Cystitis and thread-worm infestation have been shown to be absent and no other physical disease can be found. Could it be psychological?

I assure my friend that it could be and agree to see the child and her rather forbidding mother. I have only a few minutes to spare but I must at least make some sort of diagnosis. I find a healthy and nice-looking girl, plump in spite of poor appetite, not unhappy, not restless, rather thoughtful.

I find she is well looked after at home. She is an only child and the parents are aggressively respectable, so that Heather is not allowed out in the street, and very seldom has anyone in to play with her. However, at school Heather has her own friends, and one must look further than these details, important though they are, for the cause of the compulsive genital-scratching.

I ask the mother to go out of the room, and find Heather eager to tell me of bad dreams which she can keep away by keeping her eyes open. She can sleep with her eyes open, she declares. It is clear that she has not only anxiety dreams, but visual hallucinations, partly awful, and partly beautiful. Her happiness, she says, is to find enough niceness in the things she sees to balance the badness. The chief thing is that she sees brown things coming out of holes. She is eager to give details of these grotesque and bad shapes and weird animals. Also there is a fairy with a fantastic name: 'She's nice, all's well when she's there, very tall; her real name's Heather.' She seemed almost surprised to realise her own real existence, being more at home in the fairy world.

The genitals feel to her to be full of these brown grotesques and she has to be always scratching them out.

I venture a question. 'How do they get inside you?'

'Well,' she says, 'I take them in with my food. You see, I'm very fond of liver and sausages and that's why they're brown mostly.'

It is not much of a guess to say that in unconscious fantasy she had eaten good and bad people, and bits of people, and that according to the love and hate involved she has been enriched and burdened respectively with intensely sweet or terrifyingly grotesque objects in her inner world. The fairy world in day-dreaming was enjoyed at a price which is the acknowledgement of the badness which, as she felt it, had to be scratched out of her genitals.

Her symptom is in effect an acknowledgement of badness, and it enables her to keep in touch with the beauty of her fairy world.

Having illustrated my meaning of oral fantasy and the special elaboration of fantasy about insides, I give some ordinary case histories, so as to show how frequently in paediatric practice appetite becomes involved.

I need no reminder that the value of all my observation depends on my ability to know the action and limits of physical disease (infection, malnutrition, etc.). On my ability to be sure that I am allowing for physical disease depends my right to become involved on the psychological side. In this connection I suggest that the study of psychology has been obscured by our lack of control over physical disease, and by our ignorance about diet, so that it was formerly very much more difficult to observe psychological factors than it is today. Medical knowledge and practice have brought about new conditions, and already we know that in less than half of the cases attending a children's hospital out-patient clinic is there any physical illness at all. One can hardly fail now, therefore, to observe emotional disorders and developmental anomalies of personality.

Also psycho-analysis has appeared on the scene, with its willingness to explore and evaluate the unconscious. So gradually we have come to the study of the psychology of the developing infant and child.

Illustrative Cases

When I come to choose cases I am in trouble. By choosing cases I seem to indicate that appetite disturbance in psychological disorder is worth reporting as such, whereas the point I want to stress is that appetite disturbance is extremely common. It must be quite rare to get a history of an ill child, or even of a normal one for that matter, that does not reveal feeding symptoms.

Of course there is in every medical out-patient session a fairly high percentage of cases in which the child is brought openly on account of under- or over-eating, or because of a wide range of appetite vagaries. We are realizing more and more that many of these children are physically sound, and that nevertheless they may be ill in feelings. There are also the various vomiting types, from the less common hysterical vomiting to the very common bilious attack, sometimes organized (with the help of the doctor's preconceived notions) into cyclical vomiting with periodic prostration. Then there are all degrees of fat intolerance, from the common phobia of the skin on milk to coeliac disease, and so on.

My object at this point is to draw attention to the details of feeding that are so often of interest in cases brought for any reason whatever: behaviour disorders, inhibitions of intellectual attainment, failures in training to accepted standards, common anxious restlessness, phobias, anxiety states, depression phases, etc.

Naturally it is impossible for me to give illustrations of all these types of cases. The three following descriptions of children show respectively symptomatic greed, a change-over from an inhibition to a compulsion, and inhibition of greed.

Case 4. First, I take a girl who is now in early puberty. She has an older sister. The difficulty is a character difficulty. From early times she has been unable to allow her older sister any friend. The two sisters get on very well together, but their relationship has been, and still more will be, spoiled by this compulsion on the part of the younger to rob the elder sister of every boy or girl or adult who comes to mean anything to her.

When the sister was six to eight years old this tendency of the little toddler was quite amusing to all concerned, but gradually a situation has arisen in which there is a serious threat to a partnership which cannot, nevertheless, be overthrown without some damage to both parties.

It is not surprising that the greedy girl's greediness is not only for people. She also over-eats, clearly as a defence against anxiety, and at times gets quite unhealthily fat. Any attempt to diet her produces restlessness and temperamental acerbity, which contrasts acutely with what one feels is the child's normal self.

The sister has a complementary tendency to be ascetic. She is depressive in type, which brings her into contrast again with her boisterous eager sister, and she has phases of lack of zest for food with a tendency to leave part of everything offered.

Case 5. The next is a brief description of the case of a boy who changed over from being inhibited to being greedy. Tom, aged fifteen, is threatened with expulsion from a public school on account of unsatisfactory character. He seems at first contact to be an exceptionally decent sort, with a poise and rhythm which are in his favour. His intelligence quotient has been given as 120, and he seems intelligent in conversation. He has a younger brother and sister.

Tom changed in character when he went to public school at thirteen years. At prep school he had been popular, and fairly honest and straight-forward.

When he went to public school he became definitely a nuisance. Here are extracts from the Housemaster's reports: 'At first unusually untidy and unwashed; destructive of furniture, etc. (cutting holes in chairs). Inattentive in school and unable to concentrate. In trouble with various masters, and punishment has had no effect on him. The Headmaster feels he has exhausted the punishments within his range.' (This headmaster is not one who easily resorts to punishments, but the boy clearly does not respond either to understanding or to punishment in the usual ways.)

Cutting a long story short, Tom suffers from character difficulties which have developed since he left the prep school. The parents report that his face has changed since then, from extra frank to uncertain and deceptive, and also they have been worried by the fact that he has had an orgy at home of damaging his own room and its furniture with a knife. This room he has always loved.

The point that is of interest here is that with this character change there has also been a change over from inhibition of greed to greediness. At the time of the character changes he started to fill out bodily, after always having been spare, having acquired a more than healthy appetite, with some compulsion to eat in excess.

This present appetite might pass as normal but it is in marked contrast to his attitude towards food, which had been constant from early infancy to the end of the prep school period. He had been uninterested in food throughout, and no one could ever bribe him with food.

To get to the start of this feeding difficulty one has to go back to a difficulty at the breast at three months, followed by six months of difficult feeding, with secondary constipation. At nine months the baby weighed only nine pounds; from this time on he did fairly well, but kept a small desire for food and a small body. So we may say this boy's illness started at three months.

A nurse who came when he was three years old describes how she found him being fed by spoonfuls by each member of the family in turn, this being the only method by which he could be got to take enough.

How familiar one becomes, in paediatrics, with this sort of picture of an infantile feeding difficulty, augury of troubles ahead!

The importance of this case, though it is all too briefly described, lies in the fact that it shows how inhibition of appetite served the boy well for 10-12 years, in his defence against anxiety. By means of his symptoms he has managed to be a more or less lovable and social being, for he can almost do without food. Without a belief in his own and other people's goodness, however, he cannot develop a full life, at least he cannot live and remain sane.

I now wish to draw attention to the extremely early age at which a human being can attempt to solve the problem of suspicion by becoming suspicious of food. The earliest months of infancy are exceedingly difficult to understand, but it is clear that at nine and ten months this mechanism (that is, using doubt about food to hide doubt about love) can be employed in full degree.

In the next case description I give the details as they appeared in the consultation. At the end of my description an appetite disorder appears.

Case 6. Simon is brought to me at the age of eight years. With him comes his brother Bill, a plump, healthy lad, whose condition puts into sharp contrast Simon's small wiry physique. These are the only two children of a professional man and his wife, a couple who enjoy themselves and each other and the family and their position, and who are naturally worried by the one son's lack of physical development and also his other symptoms: lack of appetite, high-strung nervous state, nightmares, and other important characteristics which the mother gradually recalls in the course of my patient history-taking.

Simon is undoubtedly highly intelligent, and at school is doing moderately well; but he could read for six months before the school knew he could read, and in other ways he does not do himself justice in his intellectual attainments.

His power of concentration is small. At school they say his brain is overactive, that he has a thousand thoughts at one moment. While he is learning to ride a bicycle he is watching an aeroplane. He does things first and thinks after, if at all.

He is honest, generous, affectionate, sensitive. His parents disagree on one thing, whether to try to make him become normal by stern measures, or to humour him and play for time.

In doing things he is slow, but should he want to be quick, then he may be especially quick, since his nature is very much an alert one. For instance, dressing is always a slow business unless for some reason he wants to be the fastest at dressing in a group. Tidying up is incredibly slow. His mother, who does not employ maids, would prefer always to clear up his messes herself, but often she feels she must insist on his clearing up his toys to some extent. He will get out twenty books to find one, but the idea of putting nineteen back does not occur to him. He says, 'Why should I?' and really does not seem to know.

He adores and admires his brother, but can be ordinarily jealous of him — for instance if Bill is ill Simon will want more and more assistance over everything, until the brother is better again.

His play seems at first sight to be rather normal, but it is not very imaginative. That is to say, play is all of ships and sailors and building, and his reading is of general knowledge, of plants and animals, and of wonderful achievements. In other words, in both play and reading there can be seen some flight from fantasy to reality, though to a fairly romantic reality. The mother seems to me to be rather scared of fantasy herself.

Direct evidence of fear of fantasy is not lacking — he was heard to say in his prayers 'Please God do not let me have nightmares'. Nightmares are chiefly of animals, and in the day he is particularly fond of animals. Through analytic work we know that anxieties about animals are often about the biting animals, and in fact animals are introduced as a relief, for in the earliest corresponding anxiety there is only a threatening mouth. Animals can be tamed, but not mouths.

The boy's lack of fear must be regarded, I think, as a symptom, especially as it has led him into danger. He had three bad accidents, to each of which he contributed something. When tiny he put a stick in his eye, a little later he became involved in the mechanism of a sewing machine, and at another time he fell badly and had a scalp wound stitched.

The remarkable thing about him is that he has known what he wants to be since one year old. At least, at one year he developed an ambition to fly. Without fear he would fly from a table at this age, endangering life and limb. He has always felt he could fly like a bird, and before he could swim he dived from a height into water without fear. There has been no attempt on the parents' part to make him brave, indeed they have regarded his bravery as a symptom from the time when he was one year old, and bird-minded.

Recently he has been up in an aeroplane, and so the urge to fly has become harnessed to the ambition to be an airman, and he is only just able to wait. In this way his symptom has metamorphosed into a vocation. I think this is a most unstable form of 'normality'.

The parents have had constant anxiety in connection with Simon's lack of certain ordinary and necessary fears, and realise that this relative lack of reality-sense makes his life a precarious one.

Theoretically we know that anxiety is not absent in this case. We could put it too simply and say he is afraid to be afraid. But there are complex mechanisms involved, and a clear statement of the psychological state would take more space than I can give here. It would be possible to say that he lives inside his own inner world, where control is magical, and he no more tries to die by flying off the table than ordinary people do when they fly in their dreams.

It is interesting to note that although at first I was told that he *never* showed fear at all, the mother remembered later that when he was six weeks to two months old he was so terrified of the crackling of paper that it was impossible to unwrap a parcel in the room where he lay. He screamed and simply could not bear it. The mother felt at the time that the intensity of his fear was abnormal, so that every precaution was taken to prevent recurrences of this trauma.

While I am describing early infancy, I will mention that he showed early likes and dislikes of people, and that this characteristic has stayed with him as a marked feature. As an example, while he liked most of those round him he hated a maid who came into the house when he was four months old and kept this up till she left when he was sixteen months old. There was nothing especially noticeable about her to account for this, and he has always just liked or disliked people, without justification from the observer's point of view. His separation of the world into 'liked' and 'disliked' has always been more subjective than objective.

Simon is supposed to be a happy boy like his brother but one soon sees that this happiness has an unreal quality. He is restless and he needs constant distraction and change. His being highly strung is made more obvious by the placidity of his brother Bill's temperament.

He was found at two years to be left-handed. This was allowed.

Simon talks a lot. It can almost be said that he talks all the time if he is not reading. Nail-biting started recently, also compulsive grunting noises which he makes while he is reading, sitting, eating, and so on. While reading aloud at school he may make these noises, or alternatively, may compulsively lift his hands up to his face.

One characteristic can best be described by examples. You are angry with Simon and say 'Go to bed early', and he says: 'Good, I'm tired', and goes up as if gratified. Or you say 'No chocolates today', and he says: 'That's good because I feel sick this morning', and again you have failed to convey to him the idea of punishment.

Another characteristic: Bill is asked to help, and he very likely goes and does what you ask him to do. Simon, on the other hand, sees in advance what you want, asks if he may do whatever is needed, but after half a minute has lost sight of the whole thing and is found doing something else.

A year ago he would not go to school. This amounted to an inhibition. When forced to go he promptly vomited. I think that the vomiting originally represented an unconscious need to be rid of bad things, but soon he was making use of vomiting to gain control over his mother. He could make himself sick quite easily. Mother could only threaten bed and watch results. She eventually took him to school and let him be sick there, after which he became able to go to school.

I now come to the *appetite disturbance*. The boy's most constant symptom has been an absence of ordinary desire for food. It may be said he has never been greedy. There is no food he really likes, nothing you could give him for a treat. He eats chocolates but forgets them and would always prefer playing about to eating. His brother's appetite is normal for his age and often huge. 'On a picnic Bill will eat till all's blue but Simon will eat one sandwich and only start a second with coaxing.' His interests are elsewhere.

From infancy the brothers have been in contrast, and from the mother's point of view 'this is curious since our Simon had such a good start, and the now more placid, generally normal Bill had a bad start'. Which brings me to the mother's main statement, that Simon was 'absolutely normal' till weaned at nine months. (Of course we know he was not absolutely normal; there was the anxiety aroused by the crackling paper, for instance.) Simon enjoyed the breast and developed physically and mentally, giving no trouble at all till weaned. He did not mind when for two months food was added and the breast contact was lessened, but when the breast was quite withdrawn he changed and he never recovered. This is a history with which everyone dealing with children is familiar. Weaning is one of several critical times of early childhood.

So Simon's condition could be called an inhibition of greed, secondary to weaning trauma, which was secondary to earlier infantile anxiety of psychotic intensity and quality.

A few odd notes may be added: when Simon was eighteen months old he and his mother went to stay at his aunt's house, not a happy home, badly run and unpractical. His own home was a happy one in which routine was reverenced. He reacted very badly to having to wait for meals (his first experience of this) and he started to stutter and to bite his nails. The stuttering ceased when he went home; the nail-biting persisted but it has never been so bad as it was during this holiday.

It ought to be mentioned that Simon was incredibly dirty and wet until seventeen months. He refused to use the pot as soon as he could clearly refuse things, and when old enough he would do it on the floor. His mother made no attempt to bring about a change through special measures. One day he himself said, 'Ah, dirty boy!' and after that he never made a mess.

Until recently Simon has been a messy eater. This is a symptom that often surprises people by clearing up for special occasions. Simon recently went away for a few weeks, ate like an ordinary child, spilt not a crumb, and did not even spot his tie. But home again he was as messy as ever. When told he could not go to a party because of his exceptional messiness he said: 'Oh, but I won't do it if I go to a party', but he does not see how illogical this sort of thing is from his mother's point of view.

Mother said 'People are coming to lunch on Sunday and you can sit over at the other table.' So he said: 'I won't make a mess on Sunday', and he didn't. 'But he was damnable,' the mother added, 'and I was glad when he became messy again, and more sweet-natured.'

He has a rather dull friend whom he despises and dislikes. When asked what he liked about going over to this friend he said: 'I had a jolly good tea.' As if to say: 'He doesn't matter, one could eat him up without remorse.' This illustrates the way that the main symptom, inhibition of greed, which had actually led to stunting of his physical frame, is a part of the boy's relation to the people of his external and internal world, the two being for him not always clearly distinguished.

In Simon's case once again can be seen the great importance of the inhibition of greed, here dating from weaning; and just as at the start the attitude towards food is an attitude towards a person, the mother, so later on the feeding symptoms vary according to the child's relation to various people.

Adult Examples

Although I give cases of children the same point could be illustrated by adult cases. Here is an example:

Case 7. A man and woman consult me because of marital difficulties. Among a mass of important detail I find the following: 'A man hates babies as someone else may hate cats, and may feel bad when one comes into the room.' He said this himself. His reaction to his wife's pregnancy was to become very antagonistic and he only became fond of his child, a boy, after several years. He would have found it easier to tolerate a girl. In this connection, in his own family there was one other child, a brother born when he was two or three years old. There is much evidence that he never dealt satisfactorily with this birth of a brother, and that for him, his own child's birth was a repetition of this event. This carries his illness (paranoid depression) back to the toddler years.

In his present attitude towards food this man shows what he was like as an infant. He is a vegetarian and feels that he is forced to eat meat by a wife who does not understand. He constantly makes his wife force him to eat what he feels he does not want; and he becomes furious, of course, if she becomes indifferent, and lets him go without. It is at meal times that he behaves oddly. The maid has forgotten to put a chair for him and so he stands, and eats a meal standing, making 'a dignified protest', without sense of humour, and this in front of his little boy.

There is confirmation from his mother's early description of him that this attitude in regard to food now is a returning of his earliest attitude to feeding.

This man's inhibition of greed, which has persisted from infancy, often breaks down into symptomatic greedy acts, which distress him as well as his wife. For instance, his son had severe measles and was put on to a milk diet. Special milk was set aside for him. My patient, the child's father, used to go secretly and drink the special milk, replacing it with ordinary milk. When his son was an infant, suffering from malnutrition, he used to go secretly and water the milk. He is always liable to secrete the best cake, the best sweet, the best of anything connected with food or drink, it being compulsive for him to have the best.

Missing is the normal greediness which is acceptable to the self, and which gives such relief of instinct tension.

THE HOSPITAL OUT-PATIENT CLINIC

In the following six case descriptions I shall give each very briefly, including only what seems necessary to convey an impression of the morning's pageant.

First I want to give an account of what a baby does as he sits on his mother's lap with the corner of the table between them and me.

A child of one year behaves in the following way. He sees the spatula[1] and soon puts his hand to it, but he probably withdraws interest once or twice, before actually taking it, all the while looking at my face and at his mother's to gauge our attitudes. Sooner or later he takes it and mouths it. He now enjoys possession of it and at the same time he kicks and shows eager bodily activity. He is not yet ready to have it taken away from him. Soon he drops the spatula on the floor; at first this may seem like a chance happening, but as it is restored to him he eventually repeats the mistake, and at last he throws it down and obviously intends that it shall drop. He looks

[1] In my clinic there was always available a metal bowl full of sterilized spatulas, shiny silvered objects set at a right-angle bend.

at it, and often the noise of its contact with the floor becomes a new source of joy for him. He will like to throw it down repeatedly if I give him the chance. He now wants to get down to be with it on the floor.

It is, on the whole, true to say that deviations from this mean of behaviour indicate deviations from normal emotional development, and often it is possible to correlate such deviations with the rest of the clinical picture. There are, of course, age differences. Children of over one year tend to short-circuit the incorporation process (mouthing the spatula) and to become more and more interested in what can be done with the spatula in play.

Case 8. A mother brings her extremely healthy-looking baby for me to see as a routine measure, three months after the first consultation. The baby, Philip, is now eleven months old, and today he pays me his fourth visit. His difficult phase is past and he is now quite well physically and emotionally.

No spatula is placed out, so he takes the bowl, but his mother prevents this. The point is that he reaches for something immediately, remembering past visits.

I place a spatula for him, and as he takes it his mother says: 'He'll make more noise this time than last', and she is right. Mothers often tell me correctly what the baby will do, showing, if any should doubt it, that our picture gained in the out-patient department is not unrelated to life. Of course the spatula goes to the mouth and soon he uses it for banging the table or the bowl. So to the bowl with many bangs. All the time he is looking at me, and I cannot fail to see that I am involved. In some way he is expressing his attitude to me. Other mothers and babies are sitting in the room behind the mother some yards away, and the mood of the whole room is determined by the baby's mood. A mother over the way says: 'He's the village blacksmith.' He is pleased at such success and adds to his play an element of showing off. So he puts the spatula towards my mouth in a very sweet way, and is pleased that I play the game and pretend to eat it, not really getting in contact with it; he understands perfectly if I only show him I am playing his game. He offers it also to his mother, and then with a magnanimous gesture turns round and gives it magically to the audience over the way. So he returns to the bowl and the bangs go on.

After a while he communicates in his own way with one of the babies the other side of the room, choosing him from about eight grown-ups and children there. Everyone is now in hilarious mood, the clinic is going very well.

His mother now lets him down and he takes the spatula on the floor. playing with it and gradually edging over towards the other small person with whom he has just communicated by noises.

You noticed how he is interested not only in his own mouth, but also in mine and in his mother's, and I think he feels he has fed all the people in the room. This he has done with the spatula, but he could not have done so if he had not just felt he had incorporated it, in the way I have described.

This is what is sometimes called 'possessing a good internalized breast' or just 'having confidence in a relationship with the good breast, based on experience'.

The point that I wish to make here is this: when in physical fact the baby takes the spatula to himself and plays with it and drops it, at the same time, physically, he incorporates it, possesses it, and gets rid of the idea of it.

What he does with the spatula (or with anything else) between the taking and the dropping is a film-strip of the little bit of his inner world that is related to me and his mother at that time, and from this can be guessed a good deal about his inner world experiences at other times and in relation to other people and things.

In classification of a series of cases one can use a scale: at the normal end of the scale there is play, which is a simple and enjoyable dramatization of inner world life; at the abnormal end of the scale there is play which contains a denial of the inner world, the play being in that case always compulsive, excited, anxiety-driven, and more sense-exploiting than happy.

Case 9. The next boy, David, is eighteen months old, and his behaviour has a special characteristic.

His mother brings him over and sits him on her lap by the table and he soon goes for the spatula I place within his reach. His mother knows what he will do, for this is part of what is wrong with him. She says: 'He'll throw it on the floor.' He takes the spatula and quickly throws it on the floor. He repeats this with everything available. The first stage of timid approach and the second of mouthing and of live play are both absent. This is a symptom with which we are all familiar, but it is pathological in degree in this case, and the mother is right in bringing him because of it. She lets him follow the object by getting down and he takes it up, drops it, and smiles in an artificial attempt at reassurance, meanwhile screwing himself into a position in which his forearms are pressed into his groins. While he does this he looks hopefully round, but the other parents in the room are anxious to distract their children from the sight which to them means something to do with masturbation. The little boy finds himself in company in which no one gives him the reassurance he so desperately needs. So here we have him on the floor, throwing away the spatula, screwing himself up in his own peculiar fashion and smiling in a way that indicates a desperate attempt to deny misery and a sense of rejection. Note the way in which this child creates an abnormal environment for himself.

I must omit the details of his development, except to say that from early times he has had loose motions, in fact he tends to pass a motion after each meal. Also, at one year old, six months ago, he started the two symptoms, compulsive groin-pushing, and a very marked compulsion to throw down whatever can be got hold of.

Is it not reasonable to suggest that there is a connection one way or the other between his post-prandial defaecation and the throwing-things-down symptom, especially as psycho-analytic experience has made one familiar with just this kind of linking of the physical and the psychological?

Of course a motion after a feed happens occasionally in every baby, its occurrence as a symptom being only a matter of degree.

This case illustrates the relationship that can be found between physical and psychological happenings, and the relative lack of richness of inner world that may go with inhibition of oral fantasy and consequent absence of the enjoyment of any sort of retention.

I do not propose to discuss here the interesting and important question as to the cause of this anxiety about objects psychically incorporated or physically eaten, except to say that it involves fantasy about the inside. The main part of such fantasy is never conscious, and sooner or later what has been conscious becomes repressed; or alternatively the fantasy remains, and the link between the fantasy and the functional experience is lost.

In this boy there is denial of the inner world which affects his external relationships and along with this there is an anxiety-driven exploitation of sensuality. But the sensuality is not oral, that is, he holds his penis and pushes his groins, while his mouth interest is in abeyance.

Here is a boy whose attitude to what is offered to him has changed.

Case 10. Norman is two years old. His mother has brought him three times before this visit, and she comes today simply because I asked her to come after the summer holiday. He has improved all round, has lost his fears, and has become willing to take almost any food she offers him.

He has passed through a phase of difficulty in emotional development, and has recovered without treatment from me, other than my management of the case and my sharing of responsibility with the mother.

At one year and seven months he started to become thin and during the next few months he had many falls. His sleep became less good and he tended to wake early. One of the most marked symptoms was that, at nineteen months, from being entirely trusting he became unwilling to go to new people — he became even unwilling to go to his mother's mother, whom he had previously trusted easily.

He would take enough food if his mother gave it to him, but at this time he became suspicious of any *new* food, even from her.

While in this phase, in spite of my technique of approach, he cried during my examination of him. He turned from a spatula placed on the table within his reach to his mother, and did not get back to it. When I offered him a paper spool he did not grasp it, and his mother said: 'I knew he wouldn't take anything, not in his present state.'

This clinical picture stayed the same for a month, but at this present visit his mother is able to report the start of a return to normal in all respects. He is now sleeping well and has become more trusting. With me he is quite happy and when I offer him a paper spool he actually snatches it from me, looks very pleased, and proceeds to investigate it as he is carried away from my presence.

It will have been noticed how in the period of suspicion the boy's attitude to food was disturbed, and also his attitude to the proffered paper spool. His mother said, 'I knew he wouldn't take anything from anyone, not in his present state.' But when he recovered he snatched my offering and enjoyed investigating it, as would any other child.

Case 11. Here is a boy of two who has a feeding inhibition. He has never been ordinarily greedy. He never took to solids or to feeding himself. Also he lies awake a lot. His play is unimaginative, lacking in richness and fantasy, and he mostly uses daddy's hammer and nails, or he digs in the garden. At eighteen months he had a phase of mud-eating out of which his mother felt she had to train him. If I wish to describe a little child, I must show you something of his oral interests. With me he adopts a fairly neutral relationship. His attitude to the spatula gives the clue to his feelings. My notes are as follows: He sees the spatula, leaves it alone; touches it 'by mistake', as it were, while performing some hand-play; at this he turns right away; suddenly he returns to it and quizzes me to gauge my attitude and quickly turns away and smacks his thighs; he looks at the object and makes a rather loud sucking noise with his mouth; during a long interval he is eating the top rim of his vest, and then in relation to something he sees about me he cuddles right into his mother's bosom; he wriggles; now he takes the spatula in his hand in a quick movement and in a moment has banged it on the table and left it lying down (previously it was on end). As if alarmed by his act he leaves it as if finally but later he again touches it in an anxious way.

Here then is a picture of conflict involving oral instinct and fantasy.
There is wide scope for work along these simple lines, and I understand

from Anna Freud that she has been making this kind of observation for some years. She has pointed out to me that there is an interesting failure of *direct* correlation between inhibition of grasping and mouthing and actual feeding inhibition, and with this I am in full agreement. The relation is an indirect one; and one which because of its unexpected features must hold much in store that has theoretical importance.

Thus an infant may put things to his mouth at home alone with mother and yet not do so when he comes to my spatula; my presence brings into the situation a link with the infant's relation to father which is perhaps at the time of the consultation in a difficult phase. This phase may be marked by symptoms such as vomiting or constipation, or some other dysfunction serious enough to cause the child to be brought to hospital.

The entry of father into the arena is illustrated by the following incident:

Case 12. A boy of fourteen months was being fed for the first time by daddy, who gave him fish. The mother reacted to this neurotically, feeling jealous for the moment, and said to her husband: 'Don't give him fish, it will make him ill.' That evening the child vomited, and following this had an interesting phobia which lasted for a few weeks. He developed a dislike of fish, and also of eggs and bananas.

By way of contrast see what the next boy does when he comes to see me.

Case 13. Lawrence is a first and only child and is two years and nine months old. He looks healthy. He had the breast for six months, then was weaned all in a day, but did well on milk from the bottle. He got easily on to solids and self-feeding, and he has always been nice and greedy. He has no feeding inhibition and so is plump and well-liking.

Lawrence on his mother's knee gets somehow on top of us and rather dominates the triangular relationship of the consultation, talking all the time in a loud voice, with a speech hesitation as part of the technique of domination. He reaches down for the spatula, takes it and makes it his own, then puts it in a bowl that is near and which contains many spatulas, pushes the bowl away and says 'Ta'; I put out a spatula on the table again and his interest quickly returns and he eagerly takes all out of the bowl and declares: 'I'm playing trains.' (His mother says this is rather like what goes on during the waking period during the night.) He now makes a procession of spatulas in pairs, makes what he calls a bridge, rearranges them in all sorts of different ways. The trains move, meet, join, separate, pass under tunnels, over bridges, and occasionally collide. The fantasy relates to the primal scene. It will be agreed that the details would have vital importance if one were trying to understand the anxiety which disturbs the child's sleep, makes him stutter, and colours his play. He enjoys himself very much, and at home he can always be left to play by himself. I touch a spatula and he says: 'Don't touch, please', indicating the acute need for personal control of what instantly might become an end-of-the-world disaster. He must dominate to maintain control.

Here is no inhibition of appetite, but special anxieties have to be dealt with, anxieties about the relationship between the parents interpreted in terms of the boy's fantasy.

Lawrence's play with the spatulas reveals the quality of his fantasies. It is these same anxieties that are dealt with *at the source* by the inhibitions of greed that have appeared in so many of my other case descriptions. Inhibition means poverty of instinctual experience, poverty of inner world development, and consequent relative lack of normal anxiety about inner objects and relationships[1].

SUMMARY

In the histories of all types of psychiatric case, there may be found appetite disorders, and these disorders may be clearly interwoven with the other symptoms.

Direct clinical contact with infants gives rich opportunity for observation and therapy, and for the application of principles learned through analysis of children and adults.

The theory of psychiatric illness must be modified to allow for the fact that in many cases the history of an abnormality reaches back to the first months or even the first weeks.

[1] For further discussion of this type of observation see Chapter IV.

The Observation of Infants
in a Set Situation[1]
[1941]

FOR ABOUT twenty years I have been watching infants in my clinic at
the Paddington Green Children's Hospital, and in a large number of cases I
have recorded in minute detail the way infants behave in a given situation
which is easily staged within the ordinary clinic routine. I hope gradually to
gather together and present the many matters of practical and theoretical
interest that can be gleaned from such work, but in this paper I wish to confine
myself to describing the set situation and indicating the extent to which it can
be used as an instrument of research. Incidentally I cite the case of an infant
of seven months who developed and emerged out of an attack of asthma while
under observation, a matter of considerable interest in psychosomatics.

I want, as far as possible, to describe the setting of the observations, and
what it is that has become so familiar to me: that which I call the 'Set Situation', the situation into which every baby comes who is brought to my clinic
for consultation.

In my clinic, mothers and their children wait in the passage outside the
fairly large room in which I work, and the exit of one mother and child is the
signal for the entrance of another. A large room is chosen because so much
can be seen and done in the time that it takes the mother and her child to
reach me from the door at the opposite end of the room. By the time the
mother has reached me I have made a contact with her and probably with the
child by my facial expression, and I have had a chance to remember the case if
it is not a new patient.

If it is an infant, I ask the mother to sit opposite me with the angle of the
table coming between me and her. She sits down with the baby on her knee.
As a routine, I place a right-angled shining tongue-depressor at the edge

[1] Based on a paper read before the British Psycho-Analytical Society, April 23rd, 1941.
Int. J. Psycho-Anal., Vol. XXII, 1941.

of the table and I invite the mother to place the child in such a way that, if the child should wish to handle the spatula, it is possible. Ordinarily, a mother will understand what I am about, and it is easy for me gradually to describe to her that there is to be a period of time in which she and I will contribute as little as possible to the situation, so that what happens can fairly be put down to the child's account. You can imagine that mothers show by their ability or relative inability to follow this suggestion something of what they are like at home; if they are anxious about infection, or have strong moral feelings against putting things to the mouth, if they are hasty or move impulsively, these characteristics will be shown up.

It is very valuable to know what the mother is like, but ordinarily she follows my suggestion. Here, therefore, is the child on mother's knee, with a new person (a man, as it happens) sitting opposite, and there is a shining spatula on the table. I may add that if visitors are present, I have to prepare them often more carefully than the mother, because they tend to want to smile and take active steps in relation to the baby — to make love to him, or at least to give the reassurance of friendliness. If a visitor cannot accept the discipline which the situation demands, there is no point in my proceeding with the observation, which immediately becomes unnecessarily complicated.

THE INFANT'S BEHAVIOUR

The baby is inevitably attracted by the shining, perhaps rocking, metal object. If other children are present, they know well enough that the baby longs to take the spatula. (Often they cannot bear to see the baby's hesitation when it is pronounced, and take the spatula and shove it into the baby's mouth. This is, however, hastening forward.) Here we have in front of us the baby, attracted by a very attractive object, and I will now describe what, in my opinion, is a normal sequence of events. I hold that any variation from this, which I call normal, is significant.

Stage 1. The baby puts his hand to the spatula, but at this moment discovers unexpectedly that the situation must be given thought. He is in a fix. Either with his hand resting on the spatula and his body quite still he looks at me and his mother with big eyes, and watches and waits, or, in certain cases, he withdraws interest completely and buries his face in the front of his mother's blouse. It is usually possible to manage the situation so that active reassurance is not given, and it is very interesting to watch the gradual and spontaneous return of the child's interest in the spatula.

Stage 2. All the time, in 'the period of hesitation' (as I call it), the baby holds his body still (but not rigid). Gradually he becomes brave enough to let his feelings develop, and then the picture changes quite quickly. The moment at which this first phase changes into the second is evident, for the child's accept-ance of the reality of desire for the spatula is heralded by a change in the inside of the mouth, which becomes flabby, while the tongue looks thick and soft, and saliva flows copiously. Before long he puts the spatula into his mouth and is chewing it with his gums, or seems to be copying father smoking a pipe. The change in the baby's behaviour is a striking feature. Instead of expectancy and stillness there now develops self-confidence, and there is free bodily movement, the latter related to manipulation of the spatula.

I have frequently made the experiment of trying to get the spatula to the infant's mouth during the stage of hesitation. Whether the hesitation corre-sponds to my normal or differs from it in degree or quality, I find that it is impossible during this stage to get the spatula to the child's mouth apart from the exercise of brutal strength. In certain cases where the inhibition is acute any effort on my part that results in the spatula being moved towards the child produces screaming, mental distress, or actual colic.

The baby now seems to feel that the spatula is in his possession, perhaps in his power, certainly available for the purposes of self-expression. He bangs with it on the table or on a metal bowl which is nearby on the table, making as much noise as he can; or else he holds it to my mouth and to his mother's mouth, very pleased if we *pretend* to be fed by it. He definitely wishes us to *play* at being fed, and is upset if we should be so stupid as to take the thing into our mouths and spoil the game as a game.

At this point, I might mention that I have never seen any evidence of a baby being disappointed that the spatula is, in fact, neither food nor a container of food.

Stage 3. There is a third stage. In the third stage the baby first of all drops the spatula as if by mistake. If it is restored he is pleased, plays with it again, and drops it once more, but this time less by mistake. On its being restored again, he drops it on purpose, and thoroughly enjoys aggressively getting rid of it, and is especially pleased when it makes a ringing sound on contact with the floor.

The end of this third phase[1] comes when the baby either wishes to get down on the floor with the spatula, where he starts mouthing it and playing with it again, or else when he is bored with it and reaches out to any other objects that lie at hand.

This is reliable as a description of the normal only between the ages of about five months and thirteen months. After the baby is thirteen months old, in-terest in objects has become so widened that if the spatula is ignored and the baby reaches out for the blotting-pad, I cannot be sure that there is a real

[1] I will discuss the significance of this phase and link it with Freud's observations on the boy with the cotton-reel (1920), towards the end of this paper (see p. 68).

inhibition in regard to the primary interest. In other words, the situation rapidly becomes complicated and approaches that of the ordinary analytic situation which develops in the analysis of a two-year-old child, with the disadvantage (relative to the analytic) that as the infant is too young to speak material presented is correspondingly difficult to understand. Before the age of thirteen months, however, in this 'set situation' the infant's lack of speech is no handicap.

After thirteen months the infant's *anxieties* are still liable to be reflected in the set situation. It is his *positive interest* that becomes too wide for the setting.

I find that therapeutic work can be done in this set situation although it is not my object in this paper to trace the therapeutic possibilities of this work. I give a case that I published in 1931, in which I committed myself to the belief that such work could be done. In the intervening years I have confirmed my opinion formed then.

This was the case of a baby girl who had attended from six to eight months on account of feeding disturbance, presumably initiated by infective gastro-enteritis. The emotional development of the child was upset by this illness and the infant remained irritable, unsatisfied, and liable to be sick after food. All play ceased, and by nine months not only was the infant's relation to people entirely unsatisfactory, but also she began to have fits. At eleven months fits were frequent.

At twelve months the baby was having major fits followed by sleepiness. At this stage I started seeing her every few days and giving her twenty minutes' personal attention, rather in the manner of what I now describe as the set situation, but with the infant on my own knee.

At one consultation I had the child on my knee observing her. She made a furtive attempt to bite my knuckle. Three days later I had her again on my knee, and waited to see what she would do. She bit my knuckle three times so severely that the skin was nearly torn. She then played at throwing spatulas on the floor incessantly for fifteen minutes. All the time she cried as if really unhappy. Two days later I had her on my knee for half-an-hour. She had had four convulsions in the previous two days. At first she cried as usual. She again bit my knuckle very severely, this time without showing guilt feelings, and then she played the game of biting and throwing away spatulas. While on my knee she became able to enjoy play. After a time she began to finger her toes.

Later the mother came and said that since the last consultation the baby had been 'a different child'. She had not only had no fits, but had been sleeping well at night — happy all day, taking no bromide. Eleven days later the improvement had been maintained, without medicine; there had been no fits for fourteen days, and the mother asked to be discharged.

I visited the child one year later and found that since the last consultation she had had no symptom whatever. I found an entirely healthy, happy, intelligent and friendly child, fond of play, and free from the common anxieties.

The fluidity of the infant's personality and the fact that feelings and unconscious processes are so close to the early stages of babyhood make it possible for changes to be brought about in the course of a few interviews. This fluidity, however, must also mean that an infant who is normal at one year, or who at this age is favourably affected by treatment, is not by any means out of the wood. He is still liable to neurosis at a later stage and to becoming ill if exposed to bad environmental factors. However, it is a good prognostic sign if a child's first year goes well.

DEVIATIONS FROM THE NORMAL

I have said that any variation from that which I have come to regard as the norm of behaviour in the set situation is significant.

The chief and most interesting variation is in the initial hesitation, which may either be exaggerated or absent. One baby will apparently have no interest in the spatula, and will take a long time before becoming aware of his interest or before summoning courage to display it. On the other hand, another will grab it and put it to his mouth in the space of one second. In either case there is a departure from the normal. If inhibition is marked there will be more or less distresss, and distress can be very acute indeed.

In another variation from the norm an infant grabs the spatula and immediately throws it on the floor, and repeats this as often as it is replaced by the observer.

There is almost certainly a correlation between these and other variations from the norm and the infant's relation to food and to people.

USE OF TECHNIQUE ILLUSTRATED BY A CASE

The set situation which I have described is an instrument which can be adapted by any observer to the observation of any infant that attends his clinic. Before discussing the theory of the infant's normal behaviour in this setting, I will give one case as an illustration, the case of a baby with asthma. The behaviour of the asthma, which came and went on two occasions while the baby was under observation, would perhaps have seemed haphazard were it not for the fact that the baby was being observed as a routine, and were it not for the fact that the details of her behaviour could be compared with that of other children in the same setting. The asthma, instead of having an uncertain relation to the baby's feelings, could be seen, because of the technique employed, to be related to a certain kind of feeling and to a certain clearly defined stage in a familiar sequence of events.

Margaret, a seven-months-old girl, is brought to me by her mother because the night before the consultation she has been breathing wheezily all night. Otherwise she is a very happy child who sleeps well and takes food well. Her relations with both parents are good, especially with her father, a night worker, who sees a lot of her. She already says 'Dad-dad', but not 'Ma-ma'. When I ask: 'Whom does she go to when she is in trouble?' the mother says: 'She goes to her father; he can get her to sleep.' There is a sister sixteen months older who is healthy, and the two children play together and like each other, although the baby's birth did arouse some jealousy in the older child.

The mother explains that she herself developed asthma when she became pregnant with this one, when the other was only seven months old. She was herself bad until a month before the consultation, since when she has had no asthma. Her own mother was subject to asthma, she also began to have asthma at the time when she started to have children. The relation between Margaret and her mother is good, and she is feeding at the breast satisfactorily.

The symptom, asthma, does not come entirely unheralded. The mother reports that for three days Margaret has been stirring in her sleep, only sleeping ten minutes at a time, waking with screaming and trembling. For a month she has been putting her fists to her mouth and this has recently become somewhat compulsive and anxious. For three days she has had a slight cough, but the wheeziness only became definite the night before the consultation.

It is interesting to note the behaviour of the child in the set situation. These are my detailed notes taken at the time. 'I stood up a right-angled spatula on the table and the child was immediately interested, looked at it, looked at me and gave me a long regard with big eyes and sighs. For five minutes this continued, the child being unable to make up her mind to take the spatula. When at length she took it, she was at first unable to make up her mind to put it to her mouth, although she quite clearly wanted to do so. After a time she found she was able to take it, as if gradually getting reassured from our staying as we were. On her taking it to herself I noted the usual flow of saliva, and then followed several minutes of enjoyment of the mouth experience.' It will be noted that this behaviour corresponded to what I call the normal.

'In the second consultation Margaret reached out to take the spatula, but again hesitated, exactly as at the first visit, and again only gradually became able to mouth and to enjoy the spatula with confidence. She was more eager in her mouthing of it than she had been at the previous occasion, and made noises while chewing it. She soon dropped it deliberately and on its being returned played with it with excitement and noise, looking at mother and me, obviously pleased, and kicking out. She played about and then threw down the spatula, put it to her mouth again on its being restored to her, made wild movements with her hands, and then began to be interested in other objects that lay near at hand, which included a bowl. Eventually she dropped the bowl, and as she seemed to want to go down we put her on the floor with the bowl and the spatula, and she looked up at us very pleased with life, playing with her toes and with the spatula and the bowl, but not with the spatula and the bowl together. At the end she reached for the spatula and seemed as if she would bring them together, but she just pushed the spatula right away in the other direction from that of the bowl. When the spatula was brought back she eventually banged it on the bowl, making a lot of noise.'

(The main point in this case relevant to the present discussion is contained in the first part of the description, but I have given the whole case-note because of the great interest that each detail could have if the subject under discussion were extended. For instance, the child only gradually came to the placing of the two objects together. This is very interesting and is representative of her difficulty, as well as of her growing ability in regard to the management of two *people* at the same time. In order to make the present issue as clear as possible I am leaving discussion of these points for another occasion.[1])

In this description of the baby's behaviour in the set situation, I have not yet said when it was that she developed asthma. The baby sat on her mother's lap with the table between them and me. The mother held the child round the chest with her two hands, supporting her body. It was therefore very easy to see when at a certain point the child developed bronchial spasm. The mother's hands indicated the exaggerated movement of the chest, both the deep inspiration and the prolonged obstructed expiration were shown up, and the noisy expiration could be heard. The mother could see as well as I did when the baby had asthma. *The asthma occurred on both occasions over the period in which the child hesitated about taking the spatula.* She put her hand to the spatula and then, as she controlled her body, her hand and her environment, she developed asthma, which involves an involuntary control of expiration. At the moment when she came to feel confident about the spatula which was at her mouth, when saliva flowed, when stillness changed to the enjoyment of activity and when watching changed into self-confidence, at this moment the asthma ceased.

[1] I refer to this later, on p. 65.

A fortnight later the child had had no asthma, except the two attacks in the two consultations.[1] Recently (that is, twenty-one months after the episode I have described), the child had had no asthma, although of course she is liable to it.[2]

Because of the method of observation, it is possible for me to make certain deductions from this case about the asthma attacks and their relation to the infant's feelings. My main deduction is that in this case there was a close enough association between bronchial spasm and anxiety to warrant the postulation of a relationship between the two. It is possible to see, because of the fact that the baby was being watched under known conditions, that for this child asthma was associated with the moment at which there is normally hesitation, and hesitation implies mental conflict. An impulse has been aroused. This impulse is temporarily controlled, and asthma coincides on two occasions with the period of control of the impulse. This observation, especially if confirmed by similar observations, would form a good basis for discussion of the emotional aspect of asthma, especially if taken in conjunction with observations made during the psycho-analytic treatment of asthma subjects.

DISCUSSION OF THEORY

The hesitation in the first place is clearly a sign of anxiety, although it appears normally.

As Freud (1926) said, 'anxiety is *about* something'. There are two things, therefore, to discuss: the things that happen in the body and mind in a state of anxiety, and the something that there is anxiety about.

If we ask ourselves why it is that the infant hesitates after the first impulsive gesture, we must agree, I think, that this is a super-ego manifestation. With regard to the origin of this, I have come to the conclusion that, generally speaking, the baby's normal hesitation cannot be explained by a reference to the parental attitude. But this does not mean that I neglect the possibility that he does so because he has learned to expect the mother to disapprove or even to be angry whenever he handles or mouths something. The parent's attitude *does* make a lot of difference in certain cases.

I have learned to pick out fairly quickly the mothers who have a rooted objection to the child's mouthing and handling objects, but on the whole I can say that the mothers who come to my clinic do not stop what they tend to regard as an ordinary infantile interest. Among these mothers are even some

[1] But the mother had re-developed it.

[2] The mother again rather made a point that she, however, had been having asthma, as she felt she had to have it unless the baby had it.

who bring their babies because they have noticed that the infants have *ceased* to grab things and put them to their mouths, recognizing this to be a symptom.

Further, at this tender age before the baby is, say, fourteen months old, there is a fluidity of character which allows a certain amount of the mother's tendency to prohibit such indulgence to be over-ridden. I say to the mother: 'He can do that here if he wants to, but don't actually encourage him to.' I have found that in so far as the children are not driven by anxiety they are able to adjust themselves to this modified environment.

But whether it is or is not the mother's attitude that is determining the baby's behaviour, I suggest that the hesitation means that the infant *expects* to produce an angry and perhaps revengeful mother by his indulgence. In order that a baby shall feel threatened, even by a truly and obviously angry mother, he must have in his mind the notion of an angry mother. As Freud (1926) says: 'On the other hand, the external (objective) danger must have managed to become internalized if it is to be significant for the ego.'

If the mother has been really angry and if the child has real reason to expect her to be angry in the consultation when he grabs the spatula, we are led to the infant's apprehensive fantasies, just as in the ordinary case where the child hesitates in spite of the fact that the mother is quite tolerant of such behaviour and even expects it. The 'something' which the anxiety is about is in the infant's mind, an idea of potential evil or strictness, and into the novel situation anything that is in the infant's mind may be projected. When there has been no experience of prohibition, the hesitation implies conflict, or the existence in the baby's mind of a *fantasy* corresponding to the other baby's *memory* of his really strict mother. In either case, as a consequence, he has first to curb his interest and desire, and he only becomes able to find his desire again in so far as his testing of the environment affords satisfactory results. I supply the setting for such a test.

It can be deduced, then, that the 'something' that the anxiety is about is of tremendous importance to the infant. To understand more about the 'something' it will be necessary to draw on the knowledge gained from the analysis of children between two and four years old. I mention this age because it has been found by Melanie Klein, and I think by all who have analysed two-year-olds, that there is something in the experience of such analyses which cannot be got from the analyses of even three-and-a-half- and four-year-old children, and certainly not from the analyses of children in the latency period. One of the characteristics of a child at the age of two is that the primary oral fantasies, and the anxieties and defences belonging to them, are clearly discernible alongside secondary and highly elaborated mental processes.

The idea that infants have fantasies is not acceptable to everyone, but probably all of us who have analysed children at two years have found it necessary to postulate that an infant, even an infant of seven months like the asthma baby whose case I have already quoted, has fantasies. These are not yet attached to word-presentations, but they are full of content and rich in emotion, and it can be said that they provide the foundation on which all later fantasy life is built.

These fantasies of the infant are concerned not only with external environment, but also with the fate and interrelationship of the people and bits of people that are being fantastically taken into him — at first along with his ingestion of food and subsequently as an independent procedure — and that build up the inner reality. A child feels that things inside are good or bad, just as outside things are good or bad. The qualities of good and bad depend on the relative acceptability of aim in the taking-in process. This in turn depends on the strength of the destructive impulses relative to the love impulses, and on the individual child's capacity to tolerate anxieties derived from destructive tendencies. Also, and connected with both of these, the nature of the child's defences has to be taken into account, including the degree of development of his capacity for making reparation. These things could be summed up by saying that the child's ability to keep alive what he loves and to retain his belief in his own love has an important bearing on how good or bad the things inside him and outside him feel to him to be; and this is to some extent true even of the infant of only a few months. Further, as Melanie Klein has shown, there is a constant interchange and testing between inner and outer reality; the inner reality is always being built up and enriched by instinctual experience in relation to external objects and by contributions from external objects (in so far as such contributions can be perceived); and the outer world is constantly being perceived and the individual's relationship to it being enriched because of the existence in him of a lively inner world.

The insight and conviction gained through the analysis of young children can be applied backwards to the first year of life, just as Freud applied what he found in adults to the understanding of children, and to the understanding not only of the particular patient as a child, but of children in general.

It is illuminating to observe infants directly, and it is necessary for us to do so. In many respects, however, the analysis of two-year-old children tells us much more about the infant than we can ever get from direct observation of infants. This is not surprising; the uniqueness of psycho-analysis as an instrument of research, as we know, lies in its capacity to discover the *unconscious* part of the mind and link it up with the conscious part and thus give us something like a full understanding of the individual who is in analysis. This is true even of the infant and the young child, though direct observation can tell us a great deal if we actually know how to look and what to look for. The proper procedure is obviously to get all we can both from observation and from analysis, and to let each help the other.

I now wish to say something about the physiology of anxiety. Is it not holding up the development of descriptive psychology that it is seldom, if ever, pointed out that the physiology of anxiety cannot be described in simple terms, for the reason that it is different in different cases and at different times? The teaching is that anxiety may be characterized by pallor and sweating and vomiting and diarrhoea and tachycardia. I was interested to find in my clinic, however, that there are really several alternative manifestations of anxiety, whatever organ or function is under consideration. An anxious child during physical examination in a heart clinic may have a heart that is thumping, or at times almost standing still, or the heart may be racing away, or just ticking over. To understand what is happening when we watch these symptoms I think we have to know something about the child's feelings and fantasies, and therefore about the amount of excitement and rage that is admixed, as well as the defences against these.

Diarrhoea, as is well known, is not always just a matter of physiology. Analytic experience with children and adults shows that it is often a process accompanying an unconscious fear of definite things, things inside that will harm the individual if kept inside. The individual may know he fears impulses, but this, though true, is only part of the story, because it is also true that he unconsciously fears specific bad things which exist somewhere for him. 'Somewhere' means either outside himself or inside himself — ordinarily, both outside and inside himself. These fantasies may, of course, in certain cases and, to some extent, be conscious, and they give colour to the hypochondriac's descriptions of his pains and sensations.

If we are examining the hesitation of an infant in my set situation, we may say that the mental processes underlying the hesitation are similar to the ones that underlie diarrhoea, though opposite in their effect. I have taken diarrhoea, but I might have taken any other physiological process which can be exaggerated or inhibited in accordance with the unconscious fantasy that happens to affect the particular function or organ. In the same way, in consideration of the hesitation of the infant in the set situation, it can be said that even if the baby's behaviour is a manifestation of fear, there is still room for the description of the same hesitation in terms of unconscious fantasy. What we see is the result of the fact that the infant's impulse to reach out and take is subjected to control even to the extent of temporary denial of the impulse. To go further and to describe what is in the infant's mind cannot be a matter of direct observation, but, as I have said, this does not mean that there is nothing in the infant's mind corresponding to the unconscious fantasy which through psycho-analysis we can prove to exist in the mind of an older child or of an adult who hesitates in a similar situation.

In my special case, given to illustrate the application of the technique, control includes that of the bronchial tubes. It would be interesting to discuss the relative importance of the control of the bronchus as an organ (the displacement of control, say, of the bladder) and control of expiration or of the breath that would have been expelled if not controlled. The breathing out might have been felt by the baby to be dangerous if linked to a dangerous idea — for instance, an idea of reaching *in* to take. To the infant, so closely in touch with his mother's body and the contents of the breast, which he actually takes, the idea of reaching in to the breast is by no means remote, and fear of reaching in to the inside of mother's body could easily be associated in the baby's mind with not breathing.[1]

It will be seen that the notion of a dangerous breath or of a dangerous breathing or of a dangerous breathing organ leads us once more to the infant's fantasies.

I am claiming that it could not have been purely by chance that the infant gained and lost asthma so clearly in relation to the control of an impulse on two separate occasions, and that it is therefore very much to the point if I examine every detail of the observations.

Leaving the special case of the asthma infant and returning to the normal hesitation of a baby in taking the spatula, we see that the danger exists in the infant's mind and can only be explained on the supposition that he has fantasies or something corresponding to them.

Now, what does the spatula stand for? The answer to this is complex because the spatula stands for different things.

That the spatula can stand for a breast is certain. It is easy to say that the spatula stands for a penis, but this is a very different thing from saying it stands for a breast, because the baby who is always familiar with either a breast or a bottle has very seldom indeed any real knowledge based on experience of an adult penis. In the vast majority of cases a penis must be the infant's fantasy of what a man might have. In other words, we have said no more by calling it a penis than that the infant may have a fantasy that there is something like a breast and yet different because it is associated more with father than with mother. The child is thought to draw on his or her own genital sensations and on the results of self-exploration in the construction of fantasy.

However, I think the truth is that what the baby later knows to be a penis, he earlier senses as a quality of mother, such as liveliness, punctuality at feed times, reliability and so on, or else as a thing in her breast equated with its

---

[1] At the sight of something particularly wonderful we sometimes say, 'It takes my breath away'. This and similar sayings, which include the idea of modification of the physiology of breathing, have to be explained in any theory of asthma that is to command respect.

sticking out or its filling up, or in her body equated with her erect posture, or a hundred other things about her that are not essentially herself. It is as if, when a baby goes for the breast and drinks milk, in fantasy he puts his hand in, or dives into, or tears his way into his mother's body, according to the strength of the impulse and its ferocity, and takes from her breast whatever is good there. In the unconscious this object of the reaching impulse is assimilated to what is later known as penis.

Besides standing for breast and penis, the spatula also stands for people, observation having clearly shown that the four-to-five-months infant may be able to take in persons as a whole, through the eyes, sensing the person's mood, approval or disapproval, or distinguishing between one person and another[1].

I would point out that in the explanation of the period of hesitation by reference to actual experience of mother's disapproval, an assumption is being made that this infant is normal or developed enough to take in persons as a whole. This is by no means always true, and some infants who seem to show an interest in and a fear of the spatula nevertheless are unable to form an idea of a whole person.

Everyday observation shows that babies from an age certainly less than the age-group we are discussing (five to thirteen months) ordinarily not only recognize people, but also behave differently towards different people.

In the set situation the infant who is under observation gives me important clues to the state of his emotional development. He may only see in the spatula a thing that he takes or leaves, and which he does not connect with a human being. This means that he has not developed the capacity, or he has lost it, for building up the whole person behind the part object. Or he may show that he sees me or mother behind the spatula, and behave as if this were part of me (or of mother). In this case, if he takes the spatula, it is as if he took his mother's breast. Or, finally, he may see mother and me and think of the spatula as something to do with the relation between mother and myself. In so far as this is the case, in taking or leaving the spatula he makes a difference to the relationship of two people standing for father and mother.

There are intermediate stages. For instance, some infants obviously prefer to think of the spatula as related to the bowl, and they repeatedly take it out of the bowl and replace it with evident interest and pleasure and perhaps excitement. They seem to find an interest in two objects simultaneously more natural than an interest in the spatula as a thing that can be taken from me, fed to mother, or banged on to the table.

Only the actual observations can do justice to the richness of variation that

[1] As Freud showed, the cotton-reel stood for the mother of the eighteen-months-old boy (see below, p. 68).

a number of infants introduce into the simple setting which can so easily be provided.

The infant, if he has the capacity to do so, finds himself dealing with two persons at once, mother and myself. This requires a degree of emotional development higher than the recognition of one whole person, and it is true indeed that many neurotics never succeed in managing a relation to two people at once. It has been pointed out that the neurotic adult is often capable of a good relation with one parent at a time, but gets into difficulties in his relationship with both together. This step in the infant's development, by which he becomes able to manage his relationship to two people who are important to him (which fundamentally means to both his parents), at one and the same time, is a very important one, and until it is negotiated he cannot proceed to take his place satisfactorily in the family or in a social group. According to my observations this important step is first taken within the first year of life.

Before he is one year old the infant may feel that he is depriving others of things that are good or even essential because of the greed roused by his love. This feeling corresponds to his fear, which may easily be confirmed by experience, that when he is deprived of the breast or bottle and of his mother's love and attention, someone else enjoys more of her company. Actually this may be father, or a new baby. Jealousy and envy, essentially oral in their first associations, increase greed but also stimulate genital desires and fantasies, thus contributing to an extension of libidinal desires and of love, as well as of hatred. All these feelings accompany the infant's first steps in establishing a relation to both parents — steps which are also the initial stages of his Oedipus situation, the direct and the inverted one. The conflict between love and hatred and the ensuing guilt and fear of losing what is loved, first experienced in relation to the mother only, is carried further into the infant's relation to both parents and very soon to brothers and sisters as well. Fear and guilt stirred by the infant's destructive impulses and fantasies (to which experiences of frustration and unhappiness contribute) are responsible for the idea that if he desires his mother's breast too much he deprives father and other children of it, and if he desires some part of his father's body which corresponds to mother's breast, he deprives mother and others of it. Here lies one of the difficulties in the establishment of a happy relation between a child and both parents. I cannot deal with the complicated matter of the interplay of the child's greed and the different ways he has of controlling this greed or of counteracting its results by restoring and reconstructing, but it can readily be seen that these things become complicated where the child's relationship is to two persons instead of to mother alone.

It will be remembered that in my case-note of the infant with asthma[1], I

[1] Page 57.

65

referred to the relation between the child's growing ability to bring the spatula and the bowl together at the end of her game, and the mixtures of wishes and fears in regard to the management of a relation to two people at once.

Now this situation, in which the infant hesitates as to whether he can or cannot satisfy his greed without rousing anger and dissatisfaction in at least one of the two parents, is illustrated in the set situation of my observations in a way that is plain for all to see. In so far as the baby is normal, one of the main problems before him is the management of two people at once. In this set situation I seem sometimes to be the witness of the first success in this direction. At other times I see reflected in the infant's behaviour the successes and failures he is having in his attempts to become able to have a relation to two people at once at home. Sometimes I witness the onset of a phase of difficulties over this, as well as a spontaneous recovery[1].

It is as if the two parents allow the infant gratification of desires about which he has conflicting feelings, tolerating his expression of his feelings about themselves. In my presence he cannot always make use of my consideration of his interests, or he can only gradually become able to do so.

The experience of daring to want and to take the spatula and to make it his own without in fact altering the stability of the immediate environment acts as a kind of object-lesson which has therapeutic value for the infant. At the age which we are considering and all through childhood such an experience is not merely temporarily reassuring: the cumulative effect of happy experiences and of a stable and friendly atmosphere round a child is to build up his confidence in people in the external world, and his general feeling of security. The child's belief in the good things and relationships inside himself is also strengthened. Such little steps in the solution of the central problems come in the everyday life of the infant and young child, and every time the problem is solved something is added to the child's general stability, and the foundation of emotional development is strengthened. It will not be surprising, then, if I claim that in the course of making my observations I also bring about some changes in the direction of health.

---

[1] I have watched from start to finish a fortnight's illness in a nine-months-old infant girl. Accompanying earache, and secondary to it, was a psychological disturbance characterized not only by a lack of appetite but also by a complete cessation of handling and mouthing of objects at home. In the set situation the child had only to see the spatula to develop acute distress. She pushed it away as if frightened of it. For some days in the set situation there seemed to be acute pain as if indicating acute colic instead of what is normally hesitation, and it would have been unkind to have kept the child for long at a time in this painful situation. The earache soon cleared up, but it was a fortnight before the infant's interest in objects became normal again. The last stage of the recovery came dramatically when the child was with me. She had become able to catch hold of the spatula and to make furtive attempts to mouth it. Suddenly she braved it, fully accepted it with her mouth and dribbled saliva. Her secondary psychological illness was over and it was reported to me that on getting home she was found to be handling and mouthing objects as she had done before her illness started.

Whole Experiences

What there is of therapeutics in this work lies, I think, in the fact that the *full course of an experience is allowed.* From this one can draw some conclusions about one of the things that go to make a good environment for the infant. In the intuitive management of an infant a mother naturally allows the full course of the various experiences, keeping this up until the infant is old enough to understand her point of view. She hates to break into such experiences as feeding or sleeping or defaecating. In my observations I artificially give the baby the right to complete an experience which is of particular value to him as an object-lesson.

In psycho-analysis proper there is something similar to this. The analyst lets the patient set the pace and he does the next best thing to letting the patient decide when to come and go, in that he fixes the time and the length of the session, and sticks to the time that he has fixed. Psycho-analysis differs from this work with infants in that the analyst is always groping, seeking his way among the mass of material offered and trying to find out what, at the moment, is the shape and form of the thing which he has to offer to the patient, that which he calls the interpretation. Sometimes the analyst will find it of value to look behind all the multitude of details and to see how far the analysis he is conducting could be thought of in the same terms as those in which one can think of the relatively simple set situation which I have described. Each interpretation is a glittering object which excites the patient's greed.

NOTE ON THE THIRD STAGE

I have rather artificially divided the observations into three stages. Most of my discussion has concerned the first stage and the hesitation in it which denotes conflict. The second stage also presents much that is of interest. Here the infant feels that he has the spatula in his possession and that he can now bend it to his will or use it as an extension of his personality[1]. In this paper I am not developing this theme. In the third phase the infant practises ridding himself of the spatula, and I wish to make a comment on the meaning of this.

In this the third phase he becomes brave enough to throw the spatula down and to enjoy ridding himself of it, and I wish to show how this seems to me to relate to the game which Freud (1920) described, in which the boy mastered his feelings about his mother's departure. For many years I watched infants in this setting without seeing, or without recognizing, the importance of the third stage. There was a practical value for me in my discovery of the importance of this stage, because whereas the infant who is dismissed in the second stage is upset at the loss of the spatula, once the third stage has been reached

[1] See Chapter XVIII.

the infant can be taken away and can leave the spatula behind him without being made to cry.

Although I have always known Freud's description of the game with the cotton-reel and have always been stimulated by it to make detailed observations on infant play, it is only in more recent years that I have seen the intimate connection between my third phase and Freud's remarks.

It now seems to me that my observations could be looked at as an extension backwards of this particular observation of Freud's. I think the cotton-reel, standing for the child's mother, is thrown away to indicate a getting rid of the mother because the reel in his possession had represented the mother *in his possession*. Having become familiar with the full sequence of incorporation, retention, and riddance, I now see the throwing-away of the cotton-reel as a part of a game, the rest being implied, or played at an earlier stage. In other words, when the mother goes away, this is not only a loss for him of the externally real mother but also a test of the child's relation to his *inside* mother. This inside mother to a large extent reflects his own feelings, and may be loving or terrifying, or changing rapidly from one attitude to the other. When he finds he can master his relation to his inside mother, including his aggressive riddance of her (Freud brings this out clearly), he can allow the disappearance of his *external* mother, and not too greatly fear her return.

In particular I have come to understand in recent years (applying Melanie Klein's work) the part played in the mind even of the infant by the fear of the loss of the mother or of both parents as valuable internal possessions. When the mother leaves the child he feels that he has lost not only an actual person, but also her counterpart in his mind, for the mother in the external world and the one in the internal world are still very closely bound up with each other in the infant's mind, and are more or less interdependent. The loss of the internal mother, who has acquired for the infant the significance of an inner source of love and protection and of life itself, greatly strengthens the threat of loss of the actual mother. Furthermore, the infant who throws away the spatula (and I think the same applies to the boy with the cotton-reel) does not only get rid of an external and internal mother who has stirred his aggression and who is being expelled, and yet can be brought back; in my opinion he also externalizes an internal mother whose loss is feared, so as to demonstrate to himself that this internal mother, now represented through the toy on the floor, has not vanished from his inner world, has not been destroyed by the act of incorporation, is still friendly and willing to be played with. And by all this the child revises his relations with things and people both inside and outside himself.

Thus one of the deepest meanings of the third phase in the set situation is that in it the child gains reassurance about the fate of his internal mother and about her attitude; a depressed mood which accompanies anxiety about the internal mother is relieved, and happiness is regained. These conclusions could, of course, never be arrived at through observation only, but neither could Freud's profound explanation of the game with the cotton-reel have been arrived at without knowledge gained through analysis proper. In the play-analyses of young children we can see that the destructive tendencies, which endanger the people that the child loves in external reality and in his inner world, lead to fear, guilt, and sorrow. Something is missing until the child feels that by his activities in play he has made reparation and revived the people whose loss he fears.

SUMMARY

In this paper I have tried to describe a way by which infants can be observed objectively, a way based on the objective observation of patients in analysis and at the same time related closely to an ordinary home situation. I have described a set situation, and have given what I consider to be a normal (by which I mean healthy) sequence of events in this set situation. In this sequence there are many points at which anxiety may become manifest or implied, and to one of these, which I have called the moment of hesitation, I have drawn special attention by giving a case of a seven-months-old baby girl who developed asthma twice at this stage. I have shown that the hesitation indicates anxiety, and the existence of a super-ego in the infant's mind, and I have suggested that infant behaviour cannot be accounted for except on the assumption that there are infant fantasies.

Other set situations could easily be devised which would bring out other infantile interests and illustrate other infantile anxieties. The setting which I describe seems to me to have the special value that any physician can use it, so that my observations can be confirmed or modified, and it also provides a practical method by which some of the principles of psychology can be demonstrated clinically, and without causing harm to patients.

Child Department Consultations[1]
[1942]

WHAT FOLLOWS is a report to the Society on the cases that came through the Child Department of the Institute of Psycho-Analysis in London over a period of one year. What I have to say is therefore not directly analytic, though I think it is of interest to analysts.

One of the reasons why the Child Department was set up was to provide a clinic for children who are brought to the Institute for consultation. It was easy to foresee the difficulties and disappointments which this part of the Child Department's work must entail, and which my description of this year's work clearly shows. These cases simply fall into line with the thousands of cases that also assail me in my position as Physician at a Children's Hospital.

Over a period of one year I took trouble over each case, and gave up time deliberately in order to do so, and in order to be able to give this report to the Society.

It will be understood that I am giving an account of the cases that were actually sent to the Child Department in the course of a year, and that I am not including an account of the cases given for analysis to students, which were all taken from other sources.

Some cases never actually came for consultation. For instance, a doctor rang up about his little daughter aged 3½ who had recently started a bad stammer. She was an only child. It appeared that the child had become very attached to an aunt who had looked after her while her mother and father were away. Grief at the aunt's departure did not appear until the child's little girl friend also left the neighbourhood. She then became depressed and started the stammer. Inquiry showed that the child's emotional development had proceeded normally till these events, and the home appeared to be reasonably stable and loving. As the child lived too far away to come for analysis without

[1] Read before the British Psycho-Analytical Society, June 3, 1942. *Int. J. Psycho-Anal.*, Vol. XXIII, 1942.

the risk of seriously tiring her physically, I answered the father's query about analysis being necessary by saying that in my opinion it was normal for a child of 3½ to show violent symptoms, and that as his child's development was satisfactory in other respects the best course would be to ignore the symptom and not look to psycho-analysis for help at present. A week later the doctor again rang up, this time to say that the child's symptom had disappeared.

It will probably be agreed that it is wrong to extol the value that analysis would have, if applied, in a case where analysis is not applicable. Parents who come to consultation are feeling guilty about their child's symptom or illness, and the way in which the doctor behaves will determine whether they will calmly return to taking responsibility which they can well take, or anxiously hand over responsibility to the doctor or clinic. It is obviously better that the parents should retain such responsibility as they can bear, and especially is this true if analysis cannot be given a chance to lessen the actual illness of the child.

Case 1. Ellen, aged ten years, living in London. A first and only child. I could not get a good history in less than an hour and I could not avoid spending four separate hours on the case. Here are a few details.

It can be taken that this child was physically, emotionally, and intellectually normal at one year. At that time, however, the mother left her husband and took the child away, after which the father only saw her at intervals. When the child was 6¼, the father arrived, unannounced, and picked his daughter up in his car as she was on her way to school. The child came away without a murmur, and was contented to be brought back to London. After this the father started divorce proceedings. When she was nine, the father remarried, this time making an excellent choice. The child's home background now became good for the first time since she was one year old.

The complaint was that Ellen was artificial. She was nice, and good, and intelligent. The only thing was that 'you could not get on to a sincere basis with her', as her father said. In addition, she was childish for her age and it was said that one could never predict from her mood on rising what might or might not happen in the course of the day. School reports showed ups and downs, and the reason for consultation was one incident of thieving which stood out as more than the common petty thieving of school children, perhaps because of the absence of shame. It was a fatal thing to arrange a treat specially for her. Whatever it was, or whoever arranged it, it failed because she became depressed or irritable. Her parents said that if she was caught off her guard she would usually be found to be sorrowful. Her real mother's moods were also unreliable.

Superficially the child was very happy with her father and especially with her excellent step-mother, to whom she clung. Yet it was easily found that she mourned the loss of her real mother, who had been anything but a satisfactory parent to her.

Analysis could not be arranged. One of the reasons for this was that no analyst capable of dealing with this case had a clinic vacancy. This, I am afraid, will be a recurring theme. I was also influenced by the value to the child of keeping on at the school where she stole the chocolates, where she had some fairly good contacts, at any rate with the staff, and where she might still make good. She was still welcome there, though as a problem child. In a letter to the school I asked that the attempt to 'cure' her, to make her normal, should be abandoned; it should be considered good if major incidents were avoided.

A special problem arises in regard to the possibility of analysing a child of this sort. I have known and know of the analysis of highly suspicious children, but nothing can get away from the great danger of the child refusing to come for treatment at an early stage.

I have to hold myself in readiness to see this child again as new crises develop.

Similar suspicion marked *Case 2*. Norah, aged 13 years, living in London. Brought by her very intelligent sister because she refused to go to school. She was the youngest of several children.

I invited Norah to pay me a few visits. She came, and drew pictures. After two visits to me she wrote me the nicest possible letter stating that she did not wish to come any more. In this case I had refrained from interpreting, because I knew that if I succeeded in getting behind the suspicion at all I should have to go on with the analysis. And I was not in a position to do so.

Knowing the child's distress, I transferred her to the Paddington Green Children's Hospital and sent on her track the Psychiatric Social Worker. The P.S.W. was welcomed, and in many regular visits she made a better contact than I had made. Eventually the P.S.W., valued friend by now, came up against another version of the absolute barrier that I had met so quickly. For an analysis to have been carried out in this case, an analyst would no doubt have had to visit the child daily, and to do the first part of the analysis in the child's home and on walks and visits to museums. Naturally the clinic does not cater for this, although many of us can draw on experiences of this kind, if we go over in our minds the unexpected things that have happened to us in private practice.

The child gained considerable benefit from the P.S.W's. visits, but did not get back to school. She has now reached the school-leaving age. She has managed to take a holiday away from her home, and seems likely to start work[1].

---

[1] Later: Norah is now at work, doing well. She appears to have successfully negotiated her difficult pubertal phase.

A wealth of hidden feeling and fantasy was discovered in the course of discussing well-known paintings and studying the child's own considerable artistic efforts, but this rich world of her fantasy was really a secret inner world, and she felt it dangerous to let even the P.S.W. (who is skilled at not forcing friendships) do more than know of its existence.

In my experience, many of these adolescent children, who seem to be failures at the time of consultation, come for help or even analysis when they are on their own, say at 18 or 20 years old; and apart from this, children who are attempting to manage the acute problems of early puberty can get value from support which comes from outside the family, especially when the family is itself in unstable equilibrium.

Case 3. Maisie, aged three years. This was an acute case. Maisie had developed extreme restlessness and seriously disturbing compulsive rocking movements and neurotic anxiety in connection with her mother being near the end of her second pregnancy. The new baby was overdue, and my contact with the child extended over the period up to the birth. Tension was greatly relieved by the actual event of the baby's birth. It would have been logical to have arranged analysis for this child at the end of that time, but no one could be found to undertake the onerous task of daily taking the child to and fro. Incidentally the child suffered severely from lack of anyone to take her out, even for a walk.

My only way of helping was to visit the child in her own home. I was given facilities for seeing the child alone, and I did not use toys. I found her to be maniacal almost to the degree of being inaccessible at first, but she heard and noted my interpretations, and came to value my visits.

Her play was clearly to do with the mastery of birth fantasies, and later of various fantasies dealing with the relation between the parents. In five visits spread over a fortnight I had a tremendous amount of material for interpretations, which I gave in the full sense of the word, making use of the transference from the beginning.

It is difficult to assess results. Naturally no permanent change in the child's personality was looked for, but I had the satisfaction of seeing the chaos of the child's fantasy world becoming organized and the maniacal behaviour developing into play, with a sequence in it, as in a satisfactory analysis. The fantasies were clearly expressed and dealt with many aspects of the child's anxiety over her mother's pregnancy, which seemed as if it would never end. Anxiety about harm to her mother was important. Much material dealt with the distinction between the bad man who puts her mother in such danger and the good man (her father was a doctor) who helps her out of danger.

Fantasies of incorporating the analyst were strong and had to do with her real need for me all the time.

The child was naturally relieved at the actual birth, and soon found a normal relation to the baby sister. She is still in need of analysis, and if someone could have been found to bring her to the clinic, I should by now have arranged for her analysis as an acute case, but not necessarily a very difficult one.

Case 4. Tommy, aged twelve years, living in London, was unsatisfactory from my point of view. This boy came with a letter from a clinic. Could he be given psycho-analytic treatment? The answer was: no, because in order to get the boy for treatment someone or some group of people would have to be found to bring him daily from a very distant part of London. Further, he was a definitely psychotic case, schizophrenic in type, and therefore only suitable for research analysis by an experienced child-analyst; and no such person would be likely to have a vacancy for a free case.

I saw the mother and the boy, and this took me about an hour. The mother was very suspicious and the lack of useful outcome from the visit increased her grudge against all sorts of clinics and hospitals.

I mention this sort of detail over and over again, because it is no good our pretending to do what we cannot do. It is no good anyone asking us to consider a case if the address is in a remote district, unless there are exceptional facilities for travel, or if the child can attend on his own. And then, of course, there is hardly ever a vacancy. Further, if there is a vacancy, a student cannot be given so difficult a case as this one was certain to be. That is why it is so futile to do consultation work, unless a wide view is taken of the duties of the consultant.

Case 5 was equally futile: Max, aged nine years, living out of London. A refugee from Germany.

The parents of this child both had knowledge of analysis and, naturally, when they saw their child in distress they decided to have him analysed. Certainly the boy needed it, but to have had him analysed I should first have had to find a hostel or school where he could live. The parents had failed to see in advance that it would not be possible to overcome this difficulty, and I fear they were very much disappointed. If at any time in the distant future we have quite a number of analysts doing child-analysis, a small home must be set up where children of various ages may live a family life of sorts and get education, while being near the clinic for analysis.

This boy had had many changes of physical background and he had reacted badly to each change. He was said to have no power of concentration, to be moody, to be suspicious of food and of children of his own age, and to be unloved. And then there was the matter of his being a Jew, this having hitherto been hidden from him. The parents badly wanted help for him. I wish they could have got it. It took me well over an hour to take his history and to get the mother to realize I had nothing to offer her.

Case 6 was a little less unsatisfactory. Tessa, aged thirteen years. Living in the suburbs.

This girl's father rang up and asked for psycho-analysis for her, because she was not doing as well as he had hoped at school. In a short interview I formed the opinion that the girl was not psychiatrically ill. There were difficulties, including an unreasonable expectation on the part of her father. He wanted her to pull the family up by becoming a doctor, but she had no enthusiasm for this. I passed on the case to a colleague, who went into details and gave advice about the schooling in the way she is fully trained to do. There was no vacancy at the time for analysis, and in any case it would have been impossible for the girl to have stayed at school and also to have travelled up to the clinic every day[1].

Case 7 was entirely different. Queenie, aged three years, living in London.

Some friends of mine who are acquainted with psycho-analysis sent this child, the daughter of their charwoman, because she had started stealing. The mother brought her to me personally to treatment in my private rooms two or three times a week over a period of six months. This was quite a difficult thing for the mother to manage, and during her next pregnancy she ceased bringing the child. It was always clear that I could not reckon on daily visits in this case, nor could I expect to be allowed to give the treatment for long. However, I just went ahead, as if I were doing analysis, recognizing the limitations, but not wanting to send away with nothing but a useless consultation a child who had been brought to the clinic.

As a matter of fact quite important work was done, for the material brought by the child enabled me to show sequence and order in it, and I obtained specific results from interpretations, just as in real analysis. The play with toys and by drawing and cutting enabled me to interpret and to show that I could tolerate penis envy and ideas of violent attacks on the mother's body and on the father's penis and on babies unborn. She told me of sexual play with her brother. The stealing stopped, and the mother, as so often happens, forgot that the child had ever stolen.

I would say that a real analysis had begun, and that sufficient work had

---

[1] On looking back I think this father intended to get into touch with the National Institute of Industrial Psychology, but did not know its correct name.

been done on the child's reaction to week-ends and holidays, and so on, to enable her to deal with the end of the treatment when the visits could no longer be arranged. What I did, though it was not analysis, could only have been done by an analyst, experienced in long, unhurried analysis, in which material can be allowed to force itself on the analyst's attention while he gradually learns to understand it.

Case 8 was a possible analytic case: Norris, aged six years. Living in the suburbs.

In this case both parents are doctors. The mother came and discussed the problems that had arisen in the boy's management, and this of course took at least an hour. It appeared that the father had been timid all his life, and hoped to find in his son all the robust qualities he had missed in himself. He had married a wife who was very forceful indeed, and this the only child of the marriage was a timid boy, almost exactly like his father. It became evident that the parents could both manage this child well if they could settle down to the idea that he was of a timid type. Actually the boy's passive-masochistic organization was near-pathological. I should have liked to have arranged analysis, and it is not yet certain that analysis is impracticable here. But although I am hoping to be able to send this case to an analyst, I find it bad to let the parents feel that analysis is their salvation. They must adjust themselves to the situation without thinking of analysis, which I shall only offer them when I know it is available. I mean that one must avoid giving the impression: 'Yes, psycho-analysis will cure him, that is to say, will make him as you want him, without any more effort on your part.' I have not yet seen the boy.

I am talking to myself here. At one time, in consultations, I always thought of psycho-analysis as the treatment of choice, and this led to my feeling I had done my bit if I had tried to bring psycho-analysis about. But consultations are of negative value unless analysis is kept completely out of the picture except in so far as it can definitely be arranged. If in addition to what is advised and to other benefits, psycho-analysis can be offered *and actually brought about*, so much the better.

The following case was definitely more satisfactory, though its satisfactoriness depended on my being able to do something immediately. I do not know how we shall one day solve this problem of always having a vacancy ready waiting. But white-hot material has a special interest of its own, and an analyst who never has room to take an acute case misses valuable experiences.

Case 9. Francis, aged eleven. This boy was brought direct to the clinic by his mother, who claimed urgent help. Francis was violent and in many ways pathological, and was also distressed about his own condition and often asking for help.

The original consultation with the mother in this case took two hours and was of great importance. I found that there were two ill people in the case, the mother as well as the boy. There is a mass of interesting detail that could be given about this case, but to give it all here would be to over-reach my present aim.

I would say that there is special interest in the way the boy's mania was related to his mother's depression: intolerance of her depression would make him maniacal. In order to help her I had to start her son's treatment immediately. The result of the first few weeks, in which he behaved like a restless adult and chose to lie on the couch rather than draw or play, was that he changed in his attitude to his real father. He recovered belief in him, following direct Oedipus interpretations of material supplied at white heat in terms of play with his sister. In his fantasy the sexual father was bad and did harm to his mother's body, so that the Gestapo were acting on his behalf when they took his father away by force, and he was strongly identi-fied with them. He soon took me on as a good father, helpful but non-sexual, and asked me to see his mother sometimes, especially as she had seemed less depressed since I had come into their lives. It is noteworthy that he did not think of me as 'in love with mummy', which would have been according to his pattern with all the men he had liked before his analysis started.

Do not be disappointed when you hear that the mother's depression re-covered so far that she arranged for the boy to go away to a boarding school. This in the circumstances was a real advance in the home situation, and meant that a father figure had returned to the home. The analysis is quite firmly planted. The boy comes to me whenever there is any holiday and makes use of treatment as fully as possible in the circumstances.

Case 10. Nellie, aged 17 years.

Nellie has a brother two years her junior. Her father had been a doctor, and he and his friends made a lot of her. But when she was four her father died, whereupon her mother and she and her brother moved to town and to an entirely different life, where the grown-ups were mostly women, and the boy was now the centre of interest. Perhaps the change of surroundings, coming on top of her father's death, was too much for her, for she stopped what till then had been a satisfactory intellectual and emotional develop-ment. At 16 she had an illness with persisting body movements, which some doctors diagnosed as chorea. Her own doctor, a friend of her late father, pronounced that this was not true chorea, because of the existence of obvious and long-standing psychological difficulties. On careful enquiry. however, I was bound to say that I regarded this as true chorea, which simplified my advice to the school. For it is easier to tell a teacher to allow for bad hand-writing because of chorea than because of emotional hold-up. The main complaints, however, could not be ascribed to chorea, and included a difficulty in making friends. The teacher wrote: 'There is a turning away from, instead of a turning out towards, in a way which is not the normal reserve of adolescence, nor just a characteristic of normal "introversion".' I saw this girl several times and she liked the interest of a new doctor; but she was terribly contented to be exactly as she was, and I did no good whatever in this case, except by pointing out that the girl was still in the convalescent stage of chorea.

Analysis could not be arranged in this case, and were an analyst willing to take her on I should advise him or her to do so only for research. At any rate this is no analysis for a student.[1]

Case 11: Nancy, aged 20. Living in London, billeted in a home county. I give the following case because, although the girl is 20, she is clinically adolescent.

Nancy came to me with a *dossier* from her Teachers' Training College which it took me half an hour to read. I had to have long interviews with her mother and to read many letters from her, and I had to see the girl herself at intervals over a period of six months, perhaps ten times. Nancy's father had died when she was six, and her mother had devoted herself to the care of her two children. There is a clever, healthy brother of 17.

It might be said in two words that Nancy was a sweet and clean and beautifully dressed girl who was in a state of delayed adolescence. The atmosphere of her otherwise excellent home, as well as her internal difficulties, made it hard for her to take the next step in her development, which was to assert herself. The best thing she had done, psychiatrically speaking, was to kick the girl who was billeted with her, a fellow-student at a training college for teachers. This 'symptom' had become magnified into so great an affair that the school had decided that they could not recommend her as a teacher on account of it, unless I was willing to take responsibility. This I was willing to do. She was supposed to be dangerously impulsive — 'might hit a child'!

It was touch and go whether Nancy would withdraw for ever from impulsive aggression and get set upon the path that leads to some kind of break-down, or would bravely face the nastiness that is there somewhere

[1] This girl wrote to say that she had passed matriculation and was learning to be a masseuse. She seemed to think her interviews with me had something to do with her improvement!

in this clean and carefully folded person just as it is in other people. I think I helped her to the latter course, but to do this I had to see her; and I also had to see her mother repeatedly in order to keep her from writing vilifying letters in defence of her perfect offspring; and further I had to go personally and find her a billet, that is to say a billet that had nothing to do with the training college. For the officials in the training college (really quite an 'advanced' institution) had fully made up their minds that the girl was dangerous. Actually she has the making of an exceptionally good teacher of tinies, if she can bear to hurt her mother by living away from her.[1]

Obviously a case for analysis, but I do no good by putting her on a waiting list. I have let her know that psycho-analysis exists, and I think that one day she will take a teaching job in London, and then apply for analysis. The tragedy is that at the moment when she applies, free psycho-analysis may not be available.

Here is a child who was able to get help from me although he could not come for analysis.

Case 12: Keith, aged 3½ years, living in the suburbs.

Keith is sent to me by a relation who is a doctor friend of mine. This doctor is a bit of a psychologist, and he said it was clear to him that the child's mother (a non-Jewish girl who had married into a clannish Jewish household) was neglecting the child. After I had gone into the case, I felt that here was a clash between two methods of child-upbringing. The mother turned out to be badly in need of support. She immediately got some help through being allowed to give me the usual detailed case history, which I cannot take in less than an hour.

The boy had been easy to feed at the breast (six months) and was easy to train at first. Difficulties started at the introduction of solids. He was always forward intellectually. As a baby he was of the passive type, contented to lie and smile. He hardly ever cried, in contrast to his new brother (nine months) who is behaving quite ordinarily. Complaints were: not sleeping, even with drugs; screaming with rage, negativistic from two years; a continuous nuisance to feed, since beginning on solids; no 'guts' in relation to other children, so that he turns any child into a bully; cannot take 'no' for an answer; also, cannot be left alone with the baby, because of jealousy that did not appear till about eight months after the baby's birth.

I saw this boy once a week, as analysis could not be arranged. As long as he could be brought, I acted with him exactly as if he were in analysis, and he produced material for analysis that had to do with the management, in

---

[1] Later: Nancy has completed her college career without further trouble, and has started in a good post. Her defences are organizing into a tendency to explore spiritualism, for which there is strong precedent in her family.

his mind, of his father and mother. As a result of the work his relation to his mother improved, he became actually demonstrative with her and said 'I love you, I want to kiss you', for the first time. He also started to sleep in a way which he had not done since he was two, and he stood up to his father's going into the army quite well. When his mother found it difficult to come any more I supported her in the idea of leaving off treatment, because the alternative would have been to say to her husband's family that the child was needing more care than she could manage to give, which would have again undermined her confidence in herself.

If I had said that nothing could be done here except analysis I should have missed a good opportunity for therapeutics, and if I had confined my work to giving the mother advice I should not have found the child's new ability to tell her he loved her, which came as a result of the treatment. The adverse external factor was the rather robust but not pathological homosexuality of the father, which this particular child could not stand till he had expressed his hostility to his father in play. He dramatized this with a toy figure, pretending to pull the figure out of his anus, and made a deliberate effort to get me to understand his meaning, naming the figure 'daddy'. He rid himself of the homosexual daddy in play, and then improved in his relations to his real father and mother.

I also helped the next girl a little.

Case 13: Gertie, aged 17, living in London.

This girl was referred by the headmistress of a High School. It was reported that she had reached no satisfactory academic standard, that she had no beauty, no friends — in fact, that she was incredibly lonely. She could give lucid answers to questions, but she had speech difficulties. For a time she had had treatment at another clinic, but without result. All this came over the telephone from the school.

It took a good hour for me to take a history from the mother, who had been successful in bringing up her son (who is four years older than Gertie). The mother was already nervy while carrying Gertie, and after the birth of the child she could not help worrying about her. She wished to wean her, but the G.P. (probably unwisely in this case) persuaded her to persevere with the breast, which she did for the full nine months.

Early signs of intelligence appeared normally, so that the child cannot be said to be backward because of brain tissue defect. During the history-taking the mother remembered that at five the girl had hit her brother on the head and made him bleed, and she thought this may have been a turning-point. From about this time Gertie failed to develop at a normal pace intellectually. The family is a clever one.

The child told me she had 'doctor fright', and indeed she had seen plenty.

We made the following list of things needing cure: pimples, tendency to fester, excessive sweating, being bad at exams, writing and speech clumsiness, difficulty over making friends, difficulty over knowing what work to do, and also her mother's hypochondriacal worrying.

What she seemed to need immediately was for a doctor to say firmly to her, in front of her mother, that she would be wise to see no more doctors. I did this. A month later she came to me to let me know that she had taken a job and was making friends and was beginning to feel more confident.

If I had put her on a waiting list for analysis, I should have been a bad doctor. I wish to be understood here. I believe that there is no therapy that is in any way comparable with analysis. But as this could not be arranged in this case the alternative was to do as I did, to act apart altogether from the existence of psycho-analysis, and to put the girl off therapy of any kind.

The next case came to me from a doctor, following a visit from me to a Child Guidance Clinic.

Case 14, a boy aged ten years, living in a home county. This boy urgently needs help, and is conscious of this need. He could, however, only be analysed if there were a house where he could stay, and from which he could attend at the clinic. I hope there will one day be such a house, because as a result of the recent advances in psycho-analysis, research on insane children can now be done.

It took me an hour to get a good history of this case, and another hour to establish the contact with the boy, contact which I needed in order to form a conclusion as to his intelligence, his emotional development, his illness, and the prognosis. I have seen the boy a dozen times, because he implored me to do so, on account of the very great psychotic anxiety to which he is liable.

His trouble started with his difficult birth, which was a month delayed, so that he was a very big baby. He was born blue, and badly cut about. He was thought to be dead, but to the doctor's surprise the baby showed signs of life after having been abandoned. The doctor said: 'Well, you've got a baby, and he's going to give you a hell of a lot of trouble'—an accurate prognosis. At five he was pronounced mentally defective at a famous children's hospital. Actually he is not intellectually backward, but he is ill in a way that interferes with his relationships. His school puts up with him as odd, and rather likes him.

He is liable to attacks of extreme terror with no external factor to account for them, and he has times of uncontrolled temper, and all sorts of insane ideas appear. For instance, he once came to me with a tank on his hands. By this I do not mean that he had a toy tank or that he had an idea of a tank in his head, I mean that he felt he really had a tank on his hands. He

81

constantly tried to get it off, by squeezing his hands between his legs, passing his hands between his closely drawn thighs. He drew a picture of what he felt like. Also, for a long time, whenever he went to the lavatory to defaecate, a certain brick would seem to him to come out of the wall and wander round.

Further details of this case would be out of place here, but it seemed good to do something more than just see the boy in consultation. While I go on seeing the boy (which at first I did weekly, though I can now increase the interval to a month), he is able to avoid giving trouble at school, and he has less severe attacks of panic. This is not because of anything specific that I do.

He is clever at carpentry and sewing, and loves the idea of farming. He studies aeroplanes in great detail from books, and shows signs of making an exceptionally interesting, restless adult with patchy brilliance.

*　　　*　　　*

My object has been, as I stated at the beginning, to report a series of consultations. There is nothing particularly interesting about the series except that it comprises all the cases sent to the Department over a period of time and presumably indicates the type of case to be expected if an attempt were made to widen the range of the Department and to establish a consultation clinic.

It may be that some of this non-analytic material has proved of interest to analysts. It is a personal opinion of mine that it is to analysts that non-analytic material is really interesting. For instance, when a mother gradually pieces together an almost complete history of her child's emotional development, who but an analyst is likely to supply what she wants, which is the true recognition that all the pieces do weld together into a whole?

Also many odd flashes of insight from parent and child remind the analyst of material patiently acquired in analytic work. I would go further and say that I have learned much that is of value in analysis from the therapeutic consultation, and from the study of other non-analytic material.

One practical point emerges. The primary aim of consultation at the Institute, I take it, is the provision of suitable cases for students, or for analysts of adults who wish to go on to do child analysis. I have never expected that this aim would be achieved, and I think my fears have been justified by this report. It is a matter which we shall have to work out gradually, but it does seem to me possible that the proper place for seeking good cases for students is a paediatric department of a hospital.

There are two possible points of view. According to one, we can encourage vast numbers of cases to impinge on the Institute, and retain a percentage on the ground that they are suitable for training purposes, letting the rest fall off as their fingers tire and when they can no longer keep a hold on the waiting-list, which is their one hope. The other is for someone to be seeing and dealing with a large number of psychiatric cases of all kinds; in this way social pressure could be met, and occasionally and as required under the training scheme, suitable cases could be transferred for analysis.

In the case of children, it is possible that the second is actually the only possible method, since the adults who bring the children are in most cases normal healthy adults; and if a child is simply put on a waiting-list the adult goes elsewhere for advice. Even a fortnight's wait for consultation is usually enough to discourage a parent or guardian. A series of children put on a waiting-list and left there would be a constant source of ill-feeling, and would all the time be seriously interfering with the relations of the Society with the external world.

As far as I can see it then, while it will remain necessary for someone to attend to the consultations at the Institute as at present, it will continue to be necessary also to draw on other clinics for good analytical material for teaching purposes, especially as the best way to start teaching child analysis is to provide a little child of three, not too ill.

It might not be out of place to give a list of conditions that must be fulfilled when I am trying to supply a student with a child patient. I have to find a child of the required sex and age, of the right diagnostic grouping and degree of illness, with a mother who is genuinely, yet not hypochondriacally, concerned about the child's disorder, whose address is within easy reach of the clinic; external circumstances must allow the mother to give up two or three hours a day to one child; the parents' faith in the doctor must carry them over the period in which there is but little encouragement to be got from the changes in the child's symptoms; and the social status of the family must allow the mother to spend money every day on trains and buses.

In only a small proportion of cases can these demands be met. At present nothing approaching what is required for training purposes is to be expected from the cases coming to the clinic direct, and I am in doubt whether it should ever be our aim to make it so.

It will be felt that there is a note of frustration in my paper. I admit this. I am always wanting to arrange for the patient to be analysed, knowing well that nothing else that can be done approaches or can be compared with the results of analysis. At the same time I am acutely aware that analysis is very seldom both applicable and available. Often the patient cannot be brought to the clinic, or too complex external circumstances would have to be managed, and usually when a case could be treated it is unsuitable for a student. It must be remembered also that it is quite rare for even one new child to be required for analysis. I may go three months without being asked to supply a case.

My sense of frustration must therefore arouse your sympathy. It is clear that the only solution is for more analysts to train, and to learn to do child analysis. We all long for this, and we also know that it is just here that it is difficult to bring about changes, and that no good can come from hurry.

Postscript (1957)

From the date of this communication up to the present time there has been no child clinic at the Institute, and therefore no waiting-list. When a child is needed for a student analyst a child is found from some other established clinic.

Happily two changes have come about in the intervening decade; there are now many clinics on which to draw when a vacancy occurs for a child analysis, and also there are now 30 instead of 2—6 analysts taking the additional training in child analysis.

Ocular Psychoneuroses of Childhood[1]
[1944]

IT IS EASY to say that a child values sight, or fears blindness, and yet at the same time fail to come to grips with the immensity of the hopes and fears involved.

The fact that ophthalmologists exist who deal especially with children shows that there is a general recognition of the fact that children require a special approach. A knowledge of the anatomy, physiology, and pathology of the eye is of little use to the clinician who cannot get in touch with his child patient; and skill in making contact with a child largely depends on the eye doctor's understanding of a child's feelings and his belief in the child's hopes and suspicions and fears. The child recognizes very quickly whether the doctor believes in him, and usually he allows examinations and even co-operates helpfully. So the doctor who believes in the feelings of children starts off as a good psychologist.

Following up this idea, an enormous quantity of successful psychotherapy is all the time being done by ordinary routine management of cases. On the other hand, harm can be done. As a glaring example, I quote the experience of a friend whose childhood was spoilt by the remark of an eye surgeon to whom she was taken when small. He said to the child's mother, in front of her: 'She is suffering from retinitis pigmentosa, and will probably go blind when she is older.' This was, of course, a wrong prognosis, but the point is the surgeon did not know that it mattered, saying this in front of a little girl. The child spent her childhood expecting to go blind, and she forced herself to read everything while she could, and was always testing her eyes. Now at the age of 50 she is beginning to believe that in spite of the doctor's words she may escape blindness. Children quite naturally feel that they are custodians of their eyes, or of any other part of their body, and if they do not keep their eyes healthy they feel they have failed in a trust.

[1] *The Transactions of the Ophthalmological Society*, Vol. LXIV, 1944.

The whole of my contribution could be about the ordinary good management of the ordinary case, but I must go on to describe psychological illness as it affects the eyes. It is chiefly to the ordinary common cases that I wish to draw attention.

Three groups of psychological symptoms have to be described. First is the group of symptoms shown by children whose personality structure is satisfactory. At the other extreme is the group of symptoms associated with personality structure defect, either primary or the result of the undoing of progress already made. In between comes the group of symptoms that cluster round depression. There is much overlapping and I cannot deal with the three groups in a clearly defined way.

PSYCHONEUROSIS

A child whose very early emotional development has proceeded normally and whose personality structure is satisfactory is in spite of this liable to all sorts of symptoms, even serious ones, and some of these may have to do with the eyes. An example would be eye-rubbing. As is well known, the start of eye-rubbing may be a blepharitis, following measles or some other infection, but there is always an added emotional cause, and in certain cases the whole thing may be psychologically determined. One warning: I am half afraid to describe psychological matters to an audience of doctors. Doctors seem to have to *treat and cure* every symptom. But in psychology this is a snare and delusion. One must be able to note symptoms without trying to cure them because every symptom has its value to the patient, and very frequently the patient is better left with his symptom. In any case one must be able to describe psychological matters without immediately having to answer the question as to how to cure what is described. To treat a patient usefully, one usually has to do a lot of work, or to share some heavy burden, and it is illogical to attack the symptom unless the underlying mental conflict is recognized and dealt with. For instance, a child may be lonely or depressed, and eye-rubbing may be an exploitation of the eye-itching that belongs normally to sleepiness as a natural defence of a child against intolerable feelings. Or it may be that someone is over-exciting the child, so that the child has to manage all sorts of exaggerations of normal sensation, including perhaps burning eyelids.

I had better mention the interference with natural good looks by glasses. Not only do many children mind having glasses, but quite a number expect to have to wear glasses as a punishment for wanting to excel in good looks. Glasses quickly acquire a meaning to the child who wears them. Glasses, just like apparatus in the mouth, or splints, or clothes, become part of the personality of the child, and a great deal can be said about glasses as a fetish, but this more obviously concerns adults. Perversions in which the eyes and glasses are important can be found sometimes in the reactions of children to glasses and to eye examinations.

Now for the eye itself. The eye's complicated function works easily when the child uses it in the ordinary way, but what if the eye is used (unconsciously) *instead of another organ* of the body? What if the eye stands for an organ that contains erectile tissue and so is capable of changing when excited? In such a case the eye becomes not only the organ of sight, but also an excitable part of the body. Then symptoms may arise. The main change is a blood supply out of proportion to the need based on usage and the result is eye-tiredness. Fears that belong to other parts of the body become dramatized in the eye, and glasses are used by children to hide the eyes which have become excited, and are therefore felt to be conspicuous. Hysterical blindness is associated with guilt about seeing, especially when the eye is doing more than seeing and is controlling. I need hardly remind you that a patient cannot be expected to be conscious of what is happening, and no good whatever can come from giving explanations or imagining that the child has only to use will-power to over-come hysterical symptoms. The treatment of such a case on psychological lines would include an investigation into the causes of displacement of interest from the normal excitable organ to the eye, which is not in itself excitable. Paralysis of accommodation can very easily dramatize the repression of sight memories, especially where there remains the attempt to control the original terrifying situation. I find that a whole lot of minor eye symptoms, blinking and tiredness that have no definite cause in refraction errors, are related to unconscious guilt over the sight of things that were presumed to be taboo.

DEPRESSION

I have come to depression, and the part that this kind of difficulty plays in producing eye troubles. In children as in adults depression can be recognized as a mood, and clinically it appears very commonly in its form of common anxious restlessness, or a denial of depression by forced activity and liveliness. Along with this, as in depression phases in adults, one can see self-destructive actions, deliberate or accidental, and also hypochondriacal worry over the body or parts of the body. Far from being a rare illness, depression is a very common state in children as well as in adults, and is not even necessarily abnormal; hypochondriacal worry joins up with normal concern. The normal aspect of depression is that one should be *able* to be concerned about one's body, to enjoy it when it is well, and to want to get it well when it is ill. Tears that are increased in sadness are also physiologically valuable, so that the dry eyes that belong to a flight from sadness predispose to conjunctival infection and irritation.

Hypochondria appears in the eye department, as elsewhere, and it is very important that the doctor should know what is happening. First he must be able to distinguish between the mother's hypochondria and the child's. Many children wear glasses, or at least frequently have their eyes tested, because of their mothers' hypochondriacal illness. There is no sharp line between this the mothers' hypochondria and the natural concern that a mother feels over her child's sight, and so the doctor should be able to allow mother her worry, and when possible to say to her, 'Share the responsibility with me, visit me at intervals; at present this child's eyes are normal'. If the doctor says to the hypochondriacal mother, 'I think the child's eyes are all right, *but* we must have a Wassermann reaction done, and a blood-count and a Mantoux, and I think the child should go and see a psychologist', the mother, far from being reassured, will be convinced that her life's work is to worry about her child's health. The child's own hypochondria requires even more careful management, and the simplest rule is that the child should hear the truth. In most cases the doctor can say what he finds to the child as well as to the mother, and what he proposes to do, and how he proposes to watch for future developments. True reassurance comes from statement of fact, not from reassuring words and tones, which carry for the child an implication that there is danger. Whereas the majority of children coming to the eye doctor are able to accept the reassurance that the eyes are either well or just needing glasses, a proportion of children are unable to accept reassurance and will feel that something is being hidden from them; rather specialized management is required in such cases, a description of which would not be appropriate here, although the subject is tremendously important.

The suicidal activities of infantile and child depression are easily missed, yet very real. The child feels there is something wrong or wicked about himself. He does not easily separate out physical from bodily phenomena, and so he is either sick, or has diarrhoea, or else he allows accidents to happen to him, or he falls, or he pulls hot tea down over him, or he rubs his eye when there is a grit in it till it is scratched and infected.

The eye sometimes becomes involved in the individual's attempt to insure against depression in a way that is best described by likening convergence to thumb-sucking. The thumb represents the breast or bottle which the anxious or lonely infant needs to keep in his mouth or just outside it. So too the child gets reassurance from recovering the position of the eyes which in early infancy enable the child to see in detail the mother's breast and face, just there within a few inches of the mouth, neither swallowed up nor gone away outside.

This state of affairs might be described as a compromise between subjective sight and objective perception. There is by no means always a squint present, but the eyes become seriously involved through the continued strain of the compulsion which often leads to a tremendous reading urge. One patient of mine who developed near sight at about eleven years describes the technique for sleep in this way: as she settles down at last to sleep she takes a book that she knows well and places it very close to her eyes, where she can read it without her strong glasses. She then reads and re-reads the familiar lines until she no longer knows she is awake. Naturally she can never turn off the light. As she wakes she has to be reading before waking, just as she reads before sleeping, only this time she hallucinates the book and the page, and the subject matter and type. When she awakes she is surprised to find the real book has fallen. I think it likely that in such a case the convergence and near accommodation have to be maintained at least during light sleep.

The whole question of rest of eyes in sleep interests me. I think that many people work their eyes a great deal in sleep, and to rest their eyes they look at an object when they are awake. At any rate, it is notorious that the group of children I am describing are slave-drivers to their eyes, and any attempt to make them stop reading with the book close to their eyes is liable to meet with failure and to make them feel hopeless and lost. This condition may start very early in a child's life, but on the other hand, it may come on during the onset of puberty, or at any time. There is no condition of the eye which makes more demands than this one does on the eye doctor.

PSYCHOSIS

The subject of squint is one which needs research from the psychological side. I have good evidence that squint can have a purely psychological cause, and I think that most ophthalmologists would agree. However, when it comes to describing the actual mechanisms *I am not on sure ground*. I have already mentioned internal squint, maintained with near accommodation as a reminder of the early relation to the breast, and as a comfort, like thumb-sucking. There is one kind of squint, usually an external squint, in which the trouble seems to be that the two eyes do not work with one aim, this being associated with a division in the personality. It is as though the individual dramatized the split in the ego in a lack of co-ordination between his eyes. Illustrating this I would quote the example of a highly intelligent woman, headmistress of a large school, who used both her eyes separately, as she had an external squint. The left eye represented her good relation with her father, who spoke only English, whereas her right eye was connected with her relation with her mother, who spoke only French. This woman's parents had very little in common, and the patient developed quite differently in relation to the one and the other. She was left-handed, and was very much interested in children in her school who were left-handed. Her left hand represented her business side and her identification with her father. Her religious feeling was associated entirely with her mother, and when signing or writing anything connected with religious matters she could only use her right hand. This gives illustration to what happens when there is a clear division in the personality. But frequently there is more serious unintegration, and in that case I think that one eye is identified with the strongest part of the personality, and that the other, a hopelessly wandering eye, represents the other parts. An external squint that is not clearly due to a physical cause is difficult to cure unless there is a reintegration of the personality. This integration may occur spontaneously or, under the influence of another strong personality, a child may achieve some kind of integration which makes it possible for the squint to disappear, at any rate temporarily. This factor should not be lost sight of when the physical side of squint treatment of one kind or another is being considered. I am not, of course, despising or criticizing the physical side, but am drawing attention to the psychological side.

A third psychological type of squint, one which can appear very early, seems to be that which accompanies an acute introversion phase, the internal squint being a dramatization of a preoccupation with internal phenomena, or inner world reality. An alternative in such a case is looking in the looking-glass, which some introverted children do a great deal.

EYE AS SYMBOL

It should be remembered that, from the psychologist's point of view, the eye is not just an organ of sight. Whereas in bodily phenomena things are taken in by the mouth and excreted by the excretory organs, in the building up of the personality a parallel taking in and giving out is done through all the organs of the body, the eyes, the skin, the ears, the nose, etc. A great deal is always being taken in by the eyes. The eyes also represent an organ of excretion. Everyone has seen a friend 'into a bus', and in a sense everything we see comes out from ourselves on to the object. I have already described a girl who hallucinated a page as she woke. There are those who read the newspapers to gain information, but many expect the paper to put out before their eyes the things they are already thinking and feeling and, in fact, they cannot be said to take much notice of the actual information supplied, except as a mild corrective to their imagination.

It would be a matter for research to find out how much the intrinsic muscles and tissues of the eye are involved in ordinary visual imagery, and in hallucinatory activity. Perhaps this has been worked out, but I do not know.

Chapter VII

Reparation in Respect of Mother's Organized Defence against Depression[1]
[1948]

THE CONCEPT of the depressive position is generally accepted as a valuable one for use in actual analytic work as well as in the attempt to describe the progress of normal emotional development. In the analyses that we do we can reach the guilt in its relation to aggressive and destructive impulses and ideas, and we can watch the urge to make reparation appear as the patient becomes able to account for, tolerate, and hold the guilt feeling. There are other roots for creativeness, but reparation provides an important link between the creative impulse and the life the patient leads. The attainment of a capacity for making reparation in respect of personal guilt is one of the most important steps in the development of the healthy human being, and we now wonder how we did analytic work before we consciously made use of this simple truth.

Clinically however we meet with a false reparation which is not specifically related to the patient's own guilt, and it is to this that I wish to refer. This false reparation appears through the patient's identification with the mother and the dominating factor is not the patient's own guilt but the mother's organized defence against depression and unconscious guilt.

It may be that by expanding my title in this way I have said enough: certainly I do not feel that the idea is original or that it needs laborious development. Nevertheless, I shall attempt to illustrate my meaning briefly.

For 25 years a pageant of clinical material has been passing in front of me in my hospital Out-Patients Department. In the course of the years there is not much change in the general pattern. One type of child I remember well from the beginning. This child is particularly delightful and often talented above the average. If a girl, she is sure to be attractively dressed and clean.

[1] Read before the British Psycho-Analytical Society, 7th January, 1948. Revised August, 1954.

The point about her is a vivacity which immediately contributes something to one's mood, so that one feels lighter. One is not surprised to learn that she is a dancer or to find that she draws and paints and writes poetry. She may write a poem or two while waiting her turn to see me. When she draws me a picture I know there will be gay colours and interesting detail and the figures will have a certain sprightliness, seeming to be alive, moving. There may easily be a strong humorous element also.

The mother brings the child because at home she is irritable, moody, at times defiant, or frankly depressed. Perhaps many doctors have failed to believe that the child is anything but delightful. The mother tells me about various aches and pains of which the child complains and which at one time or another have been diagnosed by doctors as rheumatic, but which are really hypochondriacal.

Early in my career a little boy came to hospital by himself and said to me, 'Please, Doctor, mother complains of a pain in my stomach', and this drew my attention usefully to the part mother can play. Also it is a fact that the child who is supposed to have a pain has often not yet decided where the pain is. If one can catch him before his mother has indicated what she is expecting, one can find him bewildered and simply wanting to say that the pain is 'inside'. What is meant is that there is a feeling that something is wrong, or that there ought to be.

Probably I get a specially clear view of this problem in a children's out-patient department because such a department is really a *clinic for the management of hypochondria in mothers*. There is no sharp dividing line between the frank hypochondria of a depressed woman and a mother's genuine concern for her child. A mother must be able to be hypochondriacal if she is to be able to notice the symptoms in her child that the doctors are always asking for in their attempt to catch disease early. A doctor who knows nothing of psychiatry or knows nothing of the contra-depressive defences, and who does not know that children get depressed, is liable to tell a mother off when she worries about a child's symptom, and to fail to see the very real psychiatric problems that exist. On the other hand, a psycho-analyst fresh from newly discovered understanding of childhood depression could easily fail to notice when it is the mother who is more ill than the child. Watching many of these cases continuously over periods of ten or even twenty years I have been able to see that the depression of the child can be the mother's depression in reflection. The child uses the mother's depression as an escape from his or her own; this provides a false restitution and reparation in relation to the mother, and this hampers the development of a personal restitution capacity because the restitution does not relate to the child's own guilt sense. Of any series of promising students a proportion fail to reach the top because of the fact that reparation is being made in respect of the mother's depression rather than in respect of depression that is personal. When there seems to be special talent and even an initial success there remains an instability associated with dependence of the child on the mother. A homosexual overlay may or may not develop. Somewhere in a book on ballet, Arnold Haskell says: 'It should be remembered that every ballet dancer has a mother.' These children I am describing certainly have their mothers and their fathers. It is of course not always the mother. Many adolescent boys and girls seeming to have a capacity for successful work unexpectedly break down when their success in work is stolen by the needs of one or other parent or both. In the attempt of the adolescent to establish a personal identity the only solution then is through failure, and this especially applies to the case of the boy who is expected to follow exactly in his father's footsteps, and who yet never will be able to challenge the father's assumption of control.

It will be seen that these children in extreme cases have a task which can never be accomplished. Their task is first to deal with mother's mood. If they succeed in the immediate task, they do no more than succeed in creating an atmosphere in which they can *start on their own lives*. It can be readily understood that this situation can be exploited by the individual as a flight from that acceptance of personal responsibility which is an essential part of individual development. Where the child has the chance to dig down to personal guilt through analysis, then the mother's (or father's) mood is also there to be dealt with. The analyst must either recognize when the signs of this appear in the transference, or the analysis must fail, because of its success. I am describing a rather obvious phenomenon.

The usual observation is that the child's mother (or father) has a dominating personality. As analysts I think we shall want to say that the child lives within the circle of the parent's personality and that this circle has pathological features. In the typical case of the delightful girl I have described, the mother's need for help in respect of the deadness and blackness in her inner world finds a response in the child's liveliness and colour.

In a large number of these cases there is not an extreme of this condition, so that the child's reparation activities *can* be personal although there is a constant threat that the mother will steal the child's success and, therefore, the underlying guilt. In such cases it is not difficult to get astonishing clinical successes by actively displacing the parent in the early part of a psychotherapy of the child. In a favourable case it is possible to take the child's side against the parents and *at the same time* to gain and keep the parents' confidence.

I was called in by a Teachers' Training College to see a student who was under threat of expulsion. She had suddenly kicked a fellow student on the ankle. I found a girl who had had a mother's depression to bear all her life, and who, at the end of her student career, had at last reached the problem

— her own life or mother's? I managed to get the mother to believe in me while I actually got in between her and her daughter. The latter was accepted back to the College, finished well, and set out on a series of jobs away from home. She has done very well and is now a senior teacher. This was a borderline case, and without my intervention she would have had to fail and break down, or else to have staged a false success, after giving up all hope of ever achieving an existence independent of her widow-mother's heavily organized mood.

One's most spectacular successes in professional work have been in this type of work. From this there is a lesson for the psycho-analyst who at the beginning of his career can easily be deceived into thinking that early success in a treatment is due to the interpretations, when really the important thing is that he has displaced a good but depressed parent. In spite of early success, the ordinary difficulties lie ahead, including the patient's discovery of his own guilt feeling. Initially the important thing is that the analyst is not depressed and the patient finds himself because the analyst is not needing the patient to be good or clean or compliant and is not even needing to be able to teach the patient anything. The patient can proceed at his own pace. He can fail if he wishes, and he is given time and a sort of local security. These external details of management are the prerequisites for the patient's discovery of his own love with the inevitable complication of aggression and guilt, that which alone makes sense of reparation and restitution. In the extreme case, the patient will come to analysis hardly having started on the task of coping with his own guilt, or not yet having reached his own aggression belonging to primitive love, and this in spite of the fact that the world has thought well of him.

Those who work with groups are much concerned with this relationship of the patient to an environmental mood. In some cases a useful comparison can be made between the group's mood, over which the patient has some control, and the mood of his mother when he was an infant, over which he had no control; as an infant he could only accept the fact of the mother's mood, and get caught in with the mother's contra-depressive defences. In other cases, the group mood cannot be entered into by the one member because of his having too strong a need to defend or fight for his own individuality.

The group can be a family. I would say that it is clearly of great value to family life when the depressive position has been reached securely enough on a personal basis by the individuals, so that the family mood is able also to have its place, being a common factor in the lives of the individual members. This is the same as any sharing of a culture. It is obviously pathological, or an impoverishment of the family or group, if an individual member cannot share in the reparation activities of a group. And, per contra, it is a serious impoverishment of the member's life if he can only take part in activities that are quite specifically group-activities. In the former case, when he cannot share, the individual must establish his own individual approach before sharing. In the latter case, where a group is necessary, he seems at first to be a useful co-operator, but eventually his co-operation breaks down; he remains to some degree in the position of the child caught up in mother's inner world, with consequent loss of personal responsibility.

It seems to me that there is a practical application of these ideas in the Psycho-Analytical Society. I refer particularly to the opinion expressed by Glover (1945, 1949). He feels that certain analysts (Melanie Klein and her pupils) are describing certain fantasies as if they were fantasies of their patients when probably these fantasies were those of the analysts themselves. Every analyst is aware of the task of disentangling his own fantasies from those of his patients, but it is generally reckoned that it is the psycho-analysts who are best able to be clear about this sort of thing. It is very difficult for me to believe that ideas that regularly appear in both my analytic and non-analytic work are subjective. Nevertheless I recognize that unless ideas can be subjective they cannot be objectively observed; (cf. Whitehead: 'The material and conditions out of which the clinical investigator has to forge ordered knowledge are a constant challenge to his capacity for conceptual thinking as well as to his powers of observation'). It is important, however, to find out what prompts the remark, such as that of Glover, that the fantasies that we report are subjective, and not truly to be found in our patients. First, the question must be asked: has the analysis of the depressive position been put forward badly, in such a way that the ideas are unacceptable on account of the way they have been presented? (Cf. Brierley, 1951.) For instance, has due recognition been given to the need for everything to be discovered afresh by every individual analyst? At any rate there must be kept clear the distinction between the value of ideas and the feeling about them roused by the way they have been presented.

Be this as it may, there remains a need to consider the problem along with the idea put forward in this paper.

It is legitimate to demand of me that if I claim to describe the fantasy of my patients, I know that patients at times do produce *the sort of things they feel I like getting*. This is the more true the more my expectations are unconscious. A patient, recently, was quite convinced that I liked anal material, and of course produced plenty for my benefit; it was some time before this came into the open, and before he reached his own true anal feeling. In the same way patients produce, and also hide, fantasy relating to the inner world because they feel a need to relieve my supposed depression, or to make it worse. In the transference a parental depression has been revived. I must be able to recognize this. When I claim to be truly objective about ideas that patients have about their insides, and about the contending of good and bad objects or forces within, I must be able to distinguish between that which is produced for me, and that which is truly personal to the patient. I believe that Jungian analysts tend to receive 'Jungian type' dreams, and Freudians but seldom receive these elaborate mystical formations.

In this scientific group we have a common pool of theory, and we offer a group or setting for reparation activity in respect of a common pool of guilt. Each member becomes affected by the Society's mood, and is free to contribute to the group's restitution urge, which relates to the group's depressive anxieties. But always this restitution in the group must wait on the more important thing, that each individual shall reach to personal guilt, and to personal depressive anxieties. Each individual member of our Society must achieve his *own* growth at his *own* pace and develop his *own* sense of responsibility based truly on personal concern about his own love impulses and their consequences.

SUMMARY

An individual's reparation urge may be related less to the personal guilt-sense than to the guilt-sense or depressed mood of a parent. The contribution of an individual to a group is affected by the relative success or failure of the individual in establishing personal rather than parental guilt as the root of reparation activities, and of constructive effort.

Chapter VIII

Anxiety Associated with Insecurity[1]
[1952]

THE FOLLOWING is a comment on a point in Dr C. F. Rycroft's paper on 'Some Observations on a Case of Vertigo' (Rycroft, 1953). In this paper Rycroft makes two statements on which I wish to comment. The two statements are:

'In my previous paper I discussed in some detail the theoretical implications of [the patient's] ability to hallucinate objects and simultaneously recognize them as illusions. Here I only wish to mention that it shows very clearly both the depth of his regression, which was to a stage before reality testing is firmly established, and the incompleteness of the regression, since part of his ego remained capable of testing reality and of contributing actively to the analysis.'

Again, 'Vertigo is a sensation which occurs when one's sense of equilibrium is threatened. To an adult it is a sensation which is usually, though by no means always, associated with threats to the maintenance of the erect posture, and there is, therefore, a tendency to think of giddiness exclusively in terms of such relatively mature anxieties as the fear of falling over or the fear of heights and to forget that infants, long before they can stand, experience threats to their equilibrium and that some of their earliest activities such as grasping and clinging represent attempts to maintain the security of feeling supported by the mother. As the infant learns to crawl and later to walk the supporting function of the mother is increasingly taken over by the ground; this must be one of the main reasons why the earth is unconsciously thought of as the mother and why neurotic disturbances of equilibrium can so frequently be traced back to conflicts about dependence on the mother.'

It seems to me that here, in this idea of the mother's function to give a feeling of security, there is room for development, and I would like Dr Rycroft

[1] Read before the British Psycho-Analytical Society, 5th November, 1952.

to write another paper on this theme to which he has obviously given attention since he refers us to Alice Balint, Hermann, and Schilder.

It should be noted that there is a relationship between the baby and the mother here that is of vital importance, and yet it is not a derivation of instinctual experience, nor of object relationship arising out of instinct experience. It antedates instinct experience, as well as running concurrently with it, and getting mixed up with it.

We are near the well-known observation that the earliest anxiety is related to being insecurely held.

Analysts — even those who see a human being in the infant from the time of birth — often speak as if the infant's life starts with oral instinctual experience and the emerging object relationship of instinctual experience. Yet we all know that an infant has the capacity to feel awful as a result of the failure of something that is quite in another field, that is to say, that of infant care. Miss Freud's emphasis on *techniques* of infant care draws us to this very matter. At least that is my opinion, and it makes me feel that there is urgent need for us to hammer away at the discussion of the meaning of anxiety when the cause is failure in the technique of infant care, as for instance, failure to give the continuous live support that belongs to mothering.

We know that this subject can take us right back to the time of birth, that is to say, to the time when the foetus is ready to be born — at about the thirty-sixth week of intrauterine life.

The question that I want to ask is this: Can anything be said about this anxiety, or is it just a physical thing, and no more? Rycroft's case would seem at first to support the view that this early anxiety is just a matter of semi-circular canals and physiology. Nevertheless we are left with elbow-room for feeling that there might be more to be discovered. The fact of physiological vertigo is undisputed, yet (as in sea-sickness) the physiological can be exploited under certain circumstances. What in fact are those circumstances?

Instead of simply asking this question I do wish to make a partial answer.

In my view there are certain types of anxiety in early infancy that are prevented by good-enough care, and these can be studied with profit. I think that the states that are prevented by good infant care are all states that group naturally under the word mad, if they are found in an adult.

A simple example would be the state of unintegration. With good infant care this state is the natural state and there is no one there to mind about it. Good care produces a state of affairs in which integration begins to become a fact, and a person starts to be there. In so far as this is true, so far does failure of care lead to disintegration instead of to a return to unintegration. Disintegration is felt to be a threat because (by definition) there is someone there to feel the threat. Also it is a defence.

Three main types of anxiety resulting from failure in technique of child care

are: unintegration, becoming a feeling of disintegration; lack of relationship of psyche to soma, becoming a sense of depersonalization; also the feeling that the centre of gravity of consciousness transfers from the kernel to the shell, from the individual to the care, the technique.

In order to make this last idea clear I must examine the state of affairs at this early state of a human life.

Let us start with the two-body relationship (Rickman, 1951), and from this go earlier to the object relationship that is still of the nature of a two-body relationship, but the object is a part object.

What precedes this? We sometimes loosely assume that before the two-body object relationship there is a one-body relationship, but this is wrong, and obviously wrong if we look closely. The capacity for a one-body relationship *follows* that of a two-body relationship, through the introjection of the object. (Implied is an external world to which the relationship is of a negative kind.)

What then precedes the first object relationship? For my own part I have had a long struggle with this problem. It started when I found myself saying in this Society (about ten years ago) and I said it rather excitedly and with heat: *'There is no such thing as a baby.'* I was alarmed to hear myself utter these words and tried to justify myself by pointing out that if you show me a baby you certainly show me also someone caring for the baby, or at least a pram with someone's eyes and ears glued to it. One sees a 'nursing couple'.

In a quieter way today I would say that before object relationships the state of affairs is this: that the unit is not the individual, the unit is an environment-individual set-up. The centre of gravity of the being does not start off in the individual. It is in the total set-up. By good-enough child care, technique, holding, and general management the shell becomes gradually taken over and the kernel (which has looked all the time like a human baby to us) can begin to be an individual. The beginning is potentially terrible because of the anxieties I have mentioned and because of the paranoid state that follows closely on the first integration, and also on the first instinctual moments, bringing to the baby, as they do, a quite new meaning to object relationships. The good-enough infant care technique neutralizes the external persecutions, and prevents the feelings of disintegration and loss of contact between psyche and soma.

In other words, without a good-enough technique of infant care the new human being has no chance whatever. With a good-enough technique the centre of gravity of being in the environment-individual set-up can afford to lodge in the centre, in the kernel rather than in the shell. The human being now developing an entity from the centre can become localized in the baby's body and so can begin to create an external world at the same time as acquiring a limiting membrane and an inside. According to this theory there was no external world at the beginning although *we as observers* could see an infant in an environment. How deceptive this can be is shown by the fact that often we think we see an infant when we learn through analysis at a later date that what we ought to have seen was an environment developing falsely into a human being, hiding within itself a potential individual.

Continuing in this same dogmatic way I want to make a comment on the clinical condition known popularly as hysteria. The term neurosis covers nearly the same ground.

It is normal for the infant to feel anxiety if there is a failure of infant-care technique. An infant at the very beginning, however, would go into an unintegrated state, or lose contact with the body, or shift over to being the socket instead of the content, *without pain.*

Inherent in growth, then, is pain, anxiety in respect of these various phenomena that result from failure of infant care. In health, the environment (taken over by the mother or nurse) makes a graduated failure, starting off with almost perfect adaptation.

There is a state of affairs in which the fear is of a madness, that is to say a fear of a *lack of anxiety at regression* to an unintegrated state, to absence of a sense of living in the body, etc. The fear is that there will be no anxiety, that is to say, that there will be a regression, from which there may be no return.

The consequence of this is a repeated testing of capacity for anxiety and temporary relief whenever anxiety is felt, the worse the better (Balint, 1955).

The analysis of the hysteric (popular term) is the analysis of the madness that is feared but which is not reached without the provision of a new example of infant care, better infant care in the analysis than was provided at the time of the patient's infancy. But, please note, the analysis does and must get to the madness, although the diagnosis remains neurosis, not psychosis.

Would Dr Rycroft agree that his patient could both remember his early infantile experiences of physiological vertigo and *also* exploit these memory traces in defence against anxieties associated with failure of infant-care technique, anxieties which would feel to the patient (though he is not mad) like a threat of madness?

Chapter IX

Symptom Tolerance in Paediatrics[1]

A CASE HISTORY
[1953]

MY THEME, which is foreshadowed in the title, might lead along two distinct paths. I mention one of these only because I may have been expected to follow it. I refer to the fact that the natural bodily processes tending towards health and towards a resolution of illness have become more than a little obscured by the recent flood of advances in chemotherapy. It is indeed difficult for a house physician at the present time to find out by experience what a child does with pneumonia with no more help than the good nursing which, thirty years ago, was the only treatment. Today, and we all agree about this, even a boil must not be allowed to take care of itself. I feel that in the best of the medical schools the teaching does include a reminder that children lived through illnesses before penicillin and that even today it is the child and the living tissues that ultimately bring about a restoration of health, not the antibiotic.

I have not followed this important trail because this theme has been developed with great competence in various addresses to medical students by physicians who remember the bad old times, and who see that from the teaching point of view the bad old times could claim some points in their favour. My theme follows another path which in the end will, I think, prove to be a related one, since again it concerns the natural tendency towards health and the use that we can make of this tendency as doctors. In the psychological field the principle that there is a natural tendency towards health or developmental maturity is one which has a particular significance. It could be said that much of physical disease is due to an invasion from the environment or to an environmental deficiency, and is not a purely developmental disorder. By contrast, psychological disorder can always be described

---

[1] Presidential address to the Section of Paediatrics, Royal Society of Medicine, February 27, 1953. *Proceedings of the Royal Society of Medicine*, Vol. 46, No. 8, August 1953.

in terms of emotional development either delayed or distorted or in some other way prevented from reaching the maturity that is due at the age which the child has reached. There is an even closer link therefore in psychological medicine between the normal and the abnormal than there is between physiology and the pathological processes of tissues and functions. In fact when there is only a disturbance of physiology then the illness is usually psychogenic.

When I was thinking over the relationship between paediatrics and child psychiatry it occurred to me that this relationship involves not only a difference between the fields but also a difference of emotional attitude between those who adopt the one or the other approach to a case. The paediatrician feels the symptom as a challenge to his therapeutic armoury. It is hoped that this will always be true. If a child has a pain, then the sooner it is diagnosed and the cause removed the better. By contrast, the child psychiatrist sees in the symptom an organization of extreme complexity, one that is produced and maintained because of its value. The child needs the symptom because of some hitch in emotional development.

(For the purposes of clear argument it is helpful to assume that our physically ill child is psychiatrically healthy, and that our psychiatrically ill child has a well body. Although this is very often not true it is a justifiable simplification for us to make just now.)

The psychiatrist is therefore not a symptom-curer; he recognizes the symptom as an SOS call that justifies a full investigation of the history of the child's emotional development, relative to the environment and to the culture. Treatment is directed towards relieving the child of the need to send out the SOS.

There is, as I have already indicated, a degree of artificiality in this statement of contrasts. The best body-doctors do also seek causes and, when possible, employ as their chief therapeutic the natural tendency of the body to be healthy. But even body-doctors who are suitably tolerant of symptoms that are physically determined and who seek first causes when faced with physical disease tend to become symptom-allergic before a syndrome of psychological aetiology. They develop an urge to cure the moment they are confronted with an hysterical conversion symptom, or a phobia that has no apparent sense in it, or a sensitivity to noise that seems quite mad, or an obsessional ritual, a regression in behaviour, a mood disorder, an antisocial tendency, or a restlessness that connotes a hopeless confusional state at the core of the child's personality.

I am convinced that symptom intolerance appears simply because the body-paediatrician does not know anything much about the science called dynamic psychology (psycho-analysis for me), and yet by this science alone can sense be made out of symptoms. Seeing that this fifty-year-old science is at least as large as physiology, and includes the whole study of the developing human personality in its setting, it is not to be wondered at if the weary postgraduate, having reached the heights of a paediatric registrarship, boggles at yet another discipline, and eschews the new training that alone qualifies for psycho-therapeutic practice.

This problem of the double training must be left to solve itself in the course of time; meanwhile we must expect and welcome the two types of approach, the physical and the psychological, and we must try to assimilate the contribution that each can make to paediatrics.

Unfortunately I must now narrow down my subject, which could be almost infinite in depth and breadth. I have chosen to discuss enuresis, although I confess I find it difficult to leave aside so very much that would interest both myself and any paediatric audience.

There are enuresis clinics run by paediatricians, and usually the avowed aim in such clinics is the cure of the symptom. Mothers and children are grateful. There is nothing to be said against such clinics except that they side-track the whole issue of aetiology, of enuresis as a symptom that means something, as a persisting infantile relationship that has value in the economy of the child. In most cases cure of the symptom does no harm, and when a cure *could* do harm the child usually manages, through unconscious processes, either to resist cure or to adopt an alternative SOS sign, one that produces transfer to another type of clinic.

While these paediatric clinics are coming and going, child psychiatrists are all the time meeting with the symptom enuresis, and often the symptom is easily seen to be quite a subsidiary phenomenon, a little bit of a huge problem of a human being engaged in trying to develop to maturity in spite of handicaps.

I shall give only one case out of the many hundreds to hand; by this one case description I shall hope to show how enuresis appeared in the course of a psychiatric illness.

I choose that of a boy for whom psycho-analysis was not available, yet whose cure (if I may call it a cure) depended, in part, on three psychothera-peutic sessions.

At these three sessions the boy was drawing all the time, and I was able to take notes except at the most critical moments when feeling was so tense that the taking of notes would have done harm.

The case, not an unusual one, is the more suitable for presentation, because the child's treatment was mainly carried out by the parents, who were able to mend their home that had been broken by the war; I hope that you will be able to see in this part of the description, where the parents did the work, a type of illness and recovery that you have watched yourselves in those of your own child patients who have been able to use a period of physical illness as an opportunity for making delayed growth in personality. This boy was lucky; he was able to get what he needed without physical illness.

EXAMPLE: A CASE WITH ENURESIS

Philip, aged nine, was one of three children in a good family. The father had been away for a long period during the war, and at the end of the war he retired from the Army and settled down to rebuild his home, starting to be a farmer in a small way. The two boys were at a well-known prep school. The headmaster of the school wrote (October 1947) to the parents to say that he must advise them to take Philip away because, although he had never thought of the boy as in any way abnormal, he had found him to be the cause of an epidemic of stealing. He said, 'I can easily deal with the epidemic if Philip is removed', and he wisely saw that Philip was ill and would not be able to respond in a simple way to corrective treatment. As a result of this letter, which came as a great shock to the parents, they consulted their general practitioner and he, on the recommendatiom of a psychiatrist, referred the case to me.

Consideration of these details shows how precarious is this matter of the referral of a psychiatrically ill child before damage is done. It was almost by chance that I was in a good position to give help at the very beginning and before a moral attitude towards the boy's delinquency had had time to become organized, and before symptom intolerance had developed to the extent of producing panic therapy.

I arranged first of all to see the mother and in a long interview I was able to take the following detailed history. This history turned out to be substantially correct, although in one important detail the exact truth did not emerge until I had an interview with the boy.

I was able to gather that the father and mother had the ability to form and to maintain a good home, but that the disturbances of the war had caused serious disruption which affected Philip more than the brother. The small sister was obviously developing normally and was able to derive full benefit from the mended home. The parents were inclined towards spiritualism but they made it clear to me that they were not trying to impose their way of thinking on the children. The mother had a dislike of psychology and claimed to know nothing about it, and this proved to be valuable to me in my management of the case, since I was able to rely on her feelings and on her native or intuitive understanding of human nature and not on her sporadic reading and thinking.

The brother was breast-fed for five months and was a straightforward personality from the beginning. He was much admired by Philip.

Philip's birth was very difficult; the mother remembers it as a long struggle.

The amniotic fluid broke through ten days before the birth, and from the mother's point of view the birth started and stopped twice before the boy was actually born, under chloroform. Philip was fed at the breast for six weeks; there was no initial loss of weight, and there was an easy transfer to the bottle. As a baby he was what is usually called bonny, until the age of two, when the war started to interfere with his life. From this age he had no nursery days at home and he developed into rather a quiet child, perhaps too easy to manage. Nursery life had to be shared with tough and strange children. At this point he became excessively catarrhal and he developed an inability to try to blow his nose. The catarrhal tendency has continued and was not favourably affected by tonsillectomy at six years. The mother is subject to asthma and she thinks that the boy occasionally had asthma of slight degree. The mother looked after Philip most of the time although with the help of a nannie, and she early noticed the difference between the two boys. Not only was Philip less healthy on account of the catarrh, but also his co-ordination was poor.

When Philip was two–four years old he and his brother were away with the mother, after which they were back in the original home. The home, however, which was broken up when he was two, was not restored until the father retired from the Army, not long before the date of the consultation. The children's possessions were necessarily scattered, never all available at one time, and any one object was liable to become lost. As compared with the brother, Philip was not demonstrative. He was, however, affectionate enough with his mother and sister. The mother felt him to be a stranger and what possessions he had were very private to him. Actual difficulties did not show, however, till he was six years old. In regard to what is called toilet training, he had been easy, and bed-wetting had never been a trouble.

When Philip was six, which the mother reminded me was the time of his tonsillectomy, he came back home with the nurse's watch. In the course of the next three years he stole another watch and he also stole money which he would always spend. Other objects were stolen and they always got damaged. He was not without money of his own and he developed a passion for book-collecting. Being very intelligent and a good reader, he actually read the books that he bought, but the buying of the books was very important to him. They were mostly small books on moths and grasses and dogs, books of classificatory type. It was noticed that he paid 15s. for a small book on ships without seeming at all to recognize that this was expensive. Along with these symptoms the parents had noticed a change in the boy's character but they could not easily describe it. The parents were really disturbed when the following incident occurred: staying at a house, on the way home from a holiday, he stole a car registration book that belonged to the people that owned the house. He did not attempt to hide it and the parents put down the theft to his undoubted love of documents of all kinds. On looking back they could see that at this time he began to become an untidy person. Moreover he became less and less interested in possessions except new books, and along with this was an exaggeration of the wish to give things away to his sister of whom he was very fond. This was in the period when he was six–eight, up to the year in which he was brought into my care.

At the birth of the sister (when he was six) the mother said that he was first of all disturbed and openly jealous but he soon became fond of her and returned to a fairly good relation with the mother, not as easy, however, as before the birth. At this time the father began to discover that his children were interesting for the first time, partly because he had a daughter and mostly because he was now able to be living in his own home more and more. Incidentally, the mother told me that both she and the father had longed for a girl for their second child. When Philip appeared they took some time to adjust to the idea of another boy. The birth of the daughter eventually brought great relief to the family and undoubtedly released Philip from a vague feeling that he was wanted in some way to be unlike what he was. I made a special note that the tonsillectomy, which had apparently brought about the change in this boy's personality, had been done soon after the birth of the sister, and later I was to discover that the birth of the sister was the more important disturbance. At this time (he was now eight) he became shy of anything that might make people laugh at him. The mother reported as an example that he had a swelling on the face caused by a sting. Rather than risk being laughed at he would be excessively tired and would stay in bed. In defence against being laughed at he developed the art of mimicry and in this way he became able to make people laugh at will. He also developed a fund of amusing stories, and in this way he further warded off derision. While telling me this the mother felt in despair as she recognized while talking how much she had been at sea in her dealings with this boy while she had not had difficulty in understanding the brother and the sister. She had the ability to be closely in touch with a normal child but not the ability to keep in touch with a child who was ill, and it was important for me to recognize this as I needed her co-operation. Later on I described what the boy needed of her not in terms of the needs of a psychiatric case but in terms of the need of a normal infant, explaining that the boy would need to be allowed to go back and to be an infant in relation to her, so making use of his newly founded home. Thus we avoided having to instruct her against her will in psychopathology.

Sleep was always disturbed by nasal obstruction. Philip would wake and require his mother to help and it is likely that he was able to use this physical difficulty, without knowing it, in order to get his mother's presence at night; had he not had the nasal obstruction the mother would have been brought to his bedside by nightmares or some phobia. He had a phobia of being hurt and after tonsillectomy he had a phobia of doctors.

When I asked what happened when he got excited, did he get ill or just jump around? — the mother said, 'When you expect him to get excited he becomes quiet and retiring and asks repeatedly, "Oh what shall I do? What is there to do?"' The mother had noticed that it was important to him that he should be alone for some part of every day. He could make use of distractions, and for instance when taken to Switzerland he soon learned to ski, but more by effort of will than by natural skill.

The mother reported that he had bouts of increased urgency and frequency of micturition which she connected with the nasal obstruction. At the school the boy was considered to be healthy and the nasal obstruction seemed to be less in evidence. I went with the mother and boy to an oto-rhinologist who gave valuable specialist advice, but also ordered a whole host of symptom relievers from which the boy had to be rescued.

At school Philip was thought to be intelligent but lazy. The headmaster gave him a bad report but in a letter to me he said that he had never thought of this boy as being in any way abnormal until the stealing started. He was not unaccustomed to laziness and expected the boy to make good in the end. From this detail I think it can be seen how a really good school can miss psychiatric illness.

Philip was fond of the country. He possessed a greyhound of his own and this turned out to be very important, playing a vital part in his cure. While he was in trouble at school he wrote a letter in which there was no indication that he was in distress.

Summary of Case History

This history which the mother was able to give me showed that the boy started life well but that there was a disturbance in the child's emotional development dating from two years. In defence against environmental uncertainty he became withdrawn and relatively unco-ordinated. At six he started a degeneration of the personality which was progressive, leading up to the major symptomatology at nine for which he was brought to me.

Management

Although I had not seen the boy I was able to begin on the arrangement of his management. It was clear that psycho-analysis was out of the question, since a daily journey to London or even a weekly one would be a disturbance of the use that the boy could make of his mended home, and it would be this mended home that would carry the major burden of the therapy.

I told the mother that this boy would need her help as it was clear that he had missed something at the age of two years and he would have to go back and look for it. She quickly understood, and said, 'Oh well, if he has to become an infant, let him come home, and as long as you help me to understand what is happening I can manage'. She proved that this was no idle boast and eventually she was able to take the credit for having brought the child through a mental illness; the home provided the mental hospital that this boy needed, an asylum in the true sense of the word.

In technical terms, the boy regressed. He went back in his emotional development in a way that I shall describe presently, and then came forward again. It was at the depth of this regression that the bed-wetting appeared which is the link between this case and the main theme of my address.

My next task was to see the boy. I needed this interview in order to know where I stood in the management of the case over the next few months (mostly by telephone), and also because the boy was ready for insight which he got in this one and a half hours and which, although not psycho-analysis, was the application of knowledge gained by me in psycho-analytic work.

First Interview with Philip

There was no initial difficulty. The boy was an attractive intelligent lad, rather withdrawn, not showing much evidence of making objective observations about me. He was evidently preoccupied with his own affairs and slightly bemused. His sister came with him and he behaved in a natural way with her, and easily left her with her mother while he and I went into the playroom. I adopted a technique which suits these cases, a kind of projection test in which I play my part. Figs. 1–8 are a sample of the drawings. It is a game in which first I make a squiggle and he turns it into something, and then he makes a squiggle and I turn it into something.

(1) *My* squiggle (Fig. 1). He turned it round and quickly called it a map of England, adding a line which was needed in the region of Cornwall.

I saw immediately from this that he was in a highly imaginative state, and that I would get results that were very personal since this squiggle could have been made into almost anything.

(2) *His* squiggle, and I delayed making it into anything myself, thus giving him a chance to display again his imaginative capacity. He immediately said it was a rope going up into the air and he indicated the air by thin strokes crossing thick strokes of the rope.

(3) *He* again made a squiggle (Fig. 2) and I quickly turned it into a face which he called a fish. Again this was an indication that he was preoccupied with his personal or inner reality and not particularly concerned with being objective.

(4) *My* squiggle (Fig. 3). It was astonishing to witness the way in which he immediately saw in it a mother and baby sea-lion. Subsequent events proved that it was justifiable to understand from this drawing that the boy had a powerful maternal identification; also that the mother-baby relationship was of especial importance to him. Moreover this picture has beauty, not indeed on account of the squiggle, but on account of his use of it.

FIG. 1

MY SQUIGGLE. HIS MODIFICATION.
HIS COMMENT—ENGLAND.

FIG. 2

HIS SQUIGGLE. MY MODIFICATION.
HIS COMMENT—A FISH.

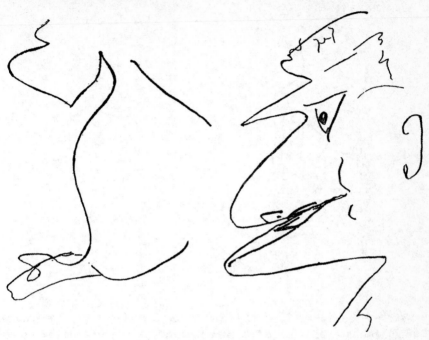

FIG. 3

MY SQUIGGLE. HIS MODIFICATION. HIS COMMENT—A SEA-LION
WITH A BABY.

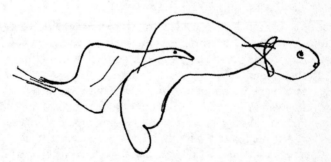

(5) *His* squiggle. Before I could make anything of it he had turned it into men roped together climbing rocks. This belonged to his recent experiences in Switzerland.

(6) *His* squiggle again, which he interpreted as a small whirlpool with waves and water. For him this was quite clear, though not so clear to me.

FIG. 4   FIG. 5

MY SQUIGGLE. HIS MODIFICATION.   DRAWING NO. 9. THE WIZARD.
HIS COMMENT—MR PUNCH WITH
TEARS IN HIS CLOTHES.

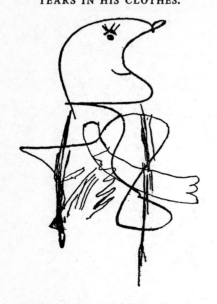

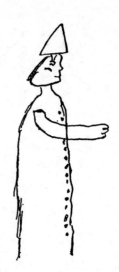

(7) *His* squiggle again, which he turned into a boot in water, again something absolutely personal to himself. I had already recognized that he was almost in what could be called a sleep-walking state, and this prepared me for the psychotic features about which I was to learn a little later on.

(8) *My* squiggle (Fig. 4). He immediately turned it into what he called Punch with tears in his clothes.

He was now very much alive in a creative sense and he said, 'There are tears in his clothes because he has been doing something with a crocodile, something dreadful, probably annoying it, and if you annoy crocodiles you are in danger of being eaten.'

(9) He was now talking about dream material and I was therefore in a position to investigate his dreams. I spoke about the frightening things that could occur to him in his thoughts, whereupon he drew Fig. 5 which he called a wizard. There was a long story with this. The wizard turned up at midnight at school. Apparently he did a lot of watching for the wizard in the night. This wizard had absolute power and magical power. He could put you underground and turn you into things. This wizard turned out to be an important clue in the understanding of the compulsion to steal.

He was now willing to tell me dreams. He was going in a car with his mother. The car was going downhill. There was a ditch at the bottom of the hill and the car was going so fast that it could not possibly stop. At the critical moment magic happened, good magic, and the car went over the ditch without falling into it.

I put into words what was implied by this and by the way that he told it to me. I said that he was frightened that in the dream he had had to use good magic because this meant that he had to believe in magic, and if there was good magic there was also bad magic. His inability to deal with reality and the necessity to employ magic was the awful thing.

He told me a further dream. He had hit his headmaster in the tummy, 'but the headmaster is nice', he said; 'he is a man you can talk to.' I asked him if he was ever sad and he was now communicating with me from very deep in his nature when he said that he certainly knew what sadness meant. He had a name for it. He called it 'dreary times'. He said that the worst sadness happened a long time ago and he then told me about his first separation from his mother. I was not sure at first what was his age at the time of the experience. He told me: 'Mother went away. I and my brother had to live by ourselves. We went to stay with my aunt and uncle. The awful thing that happened there was that I would see my mother cooking in her blue dress and I would run up to her but when I got there she would suddenly change and it would be my aunt in a different coloured dress.'

He was telling me that he was often hallucinating his mother, employing magic but constantly suffering from the shock of disillusionment. I spoke to him about the awfulness of finding things you thought real were not real. He then drew a mirage (10) and took a holiday from the subject of hallucinations by giving the scientific explanation of a mirage. His uncle had told him all about it. 'You see lovely blue trees when there are really no trees there.'

He also said that he was very fond of beautiful things. 'Now my brother, he thinks of nothing but ships and of sailing, and that is quite different. I love beauty and animals and I like drawing.' I pointed out to him that the beauty of the mirage had a link with his feelings about his mother, a fact which I deduced from the blue colour of the mirage and of the mother's frock.

My notes at this point become less clear as the situation had become very tense and the boy had become deeply serious and thoughtful. He told me quite spontaneously about his depression, or what he called dreary times. It now turned out that the worst dreary time had occurred when he was nearly six and I was now able to see the importance of the birth of the sister. By his mother's going away he had meant that she had gone to a nursing home to have the child. It was then that he and his brother stayed with the aunt and uncle and although the brother was able to manage easily, Philip only just managed to keep the thread of experience unbroken. He was not only hallucinating but also he was needing to be told exactly what to do and his uncle, recognizing this, had deliberately adopted a sergeant-major attitude and by dominating the boy's life he had counteracted the emptiness which resulted from the loss of the mother. There was one other thing that kept him going, which was that his brother, who was a great help, constantly said: 'It will end; it will end.'

The boy now had the first opportunity he had ever had for talking about his real difficulty at the time, which was to come to terms with the mother's capacity to have a baby, which made him acutely jealous of her. The picture of the mother and baby sea-lion showed how much he had idealized the mother-infant relationship. The fact that the baby had turned out to be a girl had been a relief to him.

He said, 'I spent all the time thinking of how soon the end would come, or else I just felt sick.' Once at school he had felt homesick, which was another kind of dreariness or depression, and he went to the headmaster. He said: 'The headmaster tried everything but he could not help.' He then compared the headmaster with me and quite openly said that, whereas the headmaster had only been able to say 'Cheer up', I had been able to give him some understanding, of which he was in great need.

We were now able to return to the wizard who turned out to have the overcoat of his soldier uncle, the one who had dominated his life, thus saving him from the emptiness of depression. He now told me that the wizard had a voice which was exactly that of the uncle. At school this voice continued to dominate him. The voice told him to steal and he was compelled to steal. If he hesitated the voice would say: 'Don't be a coward; remember your name.' 'In our family there are no cowards.' He then told me about the main episode for which he had been expelled. A boy had said to him, 'Oh well, there's nothing very much about what you've done; anybody might have stolen pound notes and things like that. It isn't as if you had stolen poison drugs from the matron's cupboard.' After this the voice of the wizard told him that he must take poison drugs from the matron's cupboard and he did this with consummate skill. It was when he was found to be in possession of dangerous drugs that he was expelled, but for him there was no shame since he had obeyed the voice and had not been a coward. Moreover I would add that in stealing he was in the direction of finding the mother that he had lost, but this is another subject which cannot be followed up here.

I have tried to give a faithful account of the interview but I cannot hope to convey the feeling of something having happened which was very real to both of us.

I was somewhat exhausted and ready to stop but he sat down to one final picture (Fig. 6).

(11) After drawing in silence he said that this was his father in a boat. Over the boat is an eagle and the eagle is carrying a baby rabbit.

In the setting it was clear that Philip was drawing not only to 'seal off' the interview but also to report progress. I started to put this into words. I said that the eagle stealing the baby rabbit represented his own wish or dream at the time of maximum distress, to steal the baby sister from the mother. He was first of all jealous of the mother for being able to have a baby by the father, and also he was jealous of the baby since he had an acute need to be a baby and to have a second chance to make use of his mother in a dependent state.

FIG. 6

DRAWING NO. 11. 'HIS FATHER IN A BOAT; OVER THE BOAT IS AN EAGLE AND THE EAGLE IS CARRYING A BABY RABBIT.'

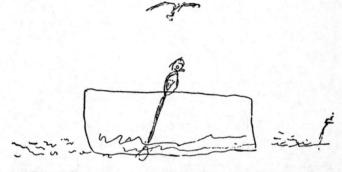

(Of course, I used language appropriate to his capacity to understand.) He took up the theme, and he said: 'And there's father, all unconcerned.' You will remember that his father had been overseas. The fact that his father was away fighting for his country is now of great importance to him, and he can boast of this at school. However in respect of his childhood needs the father was neglecting his son's urgent need for a father actually on the spot, friendly, strong, understanding, and taking responsibility. But for his uncle and his brother he would have been sunk when his relation to his mother was interrupted by the separation and by his jealousy of her. The boy was now ready to go.

Second Interview

I saw him again within a week and I shall not need to give a detailed account. I show his drawing, however (Fig. 7), through which he announced that the wizard and his voice had gone since the first interview. In this drawing of the wizard's house I am in the wizard's house with a gun, and the wizard is retreating. The smoke indicates that the wizard's wife is in the kitchen cooking. I go in and take the magic from her. You will remember his need to find his mother cooking—the alternative was the witch, and the cauldron, and the magic spells of the woman of early infancy, who is terrible to think of in retrospect, because of the infant's absolute dependence. This already has some

113

FIG. 7
THE WIZARD'S HOUSE.

FIG. 8
A 'FUNNY' PICTURE OF THE
WIZARD.

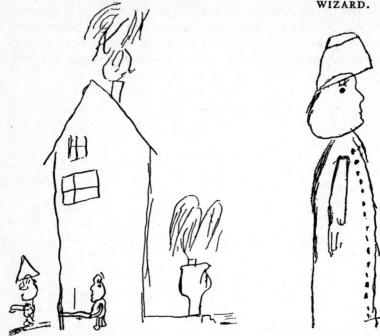

flavour of fantasying, of operation at a less deep level; and indeed the tenseness of the atmosphere of the first interview was missing. I was no longer within the inner circle of the child's personal and magical world, but a person listening to him talking and hearing about his fantasies.

Two more drawings:

One shows the wizard going down the school corridors. After this he told me again about the hallucination of the mother who changed to the aunt when he put what he saw to the test. Also here there was an important bit about the way in which the wizard's candle belonged to genital erection and to ideas of fellatio and ideas of burning hair. I had to be able to take this, along with the magic and whatever else might turn up, else I would suddenly intrude myself, as much by any display of prudery or blindness as by an active introduction of my own ideas. But this was not to be an analysis and I had to avoid giving understanding in relation to the repressed unconscious.

The last drawing of the second series (Fig. 8) shows the wizard again. This time the wizard is being laughed at. It is a 'funny' picture. It will be remembered that it was part of the child's illness that he expected to be laughed at; the object of the derision had now been got outside the house (himself), and in the place of the wizard was his highly subjective idea of me. I was simply a person who fits in and understands, and who verbalizes the material of the play. In verbalizing I talk to a conscious self and acknowledge the PLACE WHERE FROM in his total personality, the central spot of his ENTITY, without which there is no HE.

Figs. 1 to 8 have been selected out of 14 drawings.

The Third Interview

This started with a drawing in which his enemy drops a knife on his greyhound. The enemy is the son of the uncle who played such an important role in his life during the depression and whose voice and Army overcoat supplied the details for the wizard that he employed to counteract his 'dreariness'. This cousin was hated because of Philip's powerful love of the cousin's father.

The third interview changed into an ordinary play hour, and I just sat and watched Philip make a complex plan with my train-set rails. Whenever he came to me subsequently he just played with the train, and I did no more psychotherapy. Indeed I must not, unless I had been able to let the treatment develop into a psycho-analytic treatment, with its reliable daily session arranged to last over a period of one, two, or three years. This was never contemplated in Philip's case.

The Illness at Home

I now come to the illness that the boy had to have during which the parents provided him with asylum. It can be briefly described. This child needed my personal help, but there are the many cases in which the psychotherapeutic session can be omitted, and the whole therapy can be carried out by the home. The loss is simply that the child fails to gain insight, and this is by no means always a serious loss.

Philip was accepted at home as a special case, an ill child needing to be allowed to become more ill. By this I mean that there had been a controlled illness and this was to be allowed to come to full development. He was to receive that which is the right of every infant at the start, a period in which it is natural for the environment to make active adaptation to his needs.

What it looked like was this: Philip gradually became withdrawn and dependent. People said he lived in a fairy world. His mother described how he did not so much get up in the mornings as change from being in bed to out of bed, this simply because someone dressed him. This is a lay method of saying that the boy was in a somnambulistic state. On a few occasions the mother tried encouraging him to get up but he was quickly reduced to tears of distress and she abandoned all encouragements. At meals he gathered the utensils around him and ate alone, although with the family. He seemed uncivilized, taking big gulps of bread, and eating the jam down first. He would eat everything that was there rather mechanically, seeming neither to want food nor to reach a stage of having had enough. All through the meal he was in a pre-occupied state.

He went downhill steadily, becoming less and less able to live in his body or interested in his appearance, but he kept in touch with the enjoyment of body by watching his greyhound for hours on end.

His gait became unco-ordinated, and towards the bottom of the regression he progressed by a hop-skip technique, arms waving like windmill sails, or by a series of lurchings, as if propelled by some crude agency living within the self, certainly not walking. While progressing in this way he made noises which his brother called 'elephant noises'. No remark was ever made about his many oddities and eccentricities and bizarre behaviour patterns. He had the cream from the one cow, and also he figuratively skimmed the cream off the homeliness of the home.

On occasions he would come out of this state for an hour or two, as when the parents gave a cocktail party, and then he quickly returned to it.

Once he went to the local 'Hop' and there his queer attitude to girls came to the fore. He danced a little, but only with a very odd and fat creature known as 'the galleon', assumed in the locality to be mentally defective. A radio thriller became an obsession during this period, and his life revolved round this and watching the dog.

Then the bottom was reached. He was always tired. He had increasing difficulty in getting up at all. He became for the first time since infancy a bed-wetter. At last I have reached the symptom which made me choose this case for description. The mother got him up, between 3 and 4 a.m. each night, but he was usually wet. He said to her: 'I dream so vividly that I have got to the pot.' Also at the time he was addicted to water, drinking to excess. Of this he said: 'It's such fun, it's delicious, it's good to drink.'

All this took about three months.

One morning he wanted to get up. This marked the beginning of his gradual recovery, and there was no looking back. The symptoms peeled off and by the summer (1948) he was ready for a return to school. This was delayed, however, till the autumn term, one year after the start of the acute phase of the illness.

There was no return, after the first psychotherapeutic interview, either of the wizard or of the voice, or of the stealing.

On the return to the same school Philip picked up quickly, and there was no difficulty about living down a reputation for thieving. Soon the headmaster was able to write the usual letter one expects, asking what was all the fuss about, the boy being perfectly healthy and normal. He seemed to have forgotten that he had expelled him a year previously.

At 12½ Philip went to a well-known public school, rather a tough one, and at 14 he was reported to be 5 ft. 5 in., broad in physique, manly by nature, always out of doors, and good at the usual games. He was reported to be one year ahead of his age group scholastically.

RECAPITULATION

I do see the point of view of the paediatrician who, not being concerned specifically with psychology, must ignore the meaning of symptoms and must try to cure them. But I do ask these doctors to give the psychologist credit for his point of view, just as the psychologist gives the paediatrician credit for special knowledge of infant physiology, the biochemistry of fluid loss, the grouping of blood, and the early diagnosis of brain tumour. The two disciplines should produce different kinds of paediatrician each with a healthy respect for the other.

If a paediatrician had been consulted in this case on account of the bed-wetting, what would it have seemed like to him had he become involved at the point of the child's maximal regression? Ordinarily the mother would not know what was going on, nor would the child. In the case of Philip there was an exceptionally favourable setting for an illness to develop to its full extent and to come to its natural end. It would have been futile to have tried to cure Philip's enuresis without dealing with the regressive need that lay behind it.

Chapter X

A Case Managed at Home[1]
[1955]

NOT EVERY CASE in child psychiatry is of direct concern to the social worker. I present the case of Kathleen because in spite of the fact that the case was managed by myself it was not primarily a treatment by psycho-therapy. The burden of the case rested on the mother and indeed on the whole family, and the successful outcome was very largely the result of the work done in the child's home over a period of a year. Management was required from me, and this meant that I had to see the mother and child for ten to twenty minutes each week for a period of months.

At the first interview I was able to come to a fairly definite conclusion as to the psychopathology of the condition and to form a tentative opinion as to the parents' ability to see the child through her illness.

The child was referred to me with a view to my arranging for her to go to a hostel, as it had not occurred to those who were initially in touch with the case that under certain conditions a spontaneous cure could take place in the course of time. The important point was that in a careful history-taking in the first interview I was able to make a graph of the symptomatology and from this it was clear that the climax of the illness had been reached and that there was already a tendency towards improvement by the time of the consultation. In the graph there was a peak of acute *neurotic* anxiety followed by increasing distress and eventually the illness altered in quality and the child became ill in a *psychotic* way. The neurotic acute phase followed a story told to her by her sister, during a period in which she was already beginning to be upset because she was due to be bridesmaid at the wedding of her favourite aunt. The period of acute psychotic disturbance corresponded roughly with the marriage.

I was interested to find that the child had started to improve, and going into

[1] *Case Conference.* Vol. 2, No. 7, November, 1955.

this in great detail I discovered that the family had turned itself into a mental hospital, giving itself a paranoid organization into which this paranoid, withdrawn child fitted admirably. At first the child was able to manage only when in actual contact with her mother, but already at the time of the consultation there was a circle of a few feet around the mother in which the child could be free from acute distress. I found that the mother, who was not an educated woman and not actually very intelligent, but an excellent manager of her home, was interested to know why she and the family had turned themselves into such a curious and abnormal state. She did in fact keep up the mental hospital atmosphere until the child was ready for the home gradually to return to normal. The gradual recovery of the home followed as the child lost her paranoid defence organization. I had the co-operation of the local authority even when I asked that no one should visit the home and for a whole year I took full responsibility, thus simplifying the mother's task.

It was management therefore rather than direct psychotherapy which brought about a return of the child to normal or near-normal. Some direct work was done with the child in the weekly visits which, however, were of necessity short as I had no vacancy for a treatment case at the time. What was done in these brief contacts was not the main part and not an essential part of the treatment, but was in fact a useful addition.

I will now attempt to describe the case in detail.

Kathleen was referred to me at six years of age, by the psychiatrist of a County Child Guidance Clinic, with a note in which it was stated: 'She has recently become negativistic, talking to herself and staring into space, and refusing to co-operate with her mother though refusing to be parted from her.'

I was able to draw on a report made locally by a P.S.W. when compiling the following case-history after I had seen the mother:

Mother: Appears to be stable. Is now desperately anxious and is at a loss how to handle patient.

Father: Alive and well.

Siblings: Pat, aged 11 years. A bright, talkative child. Patient, aged six years. Sylvia, aged 20 months. A very attractive child.

Kathleen had been fed at the breast for three months; she then took the bottle easily and went on to solids and to feeding herself without difficulty. She started using words when about twelve months and talked early. She was walking at sixteen months; clean habits were established normally. The mother was able to compare this child's infantile development with that of the other two children and there was no question of her being backward.

There had been no important physical illness. She had been through an operation on her thumb in hospital and had not appeared to be frightened by this experience. Recently she had complained of headaches and had looked pale. In infancy she had had screaming attacks which were a little beyond what is normal, and the parents had always had to be rather more careful with this child's management than with that of the others. They found that she needed more close adaptation. In other words, she was of sensitive type. It was found that she needed to have her questions answered quickly, otherwise she was liable to develop violent temper attacks. She was always highly strung and needed tactful handling. It could be said, however, that she was within normal limits — intelligent, happy, able to play, and able to make good contacts.

When she went to school at the age of five she did not like it very much but was quite reasonable. She was pleasant and friendly and was 'able to deal with frustration by thinking things out'. She was up to standard in her work until a few weeks before the consultation, when she began to deteriorate.

At home the child liked to help her mother in the house and was quite good at it from the age of about four years. She enjoyed playing with her little sister, she was very keen on keeping her books in good condition and disliked having them messed or torn by the younger child. She was fond of her dolls. She loved going to Sunday School. She seemed fond of her little sister and liked to do things for her.

Kathleen belongs to a family of ordinary working-class people. The father is a collector of old iron and has quite a good business. He started with a plot of land, acquired a caravan for his family's home, and eventually was able to have a little country cottage and a small car. The mother is a nice woman, not very clever, but able to manage her life sensibly on the basis of not attempting more than she knows she can manage. She comes of a family of limited intelligence and on the father's side there is an epileptic uncle.

A few weeks before the first consultation Kathleen was due to be bridesmaid at the wedding of a favourite aunt. This wedding was looming up at the time of the onset of her illness. She would say to her aunt: 'It is my wedding and not yours.' This was not just a playful remark, and indeed it marked the beginning of her distress. She could see herself in her aunt's place but could not deal with the wedding as an observer. At this time she also began, at first in a mild way, to have delusions of persecution, and she tried to make everyone keep smiling because something nasty about faces was always expected. Soon it was not enough that people smiled. Then, more rapidly, there came a marked change, so that her teacher reported that during the past few weeks she had taken no notice when spoken to, even when her name had been called several times. She would sit staring in front of her, totally preoccupied. Once or twice she had refused to remove her hat and coat at school. Now her crayoning was less careful, sometimes she would scribble instead of writing, and she would make some of her letters wrongly, whereas previously this had not been a feature.

Onset of Acute Illness

At this point her 11-year-old sister, who was in fact affected by the coming wedding in the same way as was Kathleen, did something which just exactly played on the conflict in this child's mind. She told her a lurid story. Kathleen was fond of the aunt and with the female side of her personality had identified herself with her aunt; but she also had to deal with another side of her personality which was much more difficult to get at, that is to say, her identification with the *man* in the wedding. She knew him and was also fond of him. On the basis of her own identification with her own mother and her love of her father she would have been able to have dealt with all this if things had gone well. Let us say, she had two potential dreams, one of herself as a bridesmaid, identified with the bride, and another of the male side of her nature in rivalry with the bridegroom. This latter rivalry had death in it, and it was therefore a very serious matter for her when her sister (also caught up in this same conflict) recounted to her a lurid story from a radio programme about a man who was killed, and about blood running all over the floor.

Her defences against the anxiety and the conflicts roused by the wedding had been working well, and her male identification had undergone repression. Now, however, there came a threat of a break-through of the intolerable dreams belonging to rivalry with the man, and she had to organize new and more primitive defences. She became withdrawn and paranoid. This reorganization needed time, and the immediate effect of the sister's story was very severe manifest anxiety. There was thus a preliminary period of acute neurotic illness; the child developed extreme fear on going to bed; she asked repeatedly whether there was blood on the floor; she repeatedly said: 'Mum, mum, will he come and murder me? Will I be all right? Are you guarding the door?' Eventually she was able to be pacified and to sleep.

After this period of acute anxiety she recovered and was fairly normal for a time, but about a week later when she returned home from school she began talking strangely about a man who had wanted to take her in the water. She said that all the children who went into the water with him got new clothes. She had become a psychotic case.

From now on she was never herself, and towards the time of the wedding she began to get very ill indeed in a way that reminds one of mental hospital illness rather than of psychoneurosis. She would sit and stare abstractedly into space and refuse to answer. One morning she looked at her sister and friend and seemed terrified, and she shouted to mother: 'Take them away.' She said that their faces looked horrible and ugly and that she couldn't stand the sight of them. She was clearly hallucinated. Once in the street she cried out: 'Take all these people away. Don't let them hang around me.' She became totally preoccupied. If asked to do a simple job, she did not seem to comprehend, and she worked herself up into a passion, saying: 'Where, what do you mean? You're mucking me about and making me lose my days again.' She would frequently cry and use very bad language and give the appearance of extreme terror. Often she said that she hated her mother and wanted to go right away. Once she doubled herself up as if in extreme pain and said to mother: 'You're talking into my tummy, you're hurting me.' Frequently she talked of a man: 'Him and me are going it. I'm going to live with him in a bungalow and you're not coming. He's going to take me.' Sometimes she would identify a man's voice on the wireless with this man. She would appear to see him, and would stare fixedly into space as if hallucinated, crying out: 'He done it.' If given sweets she would hold them in her hand as if uncertain what to do with them.

She was now uninterested in play of any kind and had given her dolls away. She didn't care if her younger sister scribbled on her books. She didn't want to go out or play with her scooter. She followed her mother around and would not let her out of her sight. She cried every night when going to bed and wanted one or other parent to stay with her. She could not stand the name of her school being mentioned and would cover her face at the sound of the word. When she was due to go out with her father she had made eight attempts without being able to make up her mind and went to her mother in distress. Following this she would not leave her mother at all. As long as she was very near her mother she was not too bad, but she could not sleep without her mother sitting with her for one or two hours. Even then she would get up at 2 a.m. and go in with her mother, remaining restless and sleepless. There were now no nightmares. (Previous to the illness she had always slept the clock round.)

For a period of time she could not stand the sight of her older sister. She was using the younger sister, however, to represent a normal aspect of herself, somewhere to carry on while she herself was so ill, just as other similar patients use a cat or a dog or a duck. Whereas she had once loved her dolls which she would keep carefully on her bed, now she had left these aside for the baby to use. Her fondness for the baby had some anxiety mixed with it now, as she would keep feeling the baby's face and saying: 'Is she all right?' This made the baby bad-tempered.

She had also given up colour drawing entirely. There was no incontinence although the mother had always had to watch out with this child to help her quickly. Sunday school, which she used to enjoy, had now become impossible as she would not leave her mother. She went once with her mother to church, but got fed up towards the end instead of enjoying it. She could not stand the people.

Course of Acute Illness

A careful examination of details showed that the disturbance started as an exaggeration of the ordinary touchiness associated with the excitement in regard to the wedding arrangements. The sudden peak of manifest anxiety followed the radio story. There was some recovery from this but after another week there developed the psychotic phase in the illness which lasted on over the time of the wedding. Gradually after another week or two the severity of the illness tended to lessen, and this improvement, although slight and gradual, was maintained steadily until the recovery of the child in the course of a full year.

I came into the picture at the time of the slight improvement after the worst phase of the illness, and I had to ask myself what had given rise to this improvement. Was it because the wedding was over or was something else happening to help? Already I had formed an opinion that it was unlikely that I would be taking this child away and putting her into a hostel because it was improbable that I would be able to find a placement able to see her through. I began to go into the question of what the home was like, and I found that the home had converted itself into a mental hospital for the child. The parents had arranged that no one should come to the door, as the child was so frightened of knocks. The milkman was told to leave the milk outside the gate instead of on the doorstep. The postman and the coalman had similar instructions. Not even relations were allowed to visit, and so on. The whole family was involved. What hostel could do all this?

I had to ask myself whether I could provide anything better than was being provided at home, and I decided that I could not. I explained to the mother the significance of what she was doing and I asked her whether she could continue. She said: 'Now you tell me what I am doing, I can go on. How long will it be?' To this I had to reply: 'I don't know, but certainly for months.'

And so I helped the mother with her task by writing to the local authorities to ask that no one should visit either from the clinic or from the school, and co-operation was complete. As the child began to recover it was the School Welfare Officer who was first *persona grata*, and it is of incidental interest that his death recently has caused quite a gap in the family, so attached had they all become to this man. Within this artificial paranoid system the child was able gradually to let go her own paranoid withdrawal. Instead of being able to endure life only when catching hold of her mother, she began to be able to be fairly normal if within a few yards of her mother. It was remarkable the way in which the children as well as the grown-ups adapted themselves to the child's needs. Quite steadily the circle in which the child felt secure enlarged until it was the size of the house, and even larger.

Contact Maintained

All this time, although this cut across the idea of the home as a closed system, the mother brought the child to my consulting-room once a week for a very brief contact. Each week I explained to the mother what was happening, and I gave the child the opportunity to be negativistic. She would refuse to come into my play-room. She looked wild and defiant, and mostly just stood by her mother and stamped and spat and cursed and used filthy language. She was just like a wild animal. Sometimes she would say: 'Shut up, I'm going to bash you', or: 'No. No. No.' It is difficult to describe the violence of her repudiation of me. After several visits the child allowed herself to make a little quick tour of the play-room before going away. In this way she knew that there were toys, and after many weeks she allowed herself even to touch one. Once, although refusing a paper spool from my hand, she looked up from the street to my window as she left, and when I threw one down she picked it up and took it home. These visits to me were accepted by the child as an excursion outside her home, the only one which she could tolerate. Gradually she came around in the course of many of these short interviews to the beginnings of an acceptance of me.

There was a long interval in which I did not see her at all because of holidays. After this I found that the child was so much improved that I did not continue the interviews but advised the parents and the school and the social workers to allow the recovery to go on taking place slowly and naturally.

There was one more episode, which came when she was supposed to stay with the married aunt and uncle. The aunt could not have her, and for a few weeks she went back, in token form, to her illness. The symptoms all became recognizable, but after a few weeks a new spontaneous recovery took place.

Within 15 months from the onset of the illness she was back at school. The teachers said that she had obviously lost some ground but they could accept her and could treat her almost as before.

Two Years Later

Nearly two years later when she was eight she said to her mother: 'I want to see Dr Winnicott and I want to take my little sister.' The visit was arranged, and when she came into my room she obviously knew what to expect to find there and she showed the toys to her sister. I could not have been certain previously that she had really noticed the toys. The sister played a completely separate game, playing normally with the toys, and I divided my attention between the two children. Kathleen's play was a construction of a very long road, using the many little toy houses that I had in my room at that time. She was clearly asking for an interpretation, and I was able to explain to her that what she was doing was joining up the past with the present, joining my house with her own, integrating past experience with the present. That was what she had come for, and also to let me know that she had used the little sister for the normal aspect of herself. Gradually during the course of her recovery she had drawn her normal self back from her little sister and had returned to normal relations with her.

I learned that at the time following the setback due to her aunt's not being able to have her to stay, the mother had felt that she *must* get the child away from herself because there had developed a relationship between them (the mother and Kathleen) which was based on the management of the illness, rather than on being a mother, and this could not be entirely broken. The mother took the risk, therefore, of sending the child away with other relations. On returning from this holiday Kathleen seemed quite normal, sleeping well, playing and sharing, and with less liability to temper attacks than she had had before the illness.

Further Follow-up

Recently I asked for a friendly visit. The mother came very willingly, bringing all three children. The elder sister, now nineteen, is clever, well educated, in a good job, and dressed in very good taste.

Sylvia, who is nine now, is developing well.

Kathleen, at 13½ years, gives a fairly normal impression, but she is rather intense, and has not the lively intelligence of her elder sister. She was very pleased to see me, and discussed life in a mature way. At school things have gone well but she is now not good at sums.[1] Otherwise she is about average. I learn that she is liked although she has not many friends. Already she has put herself down to be trained as an embroideress and her teachers say that they have every reason to think that she will do that and will do it well.

And so it can be said that she has made a recovery. I helped in my own way. The parents did the main work and to do this they did not have to be clever. They had to feel it was worth while making a temporary special adaptation to the needs of their ill child.

Theoretical Considerations

Let me compare the neurotic illness with the psychotic development. Certain conflicts between her identification on the male side (homosexual) were unavailable to her consciousness, so she was unable to work out a satisfactory relationship between her male self and the prospective uncle. Hence the potential trauma of the wedding situation. The lurid story had brought this conflict out into the open so that she had severe anxiety. Personal psychotherapy could have helped at this stage. As the wedding approached the child developed a more serious defence. She developed a psychosis, became withdrawn, and preoccupied with the care of herself within herself. This put her in a vulnerable position, as she had no time left for dealing with the external world. In other words, she became paranoid.

[1] An Intelligence Test done at 13 years 10 months gave a result of I.Q. 91.

I was called in when this more psychotic defence organization had become established. If I had been in a position to give the child treatment in a deeper way, instead of just letting her come and spit, my room would have gradually developed the same mental hospital atmosphere which in fact developed at home. But I did not need to give this treatment. The parents supplied a setting in which she could be. She could be identified with her own (modified) home because it took on the shape of her own defences.

SUMMARY

Here was a case of child psychiatry in which a working-class family were enabled to see a child through a psychotic illness of 15 months' duration. They were helped by a minimum of personal attention to the child, and by management. The amount of my time actually spent on this case was not more than a few hours, spread over several months.

Perhaps this case may help in the Child Care Worker's attempt to understand what is going on when children make positive use of foster or adoptive parents, or of a residential school (cf. Clare Britton, 1955).

PART 3

Chapter XI

The Manic Defence[1]
[1935]

IN MY OWN particular case a widening understanding of Mrs Klein's concept at present named 'The Manic Defence' has coincided with a gradual deepening of my appreciation of inner reality. Three or four years ago I was contrasting 'fantasy' and 'reality', which led my non-psycho-analytic friends to tell me that I was using the word fantasy in a way that was different from the ordinary use of the term. I replied to their objections that the misuse was inevitable; for (as in the psycho-analyst's use of the word anxiety) the invention of a new word would have been less easily justified than the treatment of an already existing word with a splash of paint.

Gradually, however, I find I am using the word fantasy more in its normal sense, and I have come to compare external reality not so much with fantasy as with an inner reality.

In a way this point that I am making is a quibble, since if there be sufficient respect for 'fantasy', conscious and unconscious, then a changeover to the use of the term 'inner reality' requires no effort. Yet there may be some for whom, as for me, the change in terminology involves a deepening of belief in inner reality.[2]

The connection between this preliminary and the title of my paper 'The Manic Defence' is that it is a part of one's own manic defence to be unable to give full significance to inner reality. There are fluctuations in one's ability to respect inner reality that are related to depressive anxiety in oneself. The effect is that on certain days in one's analytic practice a patient who employs chiefly manic defences will present material which defies interpretation at the time;

[1] Read before the British Psycho-Analytical Society on 4th December, 1935.

[2] The term 'psychic reality' does not involve any placing of the fantasy; the term 'inner reality' presupposes the existence of an inside and an outside, and therefore of a limiting membrane belonging to what I would now call the 'psyche-soma' (1957).

129

yet the notes of that hour's associations may make quite understandable reading the following day.

The new understanding invites one to restate the 'Flight to Reality' (Searl, 1929), as a flight from internal reality rather than from fantasy. Internal reality is to be itself described in fantasy terms; yet it is not synonymous with fantasy since it is used to denote the fantasy that is personal and organized, and related historically to the physical experiences, excitements, pleasures, and pains of infancy. Fantasy is part of the individual's effort to deal with inner reality. It can be said that fantasy[1] and day-dreams are omnipotent manipulations of external reality. Omnipotent control of reality implies fantasy about reality. The individual gets to external reality through the omnipotent fantasies elaborated in the effort to get away from inner reality.

In the last paragraph of her paper ('The Flight to Reality', 1929) Miss Searl writes: '. . . in danger (the child) wants to keep the ideally loving and loved parents always with it, with no fear of separation; at the same time it wants to destroy in hate the unkind strict parents who leave it exposed to the awful dangers of unsatisfied libidinal tensions. That is, in omnipotent fantasy it eats up both loving and strict parents. . . .'

I feel that what is omitted here is recognition of the relation to the objects which are felt to be inside. It would seem that what we meet with is not merely a fantasy of incorporation of good and bad parents; we meet with the fact of which the child is largely unconscious that, for the same reasons that have been operative in the child's relation to the external parents, sadistic attacks *are going on inside* the child, attacks against the good or mutually loving parents (because by being happy together they frustrate), attacks against the parents made bad by hate, defence against the bad objects that now threaten the ego too, and also attempts to save the good from the bad, and to use the bad to counteract the bad; and so on.

Omnipotent fantasies are not so much the inner reality itself as a defence against the acceptance of it. One finds in this defence a flight to omnipotent fantasy, and flight from some fantasies to other fantasies, and in this sequence a flight to external reality. This is why I think one cannot compare and contrast fantasy and reality. In the ordinary extrovert book of adventure we often see how the author made a flight to day-dreaming in childhood, and then later made use of external reality in this same flight. He is not conscious of the inner depressive anxiety from which he has fled. He has led a life full of incident and adventure, and this may be accurately told. But the impression left on the reader is of a relatively shallow personality, for this very reason, that the author adventurer has had to base his life on the denial of personal internal reality. One turns with relief from such writers to others who can tolerate depressive anxiety and doubt.

[1] I would now use the term 'fantasying' (1957).

It is possible to trace the lessening of manic defence in the behaviour and in the fantasies of a patient during his analysis. As the depressive anxieties become less as the result of analysis, and the belief in good internal objects increases, manic defence becomes less intense and less necessary, and so less in evidence.

It should be possible to link the lessening of omnipotent manipulation and of control and of devaluation to normality, and to a degree of manic defence that is employed by all in everyday life. For instance, one is at a music-hall and on to the stage come the dancers, trained to liveliness. One can say that here is the primal scene, here is exhibitionism, here is anal control, here is masochistic submission to discipline, here is a defiance of the super-ego. Sooner or later one adds: here is LIFE. Might it not be that the main point of the performance is a denial of deadness, a defence against depressive 'death inside' ideas, the sexualization being secondary.

What about such things as the wireless that is left on interminably? What about living in a town like London with its noise that never ceases, and lights that are never extinguished? Each illustrates the reassurance through reality against death inside, and a use of manic defence that can be normal.

Again, in order to account for the existence of the Court and Personal column of our newspapers we must postulate a general need for reassurance against ideas of illness and death in the Royal Family and among the aristocracy; such reassurance can be given by reliable publication of facts. But there is no possible reassurance against the destruction and disorganization of the corresponding figures in the inner reality. Of 'God Save the King' it is not enough to say that we want to save the King from the unconscious hate we bear him. We might say that in unconscious fantasy we do kill him, and we wish to save him from our fantasy, but this strains the word fantasy. I prefer to say that in our inner reality the internalized father is all the time being killed, robbed, and burnt and cut up, and we welcome the personalization of this internalized father by a real man whom we can help to save. Court mourning is a compulsory order which pays a tribute to the normality of mourning. In manic defence mourning cannot be experienced.

In these Court and Personal columns the movements of the aristocracy are reported and predicted, and here can be seen in thin disguise the omnipotent control of personages who stand for internal objects.

The truth is, one can scarcely discuss *in the abstract* whether such devices are a normal reassurance through reality or an abnormal manic defence; one *can* discuss, however, the use of the defence that we meet with in the course of the analysis of a patient.

In manic defence a relationship with the external object is used in the attempt to decrease the tension in inner reality. But it is characteristic of the manic defence that the individual is unable fully to believe in the liveliness that denies deadness, since he does not believe in his own capacity for object love; for making good is only real when the destruction is acknowledged.

It might be that some of our difficulty in agreeing on a term for what is at present called the manic defence is directly to do with the nature of the manic defence itself. One cannot help noting that the word 'depression' is not only used but used quite accurately in popular speech. Is it not possible to see in this the introspection that goes with depression? The fact that there is no popular term for the manic defence could be linked with the lack of self-criticism that goes with it clinically. By the very nature of the manic defence we should expect to be unable to get to know it directly through introspection, at the moment when that defence is operative.

It is just when we are depressed that we *feel* depressed. It is just when we are manic-defensive that we are *least likely to feel* as if we are defending against depression. At such times we are more likely to feel elated, happy, busy, excited, humorous, omniscient, 'full of life', and at the same time we are less interested than usual in serious things and in the awfulness of hate, destruction, and killing.

I do not wish to maintain that in the analyses of the past[1] the deepest unconscious fantasies, which (following Freud) I am here calling 'inner reality', have not been reached. In learning the psycho-analytic technique we are taught to interpret *within the transference*. Full analysis of the transference gives analysis of the inner reality. But an understanding of the latter is necessary for a clear understanding of the transference.

CHARACTERISTICS OF THE MANIC DEFENCE

I now come to a rather closer examination of the nature of the manic defence. Its characteristics are omnipotent manipulation or control and contemptuous devaluation; it is organized in respect of the anxieties belonging to depression, which is the mood that results from the coexistence of love and greed and hate in the relations between the internal objects.

The manic defence shows in several different but interrelated ways, namely:
  Denial of inner reality.
  Flight to external reality from inner reality.
  Holding the people of the inner reality in 'suspended animation'.
  Denial of the *sensations* of depression — namely the heaviness, the sadness — by specifically opposite sensations, lightness, humorousness, etc.
  The employment of almost any opposites in the reassurance against death, chaos, mystery, etc., ideas that belong to the *fantasy content* of the depressive position.

Denial of Inner Reality. I have already referred to this in accounting for my

[1] i.e. in psycho-analysis before Klein.

own delay in recognizing the deepest unconscious fantasies. Clinically we see not so much the denial as the elation that is related to the denial, or a sense of unreality about external reality, or unconcern about serious things.

There is a type of partial recognition of internal reality that is worth mentioning in this setting. One may meet with an astoundingly deep recognition of certain aspects of internal reality in people who nevertheless do not acknowledge that the people who inhabit them are a part of themselves. An artist feels as if a picture was painted by someone acting from inside him, or a preacher feels as if God speaks through him. Many who live normal and valuable lives do not feel they are responsible for the best that is in them. They are proud and happy to be the agent of a loved and admired person, or of God, but they deny their parenthood of the internalized object. I think more has been written about bad internalized objects similarly disowned than about the denial of good internal forces and objects.

There is a practical point here, for in the analysis of the most satisfactory type of religious patient it is helpful to work with the patient as if on an agreed basis of recognition of internal reality, and to let the recognition of the personal origin of the patient's God come automatically as a result of the lessening of anxiety due to the analysis of the depressive position. It is necessarily dangerous for the analyst to have it in his mind that the patient's God is a 'fantasy object'. The use of that word would make the patient feel as if the analyst were undervaluing the good object, which he is not really doing. I think something similar would apply to the analysis of an artist in regard to the source of his inspiration, and also the analysis of the inner people and imaginary companions to whom our patients are able to introduce us.

Flight to External Reality from Internal Reality. There are several clinical types of this. There is the patient who makes external reality express the fantasies. There is the patient who day-dreams, omnipotently manipulating reality, but knowing it is a manipulation. There is the patient who exploits every possible physical aspect of sexuality and sensuality. There is the patient who exploits the internal bodily sensations. Of the last two, the former, the compulsive masturbator, abates psychic tension by the use of the satisfaction to be got from auto-erotic activity and from compulsive heterosexual or homosexual experiences, and the latter, the hypochondriac, comes to tolerate psychic tension by denial of fantasy content.

Suspended Animation. In this aspect of the defence, in which the patient controls the internalized parents, keeping them between life and death, the dangerous internal reality (with its threatened good objects, its bad objects and bits of objects, and its dangerous persecutors) is to some extent acknowledged (unconsciously) and is being dealt with. The defence is unsatisfactory because omnipotent control of the bad internalized parents also stops all good relationships, and the patient feels dead inside and sees the world as a colourless place. My second case illustrates this.

Denial of Certain Aspects of the Feelings of Depression

Use of Opposites in Reassurance. These two can be taken together. To illustrate my meaning, I give a series of opposites commonly exploited in their omnipotent fantasies and in omnipotently controlled external reality by patients who are in a state of manic defence. Some are more commonly employed in the service of gaining reassurance through external reality, so that omnipotence and devaluation are relatively little in evidence.

Empty	..	Filling
Dead	..	Alive, growing
Still	..	Moving
Grey	..	Coloured
Dark	..	Light, luminous
Unchanging	..	Altering constantly
Slow	..	Fast
Inside	..	Outside
Heavy	..	Light
Sinking	..	Rising
Low down	..	High up
Sad	..	Making laugh, happy
Depressed	..	Light-headed, on top of the world
Serious	..	Comic
Separated	..	Joined
Separating	..	Being joined
Formless	..	Formed, proportioned
Chaos	..	Order
Discord	..	Harmony
Failure	..	Success
In bits	..	Integrated
Unknown and mysterious	..	Known and understood

Here the key words are dead and alive — moving — growing.

Depressive — Ascensive

I wish to dwell for a few minutes on one of these defences which specially interests me.

While looking round for a word that might describe the total of defences against the depressive position I met the word 'ascensive'. Dr J. M. Taylor suggested it to me as one opposite of depressive, and it is better than the word buoyant which is familiar as an opposite of depressed in Stock Exchange reports.

It seems to me that this word, ascensive, can be usefully employed in drawing attention to the defence against an aspect of depression which is implied in such terms as 'heaviness of heart', 'depth of despair', 'that sinking feeling', etc.

One has only to think of the words 'grave', 'gravity', 'gravitation', and of the words 'light', 'levity', 'levitation'; each of these words has double meaning. Gravity denotes seriousness, but is also used to describe a physical force. Levity denotes devaluation and joking as well as lack of physical heaviness. In children's play I have always found that balloons, aeroplanes and magic carpets include a manic defence significance, sometimes specifically and sometimes incidentally. Also light-headedness[1] is a common symptom of an impending depressive phase, being a defence against heaviness, the head as if filled with gas, tending to raise the patient above his troubles. In this connection it is interesting to note that in laughter we show ourselves and our fellows that we have plenty of air, and to spare, whereas in sighing and sobbing we demonstrate a relative lack of it by our rationed in-breathing attempts.

The word ascensive brings into the foreground the significance of the Ascension in the Christian religion. I think that I should once have described the Crucifixion and Resurrection as a symbolic castration with subsequent erection in spite of corporeal insult. If I had offered this explanation to a Christian, I should have met with protest not only on account of the general disallowal of unconscious sexual symbolism; at least part of the resultant indignation would have been *justified*[2] by my having left out the depressive-ascensive significance of the myth. Each year the Christian tastes the depths of sadness, despair, hopelessness, in the Good Friday experiences. The average Christian cannot hold the depression so long, and so he goes over into a manic phase on Easter Sunday. The Ascension marks recovery from depression.

Many find sadness near enough at hand without the help of religion and can even tolerate being sad without the support that shared experience affords, but it has sometimes struck me, when I have heard people in analysis jeering at religion, that they are showing a manic defence in so far as they fail to recognize sadness, guilt, and worthlessness and the value of reaching to this which belongs to personal inner or psychic reality.

MANIC DEFENCE AND SYMBOLISM

The subject that I have chosen is certainly one capable of very wide treatment. A matter that interests me very much is the theoretical relation between

[1] cf. elation.

[2] This idea has been expressed by Brierley (1951, Chapter 6).

manic defence phenomena and symbolism. For instance, rising has a phallic, that is to say, erection significance, as is obvious, but this is not the same as its ascensive or contra-depressive significance. Balloons are employed in fantasies and games as symbolic of the mother's body or breasts, of the flatus pregnancy, flatus erection, flatus; they are *also* employed as contra-depressive symbols. In regard to feelings they are contra-depressive, whatever the object they displace.

Falling has a sexual, or a passive-masochistic significance; it *also* has a depressive significance; and so on.

A woman may envy a man, desire to be a man, hate being a woman, because being herself liable to depressive anxiety she has come to identify man with erection and so with the ascensive manic defence.

These and other relations between manic defences and sexual symbolism must be left for later study.

CLINICAL EXAMPLES

It would be easy to give relevant details from this or any week's material, of each of the ten patients who are at present under my care.

I have selected four case fragments. The first two patients are of the asocial type, the third is a severe obsessional, and the fourth a depressive.

The first, Billy, is five years old and has been with me for four terms. When he came to me at three and a half he was restless, interested chiefly in money and ice-creams, and acquisitive to a degree without being able to enjoy what he had acquired. He had started to steal money, and I think that without analysis he would have been a delinquent, especially as he has to live in a home in which he is the only child of estranged parents. His behaviour in the early stages of the analysis was consistent with a diagnosis: 'asocial, potential delinquent.'

I quote three games, chosen at random and yet I think fairly, to illustrate the changes that have occurred during analysis. There was an interval of some months between the first and second stage and between the second and third.

In the earliest stage, before the first of the three games, one could scarcely describe his activities as games — at best there had been wild attacks on pirates.

In the first game he stands at the mouth of a cannon, which I let off. He is carried high up and swiftly over the continents to Africa. On his way he knocks down various people with a stick — and in Africa he deals from above with natives who are occupied in various ways — sending them from the tops of trees to the bottoms of wells, and cutting off the head of the chief.

In an hour in which this game was dominant he was tremendously excited, and I was not surprised when after the end of the hour, in letting himself down from my room on the second floor in the lift, he went to the basement — the well of the lift — in error, and became terrified. I had on that day followed him (secretly) because of his exalted condition, and so was able to help him out of his difficulty; he was immensely reassured by finding I had appreciated his abnormal state and so had been at hand when he was in distress.

This hour followed a scene at home with his mother which, of course, was largely brought about by his own ambivalence that was becoming open. It also marked the climax of his so-called 'manic' behaviour and was related in time to the analysis of the depressive position and to the arrival of the feeling of sadness and hopelessness. With the arrival of sadness, the restitution of constructive play first became possible.

The game which reminded me of the one I have just described concerned a series of journeys in an aeroplane. This was after an interval of some months. We again fly to Africa, and we expect enemies. We look down on the world and laugh at its insignificance. But a feature of the trip is a most amazing set of safety precautions. We have two books of instructions on how to fly an aeroplane or a seaplane. We have two engines as well as a helicopter plane in case the engines fail — also a parachute each. We have an under-carriage with wheels but also a couple of floats in case we accidentally come down on water. We have a good store of food and also a bag of gold in case we run short of food or spare parts. In many other ways, too, we insure ourselves against a failure of our attempt to get above our troubles.

In this, the second game, an obsessional mechanism was clearly used, and the persecutors were raised in status, being aeroplanes of another country, capable of becoming allied aeroplanes in a war with a third country. (This was shown in further games.) Devaluation was decreased, and omnipotence lessened; but the being above was not only to be explained along the lines of our being in a position to drop faeces on to those below — it retained an ascensive or contra-depressive feel.

To compare with these two games I give a still later game.

We build a ship and set out for a pirate land. In this game (of which I give the main details only) we forget our aim, as it is a very beautiful day. We lie about basking in the sun on deck and enjoying companionship in a happy unselfconscious way. From time to time we dive into the sea and swim about lazily. There are some sharks and crocodiles, which occasionally remind us rudely of their persecuting quality, but the boy has a gun that shoots even under the water, so that we are not much worried.

We take on board a little girl whom we save from drowning and we make for her a switchback for her doll. The captain gives some trouble. Every now and again the engines stop and after a search it is found that the captain has put muck into the works. What a captain! He takes out the muck and we go on again, enjoying the benevolence of the sunshine and water.

A comparison of this play fragment with the other two games shows a lessening in persecution anxiety (the pirates having in the past given constant and serious trouble), a becoming good of bad objects (the sea used to be teeming with crocodiles and almost entirely bad), a belief in goodness and kindness (the sunshine and general holiday feeling), a linking up of fantasy and physical experiences (the gun that can shoot under water), the manageable quality of the captain's treachery which he himself makes good (removal of the muck from the engines), the new object relations (especially shown in the new inclusion of a good object in the shape of a little girl, saved from the sea and made happy with well-controlled ups and downs), and also a lessening of obsessional over-insurance against risk. Devaluation is not a feature of the game.

The manic defence comes in to the extent that dangers are forgotten, but the fact that there is some increase in the goodness of the internal objects makes the manic defence less strong and brings about the other changes. There is manic defence in that he deals with danger in a manic way, shooting at persecutors inside the body (under the water), nevertheless a stronger relation to external reality is seen, for instance, in the relation of the shooting under water to passing water in the bath.

I play the role of imaginary brother, but also of a mother.

Clinically Billy has changed to a much more normal child. At school he is learning well, and enjoying his relation to other children and to the teachers. At home he is not quite normal; he still demands money and is liable to be noisy and especially to have moments of unreasonable behaviour just as dinner is starting. But he has a delightful personality, a developing understanding of the difficulties of his parents, who remain cool towards each other. The mother is very ill herself, depressive and a drug-addict.

*   *   *

David (aged eight), another asocial child, came to me at the beginning of this term as an alternative to being expelled from school on account of 'sex and lavatory obsession' and some vaguely defined actions in regard to certain boys and girls. He is the only child of a talented but depressive father who sometimes lies in bed for several days for no clear reason, and of a mother who is — as she herself recognizes — highly neurotic as well as worried about the real home situation. The mother gives me excellent support.

Like most delinquent children, David is immediately liked for a short period by everyone with whom he does not come too much in contact. Actually, since the treatment started, there have been no unpleasant happenings outside, but I am told that he is tiring to have in one's company for long, needing and asking to be kept occupied. His knowledge of the facts of external reality is remarkable, though typical of the delinquent.

In an early hour he said to me: 'I hope I am not tiring you.' And this, coupled with my having been told by the parents of his always tiring them out, and also with my experience of a similar case (treated before I understood much about inner reality), led me to be prepared for an exhausting case.

Once, when I was describing the treatment of a delinquent child at a seminar, Dr Ernest Jones remarked that a practical point arose out of the case, namely: is it impossible to avoid getting exhausted in dealing with a delinquent? For, if so, there was a serious limitation to treatment of such cases. At that time, however, a delinquent child had been treated by Dr Schmideberg without too serious difficulty in the management of the analysis, so that I feel that what Dr Jones had in his mind at that time was that it was my technique that was at fault.[1]

The aim to tire me out soon asserted itself but before this a good deal of analysis had been possible. Chiefly, the little toys had enabled David to give me and himself a wealth of fantasy, and in great detail[2].

After a few days David fled from the anxieties belonging to deep fantasies to an interest in the world outside, the streets as seen from the window, and in the world outside my door — especially the lift. The inside of the room had become his own inside, and if he were to deal with me and the contents of my room (father and mother, witches, ghosts, persecutors, etc.) he had to have the means to control them. First he had to tire them out, as he feared he could not control them — and I felt that in this he showed some distrust of omnipotence. I had proof at this stage of a suicidal impulse. Along with the need to tire me out, there developed a desire to save me from exhaustion, so that as a slave driver he took immense care that his slave should not become exhausted. He provided me with compulsory rest periods.

Soon it became clear *that it was he who was becoming exhausted*, and the problem of the analyst becoming tired was gradually solved by the interpretations in regard to his own exhaustion in the control of the internalized parents who were exhausting each other as well as him.

I was fortunate enough to have him in my room at 11 a.m. on Armistice Day. The matter of Armistice Day observance interested him vastly; it was not so much that his father had fought in the war as that he had already developed (before analysis and in relation to the analysis) an interest in the streets and the traffic, as providing a not hopelessly uncontrollable sample of inner reality.

[1] I now see that there was a very real problem implicit in Dr Jones's remark, and I have developed the theme. (See Chapter XXII).

[2] Mrs Klein's introduction of the use of a few very small toys was a brilliant plan, because these toys give the child support in regard to contemptuous devaluation and make omnipotent mastery almost a fact. The child is able to express deep fantasies by means of the little toys at the outset of a treatment and so to start with some belief in his own inner reality.

He came full of the pleasure of buying a poppy from a lady, and at 11 o'clock he was interested in every detail of the street events. Then came the long awaited two minutes' silence. It was a particularly complete silence in my neighbourhood, and he was absolutely delighted. 'Isn't it lovely!' For two minutes in his life he felt as if he was not tired, as he need not tire out the parents, since there had come along an omnipotent control imposed from outside and accepted as real by all.

Of interest was his fantasy that during the silence the ladies went on selling flowers;[1] the only permitted activity; a more manic, internal omnipotence would have stopped everything (the good included).

Analysis of the depressive position and of the manic defence has lessened his feverish pleasure in the analysis. Moments of intense tiredness, sadness, and hopelessness have come along, and he has shown indirect evidence of guilt feelings. He has had a few weeks with games in which I have had to become very frightened, and alternatively guilty, and in which I have the most terrible nightmares. This week he has even played at being frightened himself, and today he really was afraid of something. He illustrated to me his resistance by getting me to teach him diving, which in fact he refuses to learn, and I have to say: 'Here you are wasting my time! How can I teach you to dive if you can't stand? I am very angry with you' — and so on and so on. All this becomes a tremendous joke, and he makes me laugh heartily and is then very pleased. But he is now aware that all this joking is part of the defence against the depressive position, and at present especially against guilt feelings; at the same time the defence is gradually being analysed.

How can he dive into the inside of the body,[2] the inner reality, unless he can stand, be sure he is alive, understand what he will find inside?

David's case illustrates the ego's danger from the bad inner objects, the boy fearing lest he will be emptied and exhausted by the inner parents who constantly empty each other.

David shows the flight from inner reality to the interest in the surface of his body, and in his surface feelings, and from these to an interest in the bodies and feelings of other children.

The progress of his analysis also illustrates the importance of an understanding of the mechanism of the omnipotent control of the internal objects, and of the relation of denial of tiredness, anxiety, and guilt feelings to denial of inner reality.

*   *   *

Charlotte (aged 30) has been with me in analysis for two months. She is

---

[1] This was his idea, not in fact true.

[2] Now I would be adding the idea of his meeting the mother's depression by diving into her inner world (1957).

clinically a depressive, with suicidal fears, but also with some enjoyment both of work and of outside activities.

Early in the analysis she reported a stock dream: she comes to a railway station where there is a train, *but the train never starts*.

Last week she dreamed a dream twice in one night. I must leave out much detail, but the gist was that in each she was going up and down the corridor of a train, looking for a carriage with a whole side unoccupied, so that she could lie down and sleep during the journey. A Mrs So and So, a woman she is fond of (and who compares with me in that she fusses over the patient, but who hastens to prescribe for piles while I do nothing to treat them), was telling her to find a place to wash.

In the first dream she found the compartment with a side unoccupied, and in the second she found the washing place. *In each dream the train started*. It was this last casual remark which reminded me of the stock dream. The piles, which had become a clinical feature at this time, draw attention, obviously, to anal excitement and fantasy, and one is not surprised to find travelling featured in the dreams. In this hour the patient described how she had walked across the park in heavy shoes, which helped her to work off her feelings, also how she had played with her nephew who had made her do gymnastic exercises on the floor.

I could point to my role of mother in the transference, with the patient's indirectly expressed urge to dirty me and kick and trample on my body, and so on, but I feel I should have missed something very important if I had not pointed out the significance of the lessening in manic defence and the new dangers inherent in the change. The train that never started to travel over the lines was a picture of the omnipotently controlled parents, parents held in suspended animation; Joan Riviere's words, 'the stranglehold of the manic defence', describe the clinical condition that the patient at that time feared. The starting of the trains indicated the lessening of this control of the internalized parents, and gave warning of the dangers inherent in this, and of the need for new defences should the advance in this direction outrun the ego development that the analysis was bringing about. There had been recent material and interpretations in regard to the taking in of me and of my room, etc.

In simple language, trains which start to move are liable to accidents.

The search for the washing place, in this setting, was probably connected with the development of the obsessional technique, and all that that means in regard to the ability to tolerate the depressive position and to acknowledge object love and dependence.

In the next hour the patient felt responsible for the kick marks on my door and the dirty marks on the furniture, and wanted to wash them off.

* * *

Mathilda (aged 39) has been in analysis four years. Clinically she was a severe obsessional. In analysis she has been a depressive with marked suicidal fears. She has been psychologically an ill person since very early childhood, no happy period being remembered at all. At four she could not be left at day school, and from about this time till late childhood her life was dominated by fear of being sick.

The word 'end' could not be mentioned in any context in the analysis, and the whole analysis could be almost described as an analysis of its end.[1]

Just now the first real contacts are being made, anal interest and desire have just arrived, having been deeply repressed.

At the beginning of the hour that I propose to describe, taken from this week's work, she tried to make me laugh, and laughed herself at the thought that by the attitude of my hands I was holding back my water with them. With this patient, as with others, I found that this effort to laugh and to make me laugh, was a signal of depressive anxiety, and a patient may show great relief at one's quick recognition of this interpretation, even bursting into tears instead of going on laughing and being funny. The patient now produced what is called a Polyfoto of herself. Her mother wanted a photo of her and she had felt that if 48 small photos were taken (as by this method) one or two might be found to be good. Also this method corresponds to a hope of putting together the bits of breast, of the parents, of oneself.[2] I was asked to choose which I liked best and also to look over all the 48. She intended to give me one. The idea was that I was to do something *outside the analysis*, and when, instead of falling into the trap (a few days before she had given me warning of such traps), I started analysing the situation, she felt hopeless, said she would not give a photo to anyone, and that she would commit suicide. We had had a good deal on the subject of looking as giving life, and I was to be seduced into a denial of her deadness by looking and seeing.

If I did not take, she felt injured, which linked up with her extreme anxiety in connection with the fantasy of having refused mother's breast (causing mother to feel bad, or injured) as opposed to feeling angry at being frustrated by mother. The end of each analytic hour was liable to feel to her like an angry refusal of analysis against which she defended herself by stressing the analyst's frustrating powers.

The interpretations brought to light the fact that she felt analysis as a weapon in my hands, and also that she *felt it more real for me to see her photo* (a 48th of her) than for me to see her herself. The analytic situation (which she has spent four years proclaiming to be the only reality for her) now seemed to her for the first time to be unreal, or at least a narcissistic

[1] This patient was able to leave analysis after ten years of regular treatment.

[2] I would now see much more in this incident, but I think I would act as I did then.

relationship, a relationship to the analyst that is valuable to her chiefly for her own relief, a taking without giving, a relationship with her own internal objects. She remembered that a day or two before she had suddenly thought, 'how awful to be really oneself, how terribly lonely'.

To be oneself means containing a relation between father and mother. If they are loving and are happy together, they rouse greed and hate in the lonely one; and, if they are bad, robbed, cruel, fighting, they are so because of the anger of the lonely one, anger rooted in the past.

This analysis has been a long one, partly because for the first two years of it I did not understand the depressive position; indeed, not till the last year did I have the feeling that the analysis was really going well.

I have quoted Mathilda chiefly to illustrate the feeling of unreality that accompanies the denial of inner reality in manic defence. The Polyfoto incident was an invitation to me to get caught up in her manic defence instead of understanding her deadness, non-existence, lack of feeling real.

SUMMARY

I have chosen to present certain aspects of the manic defence and of its relations to the depressive position. In doing so I have invited discussion on the term inner reality, and its meaning as compared with the meaning of the terms fantasy and external reality.

My own increased understanding of manic defence and increased recognition of inner reality have made a great difference to my psycho-analytic practice.

I hope that my case material has given some indication of the way in which the manic defence is in one way or another a mechanism that is commonly employed and that has to be constantly in the analyst's mind, like any other defence mechanism.

It is not enough to say that certain cases show manic defence, since in every case the depressive position is reached sooner or later, and some defence against it can always be expected. And, in any case, the analysis of the end of an analysis (which may start at the beginning) includes the analysis of the depressive position.

It is possible for a good analysis to be incomplete because the end has come without itself being fully analysed; or it is possible for an analysis to be a prolonged one, partly because the end, and the successful outcome itself, become tolerable to a patient only when they have been analysed, that is, after the completion of analysis of the depressive position, and of the defences that may be employed against it, including the manic defence.

The term manic defence is intended to cover a person's capacity to deny the depressive anxiety that is inherent in emotional development, anxiety that belongs to the capacity of the individual to feel guilt, and also to acknowledge responsibility for instinctual experiences, and for the aggression in the fantasy that goes with instinctual experiences.

Chapter XII

Primitive Emotional Development[1]
[1945]

IT WILL BE CLEAR at once from my title that I have chosen a very wide sub-ject. All I can attempt to do is to make a preliminary personal statement, as if writing the introductory chapter to a book.

I shall not first give an historical survey and show the development of my ideas from the theories of others, because my mind does not work that way. What happens is that I gather this and that, here and there, settle down to clinical experience, form my own theories and then, last of all, interest myself in looking to see where I stole what. Perhaps this is as good a method as any.

About primitive emotional development there is a great deal that is not known or properly understood, at least by me, and it could well be argued that this discussion ought to be postponed five or ten years. Against this there is the fact that misunderstandings constantly recur in the Society's scientific meetings, and perhaps we shall find we do know enough already to prevent some of these misunderstandings by a discussion of these primitive emotional states.

Primarily interested in the child patient, and the infant, I decided that I must study psychosis in analysis. I have had about a dozen psychotic adult patients, and half of these have been rather extensively analysed. This hap-pened in the war, and I might say that I hardly noticed the blitz, being all the time engaged in analysis of psychotic patients who are notoriously and maddeningly oblivious of bombs, earthquakes, and floods.

As a result of this work I have a great deal to communicate and to bring into alignment with current theories, and perhaps this paper may be taken as a beginning.

By listening to what I have to say, and criticizing, you help me to take my

[1] Read before the British Psycho-Analytical Society, November 28, 1945. *Int. J. Psycho-Anal.*, Vol. XXVI, 1945.

next step, which is the study of the sources of my ideas, both in clinical work and in the published writings of analysts. It has in fact been extremely difficult to keep clinical material out of this paper, which I wished nevertheless to keep short so that there might be plenty of time for discussion.

First I must prepare the way. Let me try to describe different types of psycho-analysis. It is possible to do the analysis of a suitable patient taking into account almost exclusively that person's personal relation to people, along with the conscious and unconscious fantasies that enrich and complicate these relationships between whole persons. This is the original type of psycho-analysis. In the last two decades we have been shown how to develop our interest in fantasy, and how the patient's own fantasy about his inner organization and its origin in instinctual experience is important as such.[1] We have been shown further that in certain cases it is this, the patient's fantasy about his inner organization, that is vitally important, so that the analysis of depression and the defences against depression cannot be done on the basis only of consideration of the patient's relations to real people and his fantasies about them. This new emphasis on the patient's fantasy of himself opened up the wide field of analysis of hypochondria in which the patient's fantasy about his inner world includes the fantasy that this is localized inside his own body. It became possible for us to relate, in analysis, the qualitative changes in the individual's inner world to his instinctual experiences. The quality of these instinctual experiences accounted for the good and bad nature of what is inside, as well as for its existence.

This work was a natural progression in psycho-analysis; it involved new understanding but not new technique. It quickly led to the study and analysis of still more primitive relationships, and it is these that I wish to discuss in this paper. The existence of these more primitive types of object relationship has never been in doubt.

I have said that no modification in Freud's technique was needed for the extension of analysis to cope with depression and hypochondria. It is also true, according to my experience, that the same technique can take us to still more primitive elements, provided of course that we take into consideration the changes in the transference situation inherent in such work.

I mean by this that a patient needing analysis of ambivalence in external relationships has a fantasy of his analyst and the analyst's work that is different from that of one who is depressed. In the former case the analyst's work is thought of as done out of love for the patient, hate being deflected on to hateful things. The depressed patient requires of his analyst the understanding that the analyst's work is to some extent his effort to cope with his own (the

[1] Chiefly through the work of Melanie Klein.

analyst's) depression, or shall I say guilt and grief resultant from the destructive elements in his own (the analyst's) love. To progress further along these lines, the patient who is asking for help in regard to his primitive, pre-depressive relationship to objects needs his analyst to be able to see the analyst's undisplaced and co-incident love and hate of him. In such cases the end of the hour, the end of the analysis, the rules and regulations, these all come in as important expressions of hate, just as the good interpretations are expressions of love, and symbolical of good food and care. This theme could be developed extensively and usefully.

Before embarking directly on a description of primitive emotional development I should also like to make it clear that the analysis of these primitive relationships cannot be undertaken except as an extension of the analysis of depression. It is certain that these primitive types of relationship, so far as they appear in children and adults, may come as a flight from the difficulties arising out of the next stages, after the classical conception of regression. It is right for a student analyst to learn first to cope with ambivalence in external relationships and with simple repression and then to progress to the analysis of the patient's fantasy about the inside and outside of his personality, and the whole range of his defences against depression, including the origins of the persecutory elements. These latter things the analyst can surely find in any analysis, but it would be useless or harmful for him to cope with principally depressive relationships unless he was fully prepared to analyse straightforward ambivalence. It is likewise true that it is useless and even dangerous to analyse the primitive pre-depressive relationships, and to interpret them as they appear in the transference, unless the analyst is fully prepared to cope with the depressive position, the defences against depression, and the persecutory ideas which appear for interpretation as the patient progresses.

I have more preparatory remarks to make. It has often been noted that, at five to six months, a change occurs in infants which makes it more easy than before for us to refer to their emotional development in the terms that apply to human beings generally. Anna Freud makes rather a special point of this and implies that in her view the tiny infant is concerned more with certain care-aspects than with specific people. Bowlby recently expressed the view that infants before six months are not particular, so that separation from their mother does not affect them in the same way as it does after six months. I myself have previously stated that infants reach something at six months, so that whereas many infants of five months grasp an object and put it to the mouth, it is not till six months that the average infant starts to follow this up by deliberately dropping the object as part of his play with it.

In specifying five to six months we need not try to be too accurate. If a baby of three or even two months or even less should reach the stage of development that it is convenient in general description to place at five months, no harm will be done.

In my opinion the stage we are describing, and I think one may accept this description, is a very important one. To some extent it is an affair of physical development, for the infant at five months becomes skilled to the extent that he grasps an object he sees, and can soon get it to his mouth. He could not have done this earlier. (Of course he may have wanted to. There is no exact parallel between skill and wish, and we know that many physical advances, such as the ability to walk, are often held up till emotional development releases physical attainment. Whatever the physical side of the matter, there is also the emotional.) We can say that at this stage a baby becomes able in his play to show that he can understand he has an inside, and that things come from outside. He shows he knows that he is enriched by what he incorporates (physically and psychically). Further, he shows that he knows he can get rid of something when he has got from it what he wants from it. All this represents a tremendous advance. It is at first only reached from time to time, and every detail of this advance can be lost as a regression because of anxiety.

The corollary of this is that now the infant assumes that his mother also has an inside, one which may be rich or poor, good or bad, ordered or muddled. He is therefore starting to be concerned with the mother and her sanity and her moods. In the case of many infants there is a relationship as between whole persons at six months. Now, when a human being feels he is a person related to people, he has already travelled a long way in primitive development.

Our task is to examine what goes on in the infant's feelings and personality before this stage which we recognize at five to six months, but which may be reached later or earlier.

There is also this question: how early do important things happen? For instance, does the unborn child have to be considered? And if so, at what age after conception does psychology come in? I would answer that if there is an important stage at five to six months there is also an important stage round about birth. My reason for saying this is the great differences that can be noticed if the baby is premature or post-mature. I suggest that at the end of nine months' gestation an infant becomes ripe for emotional development, and that if an infant is post-mature he has reached this stage in the womb, and one is therefore forced to consider his feelings before and during birth. On the other hand a premature infant is not experiencing much that is vital till he has reached the age at which he should have been born, that is to say some weeks after birth. At any rate this forms a basis for discussion.

Another question is: psychologically speaking, does anything *matter* before five to six months? I know that the view is quite sincerely held in some quarters that the answer is 'No'. This view must be given its due, but it is not mine.

The main object of this paper is to present the thesis that the early emotional development of the infant, before the infant knows himself (and therefore others) as the whole person that he is (and that they are), is vitally important: indeed that here are the clues to the psychopathology of psychosis.

EARLY DEVELOPMENTAL PROCESSES

There are three processes which seem to me to start very early: (1) integration, (2) personalization, and (3), following these, the appreciation of time and space and other properties of reality — in short, realization.

A great deal that we tend to take for granted had a beginning and a condition out of which it developed. For instance, many analyses sail through to completion without time being ever in dispute. But a boy of nine who loved to play with Ann, aged two, was acutely interested in the expected new baby. He said: 'When the new baby's born will he be born before Ann?' For him time-sense is very shaky. Again, a psychotic patient could not adopt any routine because if she did she had no idea on a Tuesday whether it was last week, or this week, or next week.

The localization of self in one's own body is often assumed, yet a psychotic patient in analysis came to recognize that as a baby she thought her twin at the other end of the pram was herself. She even felt surprised when her twin was picked up and yet she remained where she was. Her sense of self and other-than-self was undeveloped.

Another psychotic patient discovered in analysis that most of the time she lived in her head, behind her eyes. She could only see out of her eyes as out of windows and so was not aware of what her feet were doing, and in consequence she tended to fall into pits and to trip over things. She had no 'eyes in her feet'. Her personality was not felt to be localized in her body, which was like a complex engine that she had to drive with conscious care and skill. Another patient, at times, lived in a box 20 yards up, only connected with her body by a slender thread. In our practices examples of these failures in primitive development occur daily, and by them we may be reminded of the importance of such processes as integration, personalization, and realization.

It may be assumed that at the theoretical start the personality is unintegrated, and that in regressive disintegration there is a primary state to which regression leads. We postulate a primary unintegration.

Disintegration of personality is a well-known psychiatric condition, and its psychopathology is highly complex. Examination of these phenomena in analysis, however, shows that the primary unintegrated state provides a basis for disintegration, and that delay or failure in respect of primary integration predisposes to disintegration as a regression, or as a result of failure in other types of defence.

Integration starts right away at the beginning of life, but in our work we can never take it for granted. We have to account for it and watch its fluctuations.

An example of unintegration phenomena is provided by the very common experience of the patient who proceeds to give every detail of the week-end and feels contented at the end if everything has been said, though the analyst feels that no analytic work has been done. Sometimes we must interpret this as the patient's need to be known in all his bits and pieces by one person, the analyst. To be known means to feel integrated at least in the person of the analyst. This is the ordinary stuff of infant life, and an infant who has had no one person to gather his bits together starts with a handicap in his own self-integrating task, and perhaps he cannot succeed, or at any rate cannot maintain integration with confidence.

The tendency to integrate is helped by two sets of experience: the technique of infant care whereby an infant is kept warm, handled and bathed and rocked and named, and also the acute instinctual experiences which tend to gather the personality together from within. Many infants are well on the way toward integration during certain periods of the first twenty-four hours of life. In others the process is delayed, or setbacks occur, because of early inhibition of greedy attack. There are long stretches of time in a normal infant's life in which a baby does not mind whether he is many bits or one whole being, or whether he lives in his mother's face or in his own body, provided that from time to time he comes together and feels something. Later I will try to explain why disintegration is frightening, whereas unintegration is not.

In regard to environment, bits of nursing technique and faces seen and sounds heard and smells smelt are only gradually pieced together into one being to be called mother. In the transference situation in analysis of psychotics we get the clearest proof that the psychotic state of unintegration had a natural place at a primitive stage of the emotional development of the individual.

It is sometimes assumed that in health the individual is always integrated, as well as living in his own body, and able to feel that the world is real. There is, however, much sanity that has a symptomatic quality, being charged with fear or denial of madness, fear or denial of the innate capacity of every human being to become unintegrated, depersonalized, and to feel that the world is unreal. Sufficient lack of sleep produces these conditions in anyone.[1]

Equally important with integration is the development of the feeling that

---

[1] Through artistic expression we can hope to keep in touch with our primitive selves whence the most intense feelings and even fearfully acute sensations derive, and we are poor indeed if we are only sane.

one's person is in one's body. Again it is instinctual experience and the repeated quiet experiences of body-care that gradually build up what may be called satisfactory personalization. And as with disintegration so also the depersonalization phenomena of psychosis relate to early personalization delays.

Depersonalization is a common thing in adults and in children, it is often hidden for instance in what is called deep sleep and in prostration attacks with corpse-like pallor: 'She's miles away', people say, and they are right.

A problem related to that of personalization is that of the imaginary companions of childhood. These are not simple fantasy constructions. Study of the future of these imaginary companions (in analysis) shows that they are sometimes other selves of a highly primitive type. I cannot here formulate a clear statement of what I mean, and it would be out of place for me to explain this detail at length now. I would say, however, that this very primitive and magical creation of imaginary companions is easily used as a defence, as it magically by-passes all the anxieties associated with incorporation, digestion, retention, and expulsion.

DISSOCIATION

Out of the problem of unintegration comes another, that of dissociation. Dissociation can usefully be studied in its initial or natural forms. According to my view there grows out of unintegration a series of what are then called dissociations, which arise owing to integration being incomplete or partial. For example, there are the quiet and the excited states. I think an infant cannot be said to be aware at the start that while feeling this and that in his cot or enjoying the skin stimulations of bathing, he is the same as himself screaming for immediate satisfaction, possessed by an urge to get at and destroy something unless satisfied by milk. This means that he does not know at first that the mother he is building up through his quiet experiences is the same as the power behind the breasts that he has in his mind to destroy.

Also I think there is not necessarily an integration between a child asleep and a child awake. This integration comes in the course of time. Once dreams are remembered and even conveyed somehow to a third person, the dissociation is broken down a little; but some people never clearly remember their dreams, and children depend very much on adults for getting to know their dreams. It is normal for small children to have anxiety dreams and terrors. At these times children need someone to help them to remember what they dreamed. It is a valuable experience whenever a dream is both dreamed *and* remembered, precisely because of the breakdown of dissociation that this represents. However complex such a dissociation may be in child or adult, the fact remains that it can start in the natural alternation of the sleeping and awake states, dating from birth.

L

In fact the waking life of an infant can be perhaps described as a gradually developing dissociation from the sleeping state.

Artistic creation gradually takes the place of dreams or supplements them, and is vitally important for the welfare of the individual and therefore for mankind.

Dissociation is an extremely widespread defence mechanism and leads to surprising results. For instance urban life is a dissociation, a serious one for civilization. Also war and peace. The extremes in mental illness are well known. In childhood dissociation appears for instance in such common conditions as somnambulism, incontinence of faeces, in some forms of squinting, etc. It is very easy to miss dissociation when assessing a personality.

REALITY ADAPTATION

Let us now assume integration. If we do, we reach another enormous subject, the primary relation to external reality. In ordinary analyses we can and do take for granted this step in emotional development, which is highly complex and which, when it is made, represents a big advance in emotional development, yet is never finally made and settled. Many cases that we consider unsuitable for analysis are unsuitable indeed if we cannot deal with the transference difficulties that belong to an essential lack of true relation to external reality. If we allow analysis of psychotics, we find that in some analyses this essential lack of true relation to external reality is almost the whole thing.

I will try to describe in the simplest possible terms this phenomenon as I see it. In terms of baby and mother's breast (I am not claiming that the breast is essential as a vehicle of mother-love) the baby has instinctual urges and predatory ideas. The mother has a breast and the power to produce milk, and the idea that she would like to be attacked by a hungry baby. These two phenomena do not come into relation with each other till the mother and child *live an experience together*. The mother being mature and physically able has to be the one with tolerance and understanding, so that it is she who produces a situation that may with luck result in the first tie the infant makes with an external object, an object that is external to the self from the infant's point of view.

I think of the process as if two lines came from opposite directions, liable to come near each other. If they overlap there is a moment of *illusion* — a bit of experience which the infant can take as *either* his hallucination *or* a thing belonging to external reality.

In other language, the infant comes to the breast when excited, and ready to hallucinate something fit to be attacked. At that moment the actual nipple appears and he is able to feel it was that nipple that he hallucinated. So his ideas are enriched by actual details of sight, feel, smell, and next time this material is used in the hallucination. In this way he starts to build up a capacity to conjure up what is actually available. The mother has to go on giving the infant this type of experience. The process is immensely simplified if the infant is cared for by one person and one technique. It seems as if an infant is really designed to be cared for from birth by his own mother, or failing that by an adopted mother, and not by several nurses.

It is especially at the start that mothers are vitally important, and indeed it is a mother's job to protect her infant from complications that cannot yet be understood by the infant, and to go on steadily providing the simplified bit of the world which the infant, through her, comes to know. Only on such a foundation can objectivity or a scientific attitude be built. All failure in objectivity at whatever date relates to failure in this stage of primitive emotional development. Only on a basis of monotony can a mother profitably add richness.

One thing that follows the acceptance of external reality is the advantage to be gained from it. We often hear of the very real frustrations imposed by external reality, but less often hear of the relief and satisfaction it affords. Real milk is satisfying as compared with imaginary milk, but this is not the point. The point is that in fantasy things work by magic: there are no brakes on fantasy, and love and hate cause alarming effects. External reality has brakes on it, and can be studied and known, and, in fact, fantasy is only tolerable at full blast when objective reality is appreciated well. The subjective has tremendous value but is so alarming and magical that it cannot be enjoyed except as a parallel to the objective.

It will be seen that fantasy is not something the individual creates to deal with external reality's frustrations. This is only true of fantasying. Fantasy is more primary than reality, and the enrichment of fantasy with the world's riches depends on the experience of illusion.

It is interesting to examine the individual's relation to the objects in the self-created world of fantasy. In fact there are all grades of development and sophistication in this self-created world according to the amount of illusion that has been experienced, and so according to how much the self-created world has been unable or able to use perceived external world objects as material. This obviously needs a much more lengthy statement in another setting.

In the most primitive state, which may be retained in illness, and to which regression may occur, the object behaves according to magical laws, i.e. it exists when desired, it approaches when approached, it hurts when hurt. Lastly it vanishes when not wanted.

This last is most terrifying and is the only true annihilation. To not want, as a result of satisfaction, is to annihilate the object. This is one reason why infants are not always happy and contented after a satisfactory feed. One patient of mine carried this fear right on to adult life and only grew up from it in analysis, a man who had had an extremely good early experience with his mother and in his home.[1] His chief fear was of satisfaction.

I realize that this is only the bare outline of the vast problem of the initial steps in the development of a relation to external reality, and the relation of fantasy to reality. Soon we must add ideas of incorporation. But at the start a simple *contact* with external or shared reality has to be made, by the infant's hallucinating and the world's presenting, with moments of illusion for the infant in which the two are taken by him to be identical, which they never in fact are.

For this illusion to be produced in the baby's mind a human being has to be taking the trouble all the time to bring the world to the baby in understandable form, and in a limited way, suitable to the baby's needs. For this reason a baby cannot exist alone, psychologically or physically, and really needs one person to care for him at first.

The subject of illusion is a very wide one that needs study; it will be found to provide the clue to a child's interest in bubbles and clouds and rainbows and all mysterious phenomena, and also to his interest in fluff, which is most difficult to explain in terms of instinct direct. Somewhere here, too, is the interest in breath, which never decides whether it comes primarily from within or without, and which provides a basis for the conception of spirit, soul, anima.

PRIMITIVE RUTHLESSNESS (STAGE OF PRE-CONCERN)

We are now in a position to look at the earliest kind of relationship between a baby and his mother.

If one assumes that the individual is becoming integrated and personalized and has made a good start in his realization, there is still a long way for him to go before he is related as a whole person to a whole mother, and concerned about the effect of his own thoughts and actions on her.

We have to postulate an early ruthless object relationship. This may again be a theoretical phase only, and certainly no one can be ruthless after the concern stage except in a dissociated state. But ruthless dissociation states are common in early childhood, and emerge in certain types of delinquency, and madness, and must be available in health. The normal child enjoys a ruthless relation to his mother, mostly showing in play, and he needs his mother because only she can be expected to tolerate his ruthless relation to her even in play, because this really hurts her and wears her out. Without this play with her he can only hide a ruthless self and give it life in a state of dissociation.[2]

---

[1] I will just mention another reason why an infant is not satisfied with satisfaction. He feels fobbed off. He intended, one might say, to make a cannibalistic attack and he has been put off by an opiate, the feed. At best he can postpone the attack.

[2] There is in mythology a ruthless figure — Lilith — whose origin could be usefully studied.

I can bring in here the great fear of disintegration as opposed to the simple acceptance of primary unintegration. Once the individual has reached the stage of concern he cannot be oblivious to the result of his impulses, or to the action of bits of self such as biting mouth, stabbing eyes, piercing yells, sucking throat, etc., etc. Disintegration means abandonment to impulses, uncontrolled because acting on their own; and, further, this conjures up the idea of similarly uncontrolled (because dissociated) impulses directed towards himself.[1]

PRIMITIVE RETALIATION

To go back half a stage: it is usual, I think, to postulate a still more primitive object relationship in which the object acts in a retaliatory way. This is prior to a true relation to external reality. In this case the object, or the environment, is as much part of the self as the instinct is which conjures it up.[2] In introversion of early origin and therefore of primitive quality the individual lives in this environment which is himself, and a very poor life it is. There is no growth because there is no enrichment from external reality.

To illustrate the application of these ideas I add a note on thumb-sucking (including fist- and finger-sucking). This can be observed from birth onwards, and therefore can be presumed to have a meaning which develops from the primitive to sophistication, and it is important both as a normal activity and as a symptom of emotional disturbance.

We are familiar with the aspect of thumb-sucking covered by the term auto-erotic. The mouth is an erotogenic zone, specially organized in infancy, and the thumb-sucking child enjoys pleasure. He also has pleasurable ideas.

Hate is also expressed when the child damages his fingers by too vigorous or continuous sucking, and in any case he soon adds nail-biting to cope with this part of his feelings. He is also liable to damage his mouth. But it is not certain that all the damage that may be done to a finger or mouth in this way is part of hate. It seems that there is in it the element that something must suffer if the infant is to have pleasure: the object of primitive love suffers by being loved, apart from being hated.

[1] Crocodiles not only shed tears when they do not feel sad — pre-concern tears; they also readily stand for the ruthless primitive self.

[2] This is important because of our relationship to Jung's analytical psychology. We try to reduce everything to instinct, and the analytical psychologists reduce everything to this part of the primitive self which looks like environment but which arises out of instinct (archetypes). We ought to modify our view to embrace both ideas, and to see (if it is true) that in the earliest theoretical primitive state the self has its own environment, self-created, which is as much the self as the instincts that produce it. This is a theme which requires development.

We can see in finger-sucking, and in nail-biting especially, a turning-in of love and hate, for reasons such as the need to preserve the external object of interest. Also we see a turning-in to self, in face of frustration in love of an external object.

The subject is not exhausted by this kind of statement and deserves further study.

I suppose anyone would agree that thumb-sucking is done for consolation, not just pleasure; the fist or finger is there instead of the breast or mother, or someone. For instance, a baby of about four months reacted to the loss of his mother by a tendency to put his fist right down his throat, so that he would have died had he not been physically prevented from acting this way.

Whereas thumb-sucking is normal and universal, spreading out into the use of the dummy, and indeed to various activities of normal adults, it is also true that thumb-sucking persists in schizoid personalities, and in such cases is extremely compulsive. In one patient of mine it changed at 10 years into a compulsion to be always reading.

These phenomena cannot be explained except on the basis that the act is an attempt to localize the object (breast, etc.), to hold it half-way between in and out. This is either a defence against loss of object in the external world or in the inside of the body, that is to say, against loss of control over the object.

I have no doubt that normal thumb-sucking has this function too.

The auto-erotic element is not always clearly of paramount importance and certainly the use of dummy and fist soon becomes a clear defence against insecurity feelings and other anxieties of a primitive kind.

Finally, every fist-sucking provides a useful dramatization of the primitive object relationship in which the object is as much the individual as is the desire for an object, because it is created out of the desire, or is hallucinated, and at the beginning is independent of co-operation from external reality.

Some babies put a finger in the mouth while sucking the breast, thus (in a way) holding on to self-created reality while using external reality.

SUMMARY

An attempt has been made to formulate the primitive emotional processes which are normal in early infancy, and which appear regressively in the psychoses.

Chapter XIII

Paediatrics and Psychiatry[1]
[1948]

I HAVE CHOSEN the subject 'Paediatrics and Psychiatry' for my address because of the nature of my work. I am a paediatrician who has swung to psychiatry, and a psychiatrist who has clung to paediatrics. In an address from the Chair it is excusable, even usual, for the speaker to draw on experience that is peculiar to himself. My position, as I am a worker in two fields, ought to qualify me to communicate something that has interest for the children's doctor and also for the doctor whose work is concerned with the insane. It is, of course, inevitable that one who works in two subjects must sacrifice some degree of expertness in each.

The researches that more or less started with the pioneer work of Freud have established the fact that in the analysis of psychoneurosis the patient's childhood turns out to have harboured the intolerable conflicts which led to repression, and to the setting up of defences, and to the interruption in the emotional development of the individual, with formation of symptoms. Naturally, therefore, research became directed towards the emotional life of children. It was soon found that the reconstruction which adult patients gave of their childhood conflicts — conflicts associated with their instinctual ideas and experiences — could be seen in children, and seen clearly in the analytic treatment of children. It was not long before it began to be wondered whether the more psychotic illness of adults might not relate to the experiences of infants. Gradually a highly complex theory of the emotional development of the human being has been worked out, so that with all our terrible and at the same time exciting ignorance, we now have useful working hypotheses, hypotheses, that is to say, that really work. There is now sufficient material available for attempts to be made to formulate things about infants which

[1] Address from the Chair to the Medical Section of the British Psychological Society on 28th January, 1948. *Brit. J. Med. Psychol.*, Vol. XXI, 1948.

concern equally the psychiatrist and the children's physician, and I want to be one of those trying to say these things.

My thesis then is that the research worker in each of the two specialities has much to gain by meeting the research worker in the other. One assumption must be made; perhaps it will not be accepted. I assume a psychological basis for mental disorder. I assume that psychiatry can be studied in cases in which the health of the brain tissue is good. Naturally if a brain is diseased or physically disturbed, or cut about, mental changes must be expected. For myself I could learn but little from a study of the personality of an individual with a disordered brain, whereas there is so much that can be studied in the brain-intact individual — and so much remains to be understood about normal emotional development and its vagaries.

I hope it will not be thought that I am ignoring heredity or G.P.I. or senile dementia, injury, encephalitis, toxic delirium, or brain tumour, or even symptomatic improvement following the induction of fits.

Let me restate my idea, that it is possible to establish a clinical link between infant development and the psychiatric states, and likewise between infant care and the proper care of the mentally sick.

To do research one must have ideas, there is a subjective initiation of a line of inquiry. Objectivity comes later through planned work, and through comparison of the observations made from various angles. In justice to those who are doing research into this matter of the emotional development of the infant I will give a catalogue of the various methods of approach to any one detail that is being studied. The following types of approach provide observations that can be compared and correlated:

1. Through direct observation of the infant-mother relationship.

An example of this is provided by Dr Middlemore's work (unfortunately cut short by her death) which is described in the book *The Nursing Couple*.

2. Direct periodical observation of an infant starting soon after birth and continuing over a period of years.

In general practice and in a paediatric out-patient department of a hospital, parents attend when trouble arises or when they need advice.

3. Paediatric history-taking.

In my own experience I have given a mother the opportunity of telling me what she knows of her infant's development in about 20,000 cases. There is always more to learn about history-taking, but with this sort of experience one becomes, I hope, more and more accurate in one's assessment of a mother's description.

4. Paediatric practice, typically the management of infant feeding and excretion.

In the course of my paper I shall give an example of the psychological aspect of infant feeding problems. One could say that in the ordinary case where there is no disease process the work on the physical side has already been done by the physiologists and biochemists, and the practical problems are largely psychological.

5. Diagnostic interview with the child.

In the first interview it is often possible, and not harmful, to do a sort of analytic treatment in miniature. If analysis is undertaken later it will regularly be found to take many months to cover the same amount of ground again. In these interviews the doctor is not so sure of his ground as he is in a long analysis, but, on the other hand, he gets a deep insight into a large number of cases, and this to some extent balances the restriction of numbers in his analytic experience. Incidentally, in psychiatry, a diagnostic interview is only fruitful if it is a therapeutic interview.

6. Actual psycho-analytic experience.

This gives a different view of the patient's infancy according to whether the child is in the 2- to 4-year-old age group, or older, or near puberty, or in adolescence. For the analyst who is doing research on the earliest processes of emotional development, the analysis of fairly normal adults can be even more profitable than the analysis of children.

7. The observation in paediatric practice of psychotic regressions appearing as they commonly do in childhood and even in infancy.

8. Observation of children in homes adapted to cope with difficulties, whether these are antisocial behaviour, confusional states, maniacal episodes, relationships distorted by suspicion, or persecution, or mental defect, or fits.

9. The psycho-analysis of schizophrenics.

This I am putting in a separate group because I think such analyses are for experienced analysts only. In my view the analysis of illness associated with depression and the defences against depression are now in the class of routine treatment and are not 'research cases'. This is also true of manic-depressive and even paranoid cases. Schizophrenics, however, are in a different class and their treatment is more of a pioneering venture.

At this point I have learned to expect a misunderstanding unless deliberate care is taken to avoid it. It has often been said to me: the idea that mad people are like babies, or small children, simply isn't true. Can I make it clear that I do not suggest that the insane are behaving like infants any more than that neurotics are just like older children. Ordinary healthy children are not neurotic (though they can be) and ordinary babies are not mad. The relationship between paediatrics and psychiatry is much more subtle than this.

The theory that I am putting forward is that in the emotional development of every infant complicated processes are involved, and that lack of forward movement or completeness of these processes predisposes to mental disorder or breakdown; the completion of these processes forms the basis of mental health.

The mental health of the human being is laid down in infancy by the mother, who provides an environment in which complex but essential processes in the infant's self can become completed. It would perhaps be a good initial study to describe the task of the ordinary good mother, in so far as we can see what is happening in this partnership. I will attempt this, but before doing so there is something that must be said about the *meaning* of the actual mother to the infant.

It is fully agreed that eventually the infant comes to feel himself as a whole person, and to hold his mother to be a whole person; soon after this stage is reached other people enter his life as people, but the complications that belong to this state of affairs need not be gone into here. There is not a general agreement as to the first age at which an infant feels mother to be a person, and so feels concerned as to the results of his real and imaginary attacks on her when under the sway of instinctual tension. This puzzle, fortunately, can be left unanswered, as at the moment we are considering a mother's care at the stage before the infant can feel concerned.

I think I see what Miss Anna Freud (1947, p. 200) is referring to when she states:

'This first "Love" of the infant is selfish and material. Its life is governed by sensations of need and satisfaction, pleasure and discomfort. The mother, as an object, plays a part in this life so far as she brings satisfaction and removes discomfort. When the infant's needs are fulfilled, i.e. when it feels warm, comfortable, with pleasant gastric sensations, it withdraws interest from the object world and falls asleep. When it is hungry, cold and wet, or disturbed by intestinal sensations, it turns for help to the outside world. In this period the need for an object is inseparably bound up with the great body needs.

'From the fifth or sixth month onward the infant begins to pay attention to the mother also at times when it is not under the influence of bodily urges.'

Dr Friedlander (1947, p. 23) wrote:

'. . . during the first weeks and even months of life the relationship of the child to the mother is a rather simple one. The mother is the instrument which satisfies the child's bodily needs. Anyone who fulfils this function will arouse the same response in the child. . . .'

However I think myself that by the seventh week or so a large proportion of infants show clearly that they have at times a contact with the woman who is their mother.

Let us attempt to study the mother's job. If the infant is to be able to start to develop into a being, and to start to find the world we know, to start to come together and to cohere, then the following things about a mother stand out as vitally important:

She exists, continues to exist, lives, smells, breathes, her heart beats. She is *there* to be sensed in all possible ways.

She loves in a physical way, provides contact, a body temperature, movement, and quiet according to the baby's needs.

She provides opportunity for the baby to make the transition between the quiet and the excited state, not suddenly coming at the child with a feed and demanding a response.

She provides suitable food at suitable times.

At first she lets the infant dominate, being willing (as the child is so nearly a part of herself) to hold herself in readiness to respond.

Gradually she introduces the external shared world, carefully grading this according to the child's needs which vary from day to day and hour to hour.

She protects the baby from coincidences and shocks (the door banging as the baby goes to the breast), trying to keep the physical and emotional situation simple enough for the infant to be able to understand, and yet rich enough according to the infant's growing capacity.

She provides continuity.

By believing in the infant as a human being in its own right she does not hurry his development and so enables him to catch hold of time, to get the feeling of an internal personal going along.

For the mother the child is a whole human being from the start, and this enables her to tolerate his lack of integration and his weak sense of living-in-the-body.

If I add that the mother continues to exist in spite of repeated attacks on her (made by the infant both in love and in anger), I am going too far ahead, reaching towards the functions of the mother relative to the infant who has instincts and the capacity to be concerned.

If we examine this admittedly incomplete description we can see that whereas some functions (such as the provision of suitable food) might be performed by anyone, much can only be done by someone who has a mother's interest; moreover, continuity cannot be well provided by a multiplicity of minders; and in any case there is the actual continuity of detail as observed by the infant, starting perhaps with the close-up of the nipple or of the face, and including the smell and the details of texture, and so on. Moreover, how can anyone who is not in the position of mother with a mother's love know the infant well enough to give well-graded enrichment, to give enough to foster growing capacity, yet not enough to engender confusion?

Here I think I come to the first statement of the paediatrician's clinical gain from psychiatric contact. If it be true or even possible that the mental health of every individual is founded by the mother in her living experience with her infant, doctors and nurses can make it their first duty not to interfere. Instead of trying to teach mothers how to do what in fact cannot be taught, paediatricians must come sooner or later to recognize a good mother when they see one and then make sure that she gets full opportunity to grow to her job;

mistakes she may, and indeed will, make, but if by these she becomes able to do better in subsequent attempts there is in the end a gain.

Mothers cannot grow if they are frightened into doing as they are told. They must first find their feelings, and while doing so they need support — support against their own fears, their superstitions, their neighbours, and, of course, against physical accident and disease which can so largely be prevented or cured nowadays. I shall have more to say later about this support-without-interference, but if I were addressing a paediatric audience I could not too often mention the great danger to mental health that occurs when an infant is insulted by rude disruption of the delicate natural processes in the infant-mother partnership.

The environment is so vitally important at this early stage that one is driven to the unexpected conclusion that schizophrenia is a sort of environmental deficiency disease, since a perfect environment at the start can at least theoretically be expected to enable an infant to make the initial emotional or mental development which predisposes to further emotional development and so to mental health throughout life. An unfavourable environment later on is a different matter, being merely an additional adverse factor in the general aetiology of mental disorder.

EARLY INFANCY

Now let me briefly indicate the task of the infant happily placed in the care of an ordinary good mother. It will be understood that the task which can be said to occupy the infant (at least from birth) is not ever a completed task, and the achievements of the first weeks and months must be many times lost and regained according to the turns of fortune.

It is not difficult to see that in the case of every infant at least these three things have to happen:

1. The infant has to make contact with reality.
2. The personality of the infant has to become integrated, and the integration has to gain stability.
3. The infant has to come to feel he lives in what we see so easily as the body of that infant, but which at first is not felt by the infant to be significant in the special way we know it is.

Three things: reality contact, integration, sense of body.

The psychiatrist will readily see in the nature of these tasks the reflection of symptoms that are his continual concern; loss of reality contact and of reality sense, disintegration and depersonalization.

In order to follow up one theme in some detail I must take only one of these three, leaving the others aside.

THE RELATIONSHIP TO EXTERNAL REALITY

I have chosen to examine the matter of the establishment of reality contact, and even so I have to confine my attention to one example, the contact that arises out of that most primitive form of love, which is called greed, and which persists as cupboard-love. Equally significant is the reality contact in quiet periods between excitements, but I must not go too far from my subject.

As soon as an object relationship is possible it is immediately a matter of significance whether the object is outside or inside the child. I assume, however, that there is a stage prior to this at which there is no relationship at all. I would say that initially there is a condition which could be described at one and the same time as of *absolute independence* and *absolute dependence*. There is no feeling of dependence, and therefore that dependence must be absolute. Let us say that out of this state the infant is disturbed by instinct tension which is called hunger. I would say that the infant is ready to believe in something that could exist, i.e. there has developed in the infant a readiness to hallucinate an object; but that is rather a direction of expectancy than an object in itself. At this moment the mother comes along with her breast (I say breast for simplification of description), and places it so that the infant finds it. Here is another direction, this time towards instead of away from the infant. It is a tricky matter whether or no the mother and infant 'click'. At the start the mother allows the infant to dominate, and if she fails to do this the infant's subjective object will fail to have superimposed on it the objectively perceived breast. Ought we not to say that by fitting in with the infant's impulse the mother allows the baby the *illusion* that what is there is the thing created by the baby; as a result there is not only the physical experience of instinctual satisfaction, but also an emotional union, and the beginning of a belief in reality as something about which one can have illusions. Gradually, through the living experience of a relationship between the mother and the baby, the baby uses perceived detail in the creation of the object expected. In the course of breast feeding a mother may repeat this performance a thousand times. She may so successfully give her child the capacity for illusion that she has no difficulty in her next task, gradual disillusioning, this being the word for weaning in the primitive setting which is my interest in this paper.

It worries some people that there is no such thing in psychology as direct union, only an illusion of relationship; but I suppose psychiatrists are so used to patients' descriptions of loss of contact with reality that they will not be among those to object. Most of us are so good at using the objectively observed and expected that we manage without hallucinations, unless we are tired or weak from physical exhaustion. For the infant this clever use of shared reality which is another aspect of objectivity is by no means established, and everything depends on the mother at the beginning.

The mother does her job in this respect by simply being devoted, that is, provided she is allowed by doctors and nurses and helpful people generally to act as she loves to do.

This is where the paediatrician comes in — in clearing the way for the mother's native feeling towards her child. In accepting the psycho-analyst's help the paediatrician, incidentally, extends the usefulness of the analyst to a circle wider than that of his analytic practice. Doctors have made it very difficult for mothers to start off well in this function, one of the most important they have to perform. It is often very difficult for a woman, when preparing to have a baby, to be sure that she will be allowed to come to terms with her infant after birth in her own way, which is the infant's way. Let me quickly turn to an exception. Professor Spence[1] of Newcastle insists that each healthy baby in the maternity homes he supervises shall be in a cradle at the side of the mother. The mother has the skilled attention she so greatly needs, and she enjoys the confidence that is inspired by first-rate medical and nursing practice. At the same time she is expected to be the best judge of the feeding technique needed by her infant. There are no rules about regular feeding, and 'the nursing couples' (to use the late Dr Middlemore's term) usually find a convenient feeding rhythm sooner or later. Contrast this with the worst case, not difficult to find, of a maternity home in which the babies are kept in cots in a separate ward, even when healthy. At feed times they are wheeled in on a trolley, tightly wound round by a shawl, and at the right moment the nurse clocks in by thrusting the screaming infant's mouth at the breast of the bewildered, frustrated, often frightened mother.

This only refers to the initial stages of the feeding experience, and it will readily be seen that these ideas can be applied at all later stages. Nevertheless, if the beginning is bad the continuation is necessarily made more difficult. Moreover, clinically, serious feeding disturbances may start at the initial stage.

The paediatrician, taking careful histories of small children, cannot but be struck by the commonness of fairly or very severe feeding inhibitions[2]. He finds that there are certain critical moments that can be enumerated. (I had a severe case in a three-year-old in analysis, a little girl whose feeding inhibitions had started at twelve months on a definite day when she was sat up at table to eat with her father and mother, that is to say, all three together.) A common time for loss of zest for food would be the near arrival of a new baby. In many cases the loss of zest for food starts in infancy. There is the inhibition in respect of self-feeding, or there is a change from eagerness to refusal of food at the time of weaning from breast or bottle or from a special person, or at the introduction of solids, and even at the thickening of feeds. The arrival of

[1] Later Professor Sir James Spence.
[2] See page 33.

teeth may be accompanied by refusal of feeds. Even in very young infants one finds the refusal of anything new, and sometimes, conversely, an interest only in the new.

Some of the inhibitions, however, start from the beginning. The infant and the mother just never 'click'. At this point the mother can be held theoretically responsible, though of course not to blame.

Ordinarily if breast feeding is difficult the baby is put on to a bottle, and there are all sorts of ways out of the difficulty when the breast milk does not come or suit. In a case of difficulty, to insist on the breast when a mother could easily feed her baby well by bottle is a mistake.

In these matters the infant's doctor is at a loss if he does not understand what is going on behind the scenes in the emotional development of the infant; and he needs, too, to know something about the psychology of nursing mothers.

It is relevant here to describe a common problem of infant feeding, as I see it. I mean as I see it *now*, for I have struggled through the phases all doctors experience, in the heartbreaking attempt to deal with feeding problems along physical lines, altering quantities, intervals, proportions of fat, protein, and carbohydrate and switching from one brand of milk to another. Well do I remember the day when I made it a rule to get a feeding going well *before* altering the brand of milk. It took me years to realize that a feeding difficulty could often be cured by advising the mother to fit in with the baby absolutely for a few days. I had to discover that this fitting in with the infant's needs is so pleasurable to the mother that she cannot do it without moral support. If I advise this I must ask my social worker to visit daily, else the mother will wilt under criticism and feel responsible for too much. Obeying a rule, she can blame others if things go wrong, but she is scared to do as she deeply wants to do. On the other hand, if all goes well she never forgets the fact that she had it in her to do the right thing for her baby, without help.

These are not clever things. They simply require an appreciation of what it is that the mother and the baby are doing together. With the human infant it is never adequate to think in terms of conditional reflexes.

I want to make it clear that I am describing the paediatrician's task in the management of infant feeding, suggesting that he works blindly unless he knows what is going on behind the scenes. There the processes of emotional development are dominant, and they are of a nature that can be found in a 'state of undoing' in schizophrenic illness.

It is here that something can be said about play. The first play at the breast is of great value in that it enables the baby to find the mother and to communicate with her so that she can be prepared to act in the right way. Without the chance of play, the baby and the mother remain strangers to each other. How important are the hands in this. At twelve weeks, an infant will sometimes feed his mother while at the breast, putting his finger in her mouth.

W. H. Davies in his poem 'Infancy' said:

> Born to the world with my hands clenched,
> I wept and shut my eyes;
> Into my mouth a breast was forced,
> To stop my bitter cries.
> I did not know — nor cared to know —
> A woman from a man;
> Until I saw a sudden light,
> And all my joys began.
>
> From that great hour my hands went forth,
> And I began to prove
> That many a thing my two eyes saw
> My hands had power to move:
> My fingers now began to work,
> And all my toes likewise;
> And reaching out with fingers stretched,
> I laughed, with open eyes.

PSYCHIATRY AND INFANT CARE

It is time I linked this with something of interest to the psychiatrist.

In the psycho-analysis of a woman (who had done well in life but who came for treatment because of an increasing dissatisfaction, and a growing feeling that nothing meant anything to her) the following happened. There was an hour in which the important thing was that I kept absolutely still and quiet and said nothing at all. The next hour the same was happening, but after a length of time I reached for a cigarette. The result of the tiny movement I made was nearly disastrous, and the situation was only saved by my patient's being able to see what was afoot. From what had gone before we both knew that she was right back in the infant-mother relationship. In the quiet my patient had been lying on her mother's lap. Just when I made the movement the patient was (in her mind) starting to reach up with her hand, and in doing so she would have found the breast, and in the course of time the mother would have responded, and the feed would have started. The two would have come to terms. It was for this very experience that this patient was unconsciously looking. As I moved, however, I broke the spell and suddenly became the nannie. (Historically she had had the breast for a period of one month and had then been handed over to a nannie and fed by bottle.) Now this meant a disruption of natural progress. The nannie, although in many ways a better mother than the real mother, because not depressed, nevertheless at the moment for a feed had to get up and fetch or even prepare the bottle, and by the time all was ready the infant had lost much of the ability to 'create' the bottle or the milk; it had become a thing coming at her, with which she had to try to come to terms.

This sort of case material leads me on to the description of other analytic studies. It is very difficult to convey to those (either paediatricians or psychiatrists) who are not doing psycho-analysis the feeling of conviction that one digs down to solid rock, by which I mean that one sees real things re-lived in this work. However, each one of us can only get a certain number of types of experience, and therefore each must inevitably rely on learning from the work of colleagues.

I have long struggled with a case which illustrates my point in that, to help this patient at all, I have had to be ready waiting when she comes. This woman is one of twins, and the different treatment afforded her as compared with her twin sister by her mother has always been a source of grievance with her. Her twin being the weak one was taken over by the mother and fed and cared for by her, and taken into the mother's bed, while my patient, being strong and large, was handed over to a nurse. This was the conscious reconstruction. Only gradually has the true early infantile situation come out in the transference. This patient comes to me from a mental hospital. She has a fairly severe degree of splitting of personality, and for the first two decades (apart from her infancy) she made an exceptionally good adjustment on a compliance basis. Then she broke down, and started on her long search for a chance to find her own self, and a relation to the world that she could feel to be real. Needless to say, she did not know what she was looking for, and at one stage, in despair, she developed rheumatoid arthritis with the unconscious aim of becoming bed-ridden and helpless, so getting her family to comply with her. Or, shall I say, she used her arthritis in that way.

Hope of getting what she needed from analysis brought with it the absolute need that I have mentioned for me to be ready for her. At one time I had to be at the front door myself, actually opening the door as the bell rang. It can be well imagined that there was an infinity of play round this detail of management. Sometimes she would telephone me on the way, otherwise not believing I existed at all. The reason why I had to take the trouble to do all this, which was very trying, was that otherwise it was no use seeing her at all; she would come, and talk and go, but would get no feeling of our having met. On the other hand, a long spell of my giving her direct access always brought its reward. In six years a great deal has happened but the basis of it all has been the provision of direct access. She is having an essential experience for the first time, although it belongs to infancy, and this fact comes out quite clearly in the detailed material that I have not time to reproduce here. In this

M 167

case there is a strong regression element, the main trauma being related to early childhood rather than to infancy, namely a long period of rigid management by an almost insane nurse.

In case it should be thought that the analyst puts these ideas into the patient's head I would give a detail out of the treatment of a boy who was an apparent mental defective, but who was really a case of childhood schizophrenia, with regression to a powerfully controlled introversion. When the boy came to me at the age of five years he spent his time over a period of two or three months simply coming towards me and going away again, testing my ability to give direct access and egress.

Gradually this boy let himself sit on my lap, and go on to make affectionate contact. In the next phase he would get right inside my coat, and out of this developed a game of sliding out on to the floor head first from between my legs. During all this period I made very few verbal interpretations. In the next phase he had so strong a need for honey — it was wartime, and honey scarce — that he strained all resources until mercifully he became able to accept malt and oil instead, of which he ate voraciously. He now covered everything with saliva and became destructive with the honey-spoon. His saliva would form a pool on the doorstep if he was kept waiting. Out of all this there came a slow but steady development which had previously ceased and had become negative.

In this experience I seemed to see a child re-living early infantile experience and out of some need in himself correcting the faulty introduction to the world, being born again. I saw one environment supplanting another. After this, analysis by verbal interpretation became not only possible but acutely necessary. But in the phase I have described my job was to provide a certain type of environment, thereby allowing the boy to do the work.

There is a direct application of all this to the care of adolescents. Here is a typical adolescent case. A box of sixteen at a public school tells his school doctor that he insists on seeing a psychiatrist. In the end he gets his own way and his parents bring him to me. I take a detailed history from the parents, and in the interview with the boy I find him depressed, and flabby. In about an hour I get nothing from him, and I do not make any effort to bring him out. As I find later, the important thing in that interview was the lack of any urge on my part to get him to respond. On parting I let him know that I was expecting to see him again sometime.

The next I hear is through the telephone. He rings me up from school and asks if I can see him tomorrow, a Saturday. I know that I must do this, as the gesture has come from him, and I put aside everything to fit in with him. On the phone I immediately say yes, before I have decided how to manage it.

These conditions bring a very different boy to my room. He makes very considerable use of me, and in an hour or two he has done an analysis in miniature. Considerable results follow this, more I think than would have been reached in weeks of a set analysis at this stage. In the next holidays I find the boy has left school on his own initiative, decided on a career, made arrangements to attend a university, and to live in London where he can have analysis over a proper period, whether from me or a colleague. I think that this is the right way for such an analysis to start, and that many treatments of schizoid types of adolescent fail because they are planned on a basis that ignores the child's ability to 'think up' — in a way, to *create* — an analyst, a role into which the real analyst can try to fit himself.

If this is true it follows that set techniques for interview defeat their aim, which, presumably, is to make a diagnosis and to initiate a therapeutic procedure. The set technique wastes the patient's ability to make one sort of contact, and with a case of schizoid type this waste of opportunity may act as a negative therapy, and may do harm.

In the analysis of a schizophrenic adolescent girl I had to adopt a procedure over a long period of time by which I saw her or dealt with analytic material over the telephone just exactly when she rang. Claustrophobia was activated if any sort of definite arrangement was made. With this proviso good analytic work was done. Eventually a regular time was achieved. If, however, I had forced a regular arrangement too early this patient would have been unable to have made a contact with me that meant anything to her. Over a long period we talked chiefly of infant management and infant feeding; as a matter of fact before coming to me this girl had been giving infants in her care just the management that she needed from me and that she failed to get from her mother. The mother had been excellent except for a tremendous need to get reassurance from her feeding activities. 'None of my children ever refused anything I offered them', she would say, and as she was a trained dietician they all waxed fat, especially my patient. But till she came to me this girl scarcely knew what it was to make contact with reality from her end.

I now wish to describe what I can see of the theoretical basis of all this. In the favourable case the expectation of the infant meets impinging reality, and at this point I would place the word 'Illusion'. In case this is not understood by someone the following story may help.

Recently, during a hot spell, an analyst had to do an extra analytic session in the lunch hour. He was tired and perhaps a little sleepy, and he had the following experience at the same time as being an ordinary competent analyst.

He could see out of his window, and on a roof some distance away he saw a man. This man was about 45 years old, and had a rather bald head. He had finished his sandwiches and had let his mid-day paper with its racing tips fall. Obviously he had allowed himself to drop off to sleep.

Dimly aware of all this the analyst would never have registered anything had it not been that there was a sequel. We all know the way in which a continuous noise may be unnoticed until it stops. Well, in this case the disturbing thing was that the man made no movement at all. After half an hour the analyst definitely registered the fact that the man ought to have woken up, and then suddenly: pop! the man's head swelled to the size of the rather large stone spherical ornament that it had been all the time. The sight of the man going to sleep was no more than an indication that my friend wanted to go to sleep himself. He had failed to confine his hallucinations to situations that could absorb them.

To return, in the favourable case impulse or expectation of the infant meets impinging reality.

What are the consequences of failure in the introduction of the shared world to the infant?[1] In the extreme of failure these two lines in a diagram would be parallel. The infant creates out of his native poverty, and the world impinges in vain. The lines never meet. In such a hypothetical case there must be mental defect even if there is normal brain capacity. Commonly there is some degree of this splitting at the earliest level, and the basis is thereby laid for the infant to have a relationship unshared by us with a self-created world, in which magic holds sway, and alongside this a compliance with mundane management from outside, convenient because life-giving, but unsatisfactory in the extreme to the infant. Later on in childhood or adult life the compliance breaks down, if it is too isolated from the other trend which contains all the child's spontaneity. These parallel paths regularly appear in our analytic work, illustrated at the simplest by the patient who said that his analytic sessions were in duplicate, a rather dull one actually with the analyst, and the operative one afterwards in relation to an imagined analyst.

PAEDIATRICIAN AND PSYCHIATRIST

The main point about this is that in investigating the phenomena of human contact and communication, the paediatrician and the psychiatrist badly need each other's help. For instance very few psychiatrists can take a reliable history from a mother about early feeding details. Yet no history of a psychotic case is complete unless the last ounce of detail of the early nursing couple experience has been obtained, if it is available to skilled inquiry. Also, the paediatrician needs the psychiatrist. On his own he will fail to recognize the psychiatrically-ill infant, for such an infant may be in bursting physical health, never defiant or difficult, indeed most delightfully acquiescent. The ill baby

[1] For a clearer description see page 152.

may in fact be especially all the time good, 'we never knew we had him, doctor', able to be left on the arm of the chair with no danger of wriggling off, and so on. Healthy babies cry, do not by any means always take willingly, they have wills of their own, they are in fact a trouble. To their own mothers healthy babies are of course more rewarding than ill babies ever can be, because along with their nuisance value they also show spontaneous love feelings, so much more encouraging than the negative virtues.

In the matter of practical management I feel that those who care for infants (I mean mothers and nursery nurses) can teach something to those who manage the schizoid regressions and confusion states of people of any age. The provision of a stable though personal environment, warmth, protection from the unexpected and unpredictable, and the serving of food in a reliable way and accurately on time (or even following the whims of the patient), these things might help the nursing of schizoid cases.

The important thing for the psychiatrist, at the moment, however, is not practice but theory. I am saying that the proper place to study schizophrenia and manic depression and melancholia is the nursery, and if this be true then some modern trends in psychiatry are like barking up the wrong tree.

It may be asked, what do ordinary people do about this matter of contact with reality? Of course as development proceeds a great deal happens that seems to get round the difficulty, for enrichment by incorporation of objects is a psychical as well as a physical phenomenon, and the same can be said of being incorporated, including the eventual contribution to the world's fertility which is the privilege of even the least of us. And especially the sexual life offers a way round, with the conception of infants, a true physical mingling of two individuals. Nevertheless, while we have life, each one of us feels the matter of crude reality-contact to be a vital one, and we deal with it according to the way in which we have had reality introduced to us at the beginning. In some of us the ability to use the objectively verifiable, to objectify the subjective, is so easy that the fundamental problem of illusion tends to get lost. Unless they are ill or tired people do not know that there is a problem of relationship with reality, or a universal liability to hallucination, and they feel that mad people must be made of different stuff from themselves. Some of us, on the other hand, are aware of a tendency in ourselves towards the subjective, which we feel to be more significant than the world's affairs, and for such the sane may seem rather dull folk, and the common round seems mundane.

One of the ways out is the dreaming of dreams, and the remembering of them. In sleep we dream all the time and when we wake we need to carry something forward from the dream world into real life, just as we need to recognize everyday affairs turning up and weaving themselves into the dreams.

Apart from this, is it not largely through artistic creation and artistic experience that we maintain the necessary bridges between the subjective and the objective? It is for this reason, I suggest, that we value tremendously the lone struggle of the creator in any art form. For us all, as for himself, the artist is repeatedly winning brilliant battles in a war to which, however, there is no final outcome. A final outcome would be finding what is not true, namely, that what the world offers is identical with what the individual creates.

I will end with an illustration which broadens the subject a little. A man dreamed he was driving a car up the curve of a hill when he saw a larger car coming at him down the curve of the hill, at speed. It was a flash dream. He swerved to the left, but he knew that if he had not wakened there would have been a terrific crash. It was a satisfactory dream, and he woke to the memory of banging his head on a pillar when walking with his mother as a little boy. This was an easy memory, an incident, never forgotten. Suddenly it occurred to him that the memory was a false one. He had been walking with his mother and it was *another* boy walking with his mother who had absent-mindedly crashed into the post and had badly hurt his head, producing a copious flow of blood.

The fact was that, because of analysis in respect of reality-contact, he had become able to understand that he envied the boy who crashed into the post. I mean, this crash seemed ever so real to him at the time it occurred, contrasting with his own growing and distressing inhibition and lack of reality-sense in his contact with his mother, secondary to the repression of his Oedipus wishes.

From this step forward in his analysis he got a new feeling about children's love of the awful phenomena of gangster films, and of crashing Spitfires and bombers, and the like[1]. I, too, realized more clearly than previously that in trying to unravel all the complex psychology of childhood behaviour it would be unwise to neglect the threat of feelings of unreality and loss of contact. I need hardly add to an audience of psychiatrists that the same applies to the study of adults.

It is those who feel that external reality lacks meaning whenever routine holds sway who need the refreshment of music or painting absolutely. Someone I know who is recovering from a long phase of loss of contact found the colour in van Gogh's pictures *painfully* real. The colour came at her as the car did in the man's dream. The colour was too much for her in a physical sense, and she had to go away and come back another day to complete the visit to the picture gallery.

[1] Today I would add horror comics (1957).

In the management of children comparable happenings can be observed. Unreality feelings show as a craving for the new. This turns up in early feeding management, in the problem of the baby who is put on one food after another, and who does well for a few days on each, and then loses interest. But the new can also hurt. It would be wise to keep in mind that for the infant the new, whether in taste, texture, sight, or sound, can come at the infant as the colour did to my friend, and physically hurt. An ordinary good mother is sparing with new things, and yet provides them according to the infant's ability to come to terms with them. In psychiatric practice, as I have already suggested, there could perhaps be room for the attempt to coax back a withdrawn person by the provision of an extremely simplified bit of the world, a world into which the patient could gradually come back without suffering painful impressions. In the analysis of borderline cases some such provision is made in the limited setting of the analytic session, and such provision is a prerequisite for the work based on the verbal interpretation.

SUMMARY

I have tried to focus attention on one process, that of the individual's contact with shared reality, and the development of this from the start of the infant's life. I have hoped to encourage a co-operation between the children's doctor and the psychiatrist in arriving at descriptive terms that have clinical meaning to each. I have made an attempt to do this in an examination of the normal establishment of reality-contact.

It was difficult to cast aside psychosomatic disorders, to turn a deaf ear to the common anxiety states, and a blind eye to depression, hypochondria, and persecution delusions. All these disorders affect the day-by-day work of the paediatrician. It was difficult to steer my course away from the pathological psychotic regressions and psychotic distortions which are much commoner in childhood than is generally supposed. Also it was difficult to choose the one process, and to ignore those of integration and body sense. However, as it is, I have had more to convey than can easily be listened to at one sitting, and I console myself that it is better to convey the idea that a thing is complex, if it is so, than to give a false impression of simplicity.

These things have been argued about by philosophers and psychologists, and psychopathologists of all schools have made their own attempts to state what they feel they see. Here is my statement, forged out of clinical work and a psycho-analytic training.

Chapter XIV

Birth Memories, Birth Trauma, and Anxiety[1]
[1949]

IN THIS PAPER I wish to present certain clinical examples illustrating fantasies and possible memories of the birth experience.

In psycho-analytic theory there has been some confusion since Freud put forward the valuable idea that the symptomatology of anxiety may be related to birth trauma. It is not clear whether birth memories are individual or racial, whether birth can be normal or whether trauma is an inherent part of birth or a variable and chance accompaniment. Also, what exactly is the nature of the trauma in terms of ego psychology? There is therefore much left over for re-search, and perhaps the following collection of ideas may be useful in stimulating thought.

It is difficult to know how to quote Freud usefully at this point. To do Freud justice one would have to write a separate paper tracing the changes in his views on the relationship between anxiety and birth trauma. This would be an excellent exercise and it has already been done, notably by Greenacre.[2] In any case it is not necessary for me to try to do justice to Freud's views here. On re-reading many of his references to the subject since writing the main part of my paper, I think I can find everything that I have suggested somewhere in his writings. Perhaps I could best quote the sentence where he says: 'Now it would be very satisfactory if anxiety, as a symbol of separation, were to be repeated on every subsequent occasion on which a separation took place, but unfortunately we are prevented from making use of this correlation by the fact that birth is not experienced subjectively as a separation from the mother, since the foetus, being a completely narcissistic creature, is totally unaware of

---

[1] Paper read before the British Psycho-Analytical Society, 18th May, 1949.

[2] This part has had to be re-written (1954) as I discovered Greenacre's work after writing and reading this contribution, although much of her work had been published and was available before the date of my contribution.

174

her existence as an object.' Again, comparing birth with weaning, he says, 'the traumatic situation of missing the mother differs in one important respect from the traumatic situation of birth. At birth no object existed and so no object could be missed. Anxiety was the only reaction that occurred, (Freud, 1926).

What interests me is precisely this subject of the foetus and the child who is being born, the 'completely narcissistic creature'; I want to know what is actually happening there. I like to think that Freud was feeling round this subject without coming to a final conclusion because of the fact that he lacked certain data which were essential to the understanding of the subject. In considering Freud's view therefore we have constantly to try to remember what he, a scientific worker in the field, would do if he were alive now and active in the psycho-analytic world, taking into consideration advances in our new understanding of infants.

The main thing really is that Freud believed in the significance of birth trauma as a scientific worker, and not only as an intuitive thinker. It is rare to find doctors who believe that the experience of birth is important to the baby, that it could have any significance in the emotional development of the individual, and that memory traces of the experience could persist and give rise to trouble even in the adult. Those who knew Freud, and I am not one of them, may have information as to his latter-day belief in the importance of the birth trauma. In *Group Psychology* Freud says: 'Thus by being born we have made the step from an absolutely self-sufficient narcissism to the perception of a changed outer world and to the beginnings of the discovery of objects'. He goes on to say '. . . and with this is associated the fact that we cannot endure the new state of things for long and that we periodically revert from it in our sleep to our former condition of absence of stimulation and avoidance of objects'. Here however he is introducing a new subject and I do not take for granted that sleep has a simple relation to intra-uterine existence. This subject needs separate discussion.

I had thought that Freud believed that in the history of every individual there were memory traces of the birth experience which determined the pattern anxiety would take throughout the life of the individual. Greenacre appears to think, however, that Freud linked anxiety with birth by a sort of collective unconscious theory, with birth as an archetypal experience. (I am using Jungian expressions here on purpose because they seem to apply.) But whatever Freud wrote or did not write he held the view that the personal experience of birth is also important to the individual if the following story is true: when he heard of an infant that was born by Caesarian section he remarked that it would be interesting to remember this fact, which might eventually be found to affect the pattern of anxiety in that individual.

Much of what I wish to contribute is already expressed by Greenacre (1945). She writes:

'In summary, it seems that the general effect of birth is, by its enormous sensory stimulation, to organize and convert the fetal narcissism, producing or promoting a propulsive narcissistic drive over and above the type of more relaxed fetal maturation process that has been existent in utero. There is ordinarily a patterning of the aggressive-libidinization of certain body parts according to the areas of special stimulation. Specifically, birth stimulates the cerebrum to a degree promoting its development so that it may soon begin to take effective control of body affairs; it contributes to the organization of the anxiety pattern, thereby increasing the defense of the infant, and it leaves unique individual traces that are superimposed on the genetically determined anxiety and libidinal patterns of the given infant.'

The matter needs study. Greenacre's two articles (1941) need much more attention that I have been able to give them so far. In the summary of the first of these two papers she says, 'The anxiety response which is genetically determined probably manifests itself first in an irritable responsiveness of the organism at a reflex level; this is apparent in intra-uterine life in a set of separate or loosely constellated reflexes which may become organized at birth into the anxiety reaction', and so on. It may be seen from this that she is asking for a reconstruction of the problem of the relation of anxiety to birth trauma in the light of the work that is being done on infant behaviour.

In the second article, which is more clinical, and more related to psycho-analytic work, Greenacre draws attention to the value to be got from correlating early infant histories with material elicited in the course of subsequent therapy. In her summary she says: 'It is clear that the consideration of these cases takes us back to the need for more observation with infants, work which appears to me the source of the richest material for psycho-analysis.' I expect she would agree, however, that there is no more important method of studying the birth trauma than the one which we have especially at our disposal, namely the psycho-analysis of adults and children. 'The other methods are also important and they include particularly the studies based on observations of infants at birth, before and immediately after birth, and also the type of investigation which can only be carried out by the neurological specialist.'

I would like to draw attention to Dr Grantly Dick Read's work (1942). He sees the birth process from the midwifery point of view, and much of his success in practice is due to the fact that he adds to his knowledge of the physical side of birth processes a belief in the importance of giving the mother confidence. He aims at preventing or overcoming the fear in the mother which he finds so seriously disturbing to her function at the time of parturition. He is sympathetic to psycho-analysis and psycho-analytic theory. Dr Read is quite willing to believe that the psychology of an individual is something which can be studied pre-natally and at the time of birth, and that the experiences at this early date are significant. In this I feel that he is ahead of many obstetricians and paediatricians.

The personal view that I am putting forward in this paper is based on analytic work.[1] My ideas fall into three groups.

The first point I want to make is that there are various types of material appearing in an analysis. When I add to them the birth trauma type of material I am not claiming that treatments can be done on birth material alone. The analyst must be prepared to expect whatever type of material turns up, *including birth material.*

The analyst must indeed expect environmental factors of all kinds. For instance, one needs to recognize and assess the type of environment that belongs to the intra-uterine experience, also the type of environment that belongs to the birth experience; likewise the mother's capacity for devotion in respect of the newborn infant, the capacity of the parental team for taking joint responsibility as the infant develops into a little child; and also the capacity of the social setting for allowing maternal devotion and parental co-operation to play their parts, and for continuing these functions and extending them, eventually enabling the individual to play his or her part in the creation and maintenance of the social setting.

In other words, no consideration of the birth trauma can have value unless a sense of proportion can be maintained. Nevertheless in a discussion of any one subject one should not be afraid *temporarily* to seem to over-estimate the importance of the subject under discussion.[2]

The second point that I want to make is that in common with other analysts I do find in my analytic and other work that there is evidence that the personal birth experience is significant, and is held as memory material. It is generally held that in psychotic states those very things are remembered that are unavailable to consciousness in more normal states. You will notice that in stating my second point I have used the word 'birth experience' instead of 'birth trauma' and I will return to this point, but first I wish to describe an episode in the analysis of an apparently defective boy whose defect was probably secondary to early psychosis, and not due to brain limitation.

This boy, who was then five, spent a month or two of his analysis testing out my ability to accept his approaches without demanding anything, and actively to adapt to his needs in a way that his mother could not do. He re-

[1] It will be observed that I am now leaving the work of other writers and am making an attempt to state my own position in my own words. I am only too happy when after making my own statement, I find that what I have said has been said previously by others. Often it has been said better, but not better for me.

[2] For instance, when I write a paper for this Society on any subject I nearly always find myself dreaming dreams which belong to that subject.

peatedly came towards me and went away again, testing out my ability to accept him. Eventually he came to sit on my lap. No words were spoken at all for the whole of this period. The further development of his relation to me took the following unexpected form. He would get inside my coat and turn upside down and slide down to the ground between my legs; this he repeated over and over again.

When he had thoroughly established this procedure which seemed to follow his decision that I could be used as the mother that he needed, he would get up from the floor and demand honey. I procured honey (and later cod-liver-oil and malt, which was easier to get during the war) and he would often scoop out as much as half a pound and eat it immediately with great relish. This was the beginning of a tremendous phase of oral activity with excessive salivation. He would make a pool on the doorstep with his saliva as he waited for me to open the door. Previously to this his oral desires only turned up as hallucinated objects (which he called Käfers) which appeared on the walls and of which he was very frightened. The interpretation which had made him able to lose these hallucinated insects was this: that they were his own *mouth*. In the next phase he became a Käfer himself and then he started on the phase of the analysis which I have described, in which he was testing me out as a mother who could actively adapt.

After this experience I was prepared to believe that memory traces of birth can persist. Of course the same thing in play has turned up in many analyses and on still more occasions in the play of normal children and in one's own play as a child.

The following case also presents certain features which help in the approach to the study of birth experience:

Miss H. is a nurse (50 years old). She had treatment from me when she was about 25, at a time when I was house physician at St Bartholomew's Hospital and had only read a book or two on psycho-analysis. This patient had a very severe neurosis, including constipation of a degree that I have never met before or since. She had been a shorthand-typist but after getting help from me she became a hospital nurse. Later on she specialized in the care of psychotic children. She has an unusual intuitive understanding of the needs of children who are in a state of regression.

In this patient's treatment, which was cathartic in quality, she would lie and sleep, and then suddenly wake in a nightmare. I would help her to wake by repeating over and over again the words that she had shouted out in the acute anxiety attack. By this means when she wakened I was able to keep her in touch with the anxiety situation and to get her to remember all sorts of traumatic incidents from her very eventful early childhood.

I never knew what to make of her reconstruction of her birth. Birth memories appeared with fantastic embellishments clearly derived from all stages of development and from the sophistication of the adolescent, if not of the adult. Nevertheless the effect seemed to me to be real in its terrific intensity. *While disbelieving the details described as memories I found myself prepared to believe in the accompanying affect.*

Recently this patient has been looking after a little girl of seven, a psychotic case (autistic) undergoing analysis. Miss H. suddenly was taken ill and without being able to let anybody know she simply did not turn up at her job, which was to take the child for treatment and to look after her during the day. I was able to visit her and found that she was just beginning to recover from an illness of a kind that was not new to her, but which had previously never been so acute. She had suddenly had to go to bed with what she called a 'blackout'. She had lain absolutely rigid and curled right up tight on her side, unable to do anything at all, and as near unconscious as may be. A doctor was called in who said he could find nothing wrong with her body. While she was in this condition she was unable to do anything about food at all. Gradually she became conscious, and allowed herself to be moved to a friendly place, and in the course of a week or ten days she was able to get about again. This nurse frequently keeps me in touch with the details of whatever case she is nursing, but previous to this occasion she had never once, since the time twenty years ago when I was treating her, asked me about herself. On this occasion, however, before going back to her job, she came to me and sat down and said, 'What about this blackout? What had it to do with?' I had no idea, and I told her so. Then she went on talking, and I gradually realized that although she was not expecting to be having a therapeutic session, nevertheless she was giving me from her unconscious the material which would enable me to explain her blackout.

I found that she had been living with this little girl of seven and had been identified extremely closely with the child as she always is with psychotic children in her charge. She told me that in order to understand the child's condition, she had been imitating her more and more, putting a hand here, and walking in this way, and that, and doing everything she saw the child do 'in order to get the feeling of the child's state of mind and body'. Now it so happened that this little girl was going through an acute anxiety state and had developed a very great fear of travelling in the Underground. Miss H. had been trying to take her in the Underground to distract her attention and to show her by experience that the Underground was not as bad as expected. A great deal of material of this kind suddenly showed me that I must say to Miss H. that she herself was reliving the birth experience along with the little girl. Here was no hysterical reconstruction. She had been actually having to re-experience the physical thing, which in her case had included a feeling of asphyxiation. Interpretation along these lines produced a most dramatic effect. Miss H. felt better, felt she understood what was going on, and went back confidently to her job. The doctor of the case said to me, 'Somehow or other Miss H. looks much better since her illness'. After this she continued to do good work with this little girl, and with a more objective understanding of the anxiety that is actually important in the little girl's case.

Hysterical patients make us feel that they are acting, but we know better than they can know that true affect is displayed and hidden in the hysterical manifestations.

In many child analyses birth play is important. In such play the material might have been derived from what has been found out by the patient about birth, through stories and direct information and observation. The feeling one gets is, however, that the child's body knows about being born.

I return to the fact that I used the words 'birth experience' instead of 'birth trauma'. This leads to the third point that I wish to make. I feel that Freud's remarks become very much more understandable when he separates birth experience from birth trauma. Greenacre emphasizes this. Possibly birth experience can be so smooth as to have relatively little significance. This is my own view at present. Contrariwise, birth experience that is abnormal over and above a certain limit becomes birth trauma, and is then immensely significant.

When there has been a normal birth experience, birth material is not likely to come into the analysis in a way that draws attention to itself. It will be there, but if the analyst does not easily think in birth terms the patient is not likely to force the issue in these terms. There will be more urgent and apposite settings for the anxiety which both patient and analyst are trying to reach.

When, however, birth experience has been traumatic it has set a pattern. This pattern appears in various details which will need to be interpreted and dealt with each in its own right, at the appropriate time.

I wish to emphasize, however, that interpretation in terms of birth trauma will not suddenly produce total and permanent relief. It is rather this, that since the birth trauma is real it is a pity to be blind to it, and in certain cases and at certain points the analysis absolutely needs acceptance of birth material in among all the other material.

It would be useful to give three categories of birth experience. The first is a normal, that is to say healthy, birth experience which is a valuable positive experience of limited significance; it provides a pattern of a natural way of life. This sense of a way of life can be strengthened by various kinds of subsequent normal experiences, and so the birth experience becomes one of a series of factors favourable to the development of confidence, sense of sequence, stability, and security, etc.

In the second category comes the common rather traumatic birth experience which gets mixed in with various subsequent traumatic environmental factors, strengthening them and being strengthened by them.

I refer at a later stage to the extreme of traumatic birth experience, which provides a third category or grade.

It will be seen that it is difficult for me to think that what happens in anxiety is determined by birth trauma, because that would mean that the individual who is born naturally has no anxiety or has no way to *show* that he is anxious. This would be absurd.

I would like to bring in at this point a discussion of the word 'anxious'. I cannot think of a baby as being anxious at birth, because there is no repression or repressed unconscious at this early date. If anxiety means something simple like fear or reactive irritability, all is well. It seems to me that the word 'anxious' is applicable when an individual is in the grips of physical experience (be it excitement, anger, fear, or anything else) which he can neither avoid nor understand; that is to say, he is unaware of the greater proportion of the reason for what is happening. By the word unaware I am referring to the repressed unconscious. Should he become rather more conscious of what is afoot, he will no longer be anxious, but instead he will be excited, afraid, angry, etc.

Freud in *Beyond the Pleasure Principle* states: '*Angst* denotes a certain condition as of expectation of danger and preparation for it, even though it be an unknown one.' But he does not seem here to express what I am trying to say, that the individual has to have reached a certain degree of maturity, with capacity for repression, before the word anxiety can be usefully applied. This is an example of the considerations which make me want to ask that the theory of a relationship between anxiety and birth trauma should be held in abeyance while work is being done on the psychology of the infant before, during, and after birth.

My present thesis is therefore a composite one, namely that the normal birth experiences are good, and can promote ego strength and stability.

I now wish to draw attention to the way in which birth trauma comes into the analytic situation, making it especially clear that talking with the patient about the birth trauma is something that is extremely likely to be sidetracking the main issue. I would doubt the value of an interpretation along birth trauma lines in the case of a patient who is not deeply regressed at the time in the analytic situation, and who is not clinically ill in the times between analytic sessions.

One of the difficulties of our psycho-analytic technique is to know at any one moment how old a patient is in the transference relationship. In some analyses the patient is most of the time his own age, and one can reach all that one needs of the childhood states by means of his memories and fantasies expressed in an adult way. In such analyses I think there will be no useful interpretation of birth trauma; or birth material will appear in dreams, which can be interpreted at all levels. An analysis, however, may be allowed to go deeper if necessary, and the patient does not have to be very ill to be at times an infant during an analytic session. At such a time there is a great deal that one has to understand without asking for an immediate description of what is happening in words.

I am referring to something which is more infantile than the behaviour of a child playing with toys. According to the predilections of the analyst and according to the diagnosis of the patient there will be variations in the wisdom or unwisdom of working with the patient on these terms. What I am trying to make clear is that if birth experiences are coming into the analytic situation there will certainly be a great deal of other evidence that the patient is in an extremely infantile state.

BIRTH EXPERIENCE

It will be understood, Freud having pointed it out, that birth experience has nothing to do with any sort of an awareness of a separation from the mother's body. We can postulate a certain state of mind of the unborn. I think we can say that things are going well if the personal development of the infant ego has been as undisturbed in its emotional as in its physical aspect. There is certainly before birth the beginning of an emotional development, and it is likely that there is before birth a capacity for false and unhealthy forward movement in emotional development; in health environmental disturbances of a certain degree are valuable stimuli, but beyond a certain degree these disturbances are unhelpful in that they bring about a *reaction*. At this very early stage of development there is not sufficient ego strength for there to be a reaction without loss of identity.

I am indebted to a patient for a way of putting this which came from an extremely deep-rooted appreciation of the position of the infant at an early stage. This patient had a depressed mother whose rigidity was marked and who continued after the child was born to hold the child always tightly for fear of dropping her. It is for this reason that the description is in terms of pressure. Together we worked out the following statement which eventually proved to be vitally important in that analysis. The understanding of this reached right down to the bottom of her difficulties and described accurately enough the extent of the regression which she had to make before starting to come forward again in her emotional development. This patient said: 'At the beginning the individual is like a bubble. If the pressure from outside actively adapts to the pressure within, then the bubble is the significant thing, that is to say the infant's self. If, however, the environmental pressure is greater or less than the pressure within the bubble, then it is not the bubble that is important but the environment. The bubble adapts to the outside pressure.' Along with the understanding of this the patient felt that for the first time, in the analysis, she was being held by a relaxed mother, that is to say, a mother alive, awake, and ready to make active adaptation through the quality of being devoted to her infant.

Before birth, and especially if there is delay, there can quite easily be repeated experiences for an infant in which, for the time being, the stress is on environment rather than on self, and it is likely that the unborn infant becomes more and more caught up in this sort of intercourse with the environment as the time for birth arrives. Thus, in the natural process *the birth experience is an exaggerated sample of something already known to the infant.* For the time being, during birth, the infant is a reactor and the important thing is the environment; and then after birth there is a return to a state of affairs in which the important thing is the infant, whatever that means. In health the infant is prepared before birth for some environmental impingement, and already has had the experience of a natural return from reacting to a state of not having to react, which is the only state in which the self can begin to be.

This is the simplest possible statement that I can make about the normal birth process. It is a temporary phase of reaction and therefore of loss of identity, a major example, for which the infant has already been prepared, of interference with the personal 'going along', not so powerful or so prolonged as to snap the thread of the infant's continuous personal process.

It will be noted that I do not at present hold that it is essentially traumatic to start breathing. The normal birth is non-traumatic by virtue of its nonsignificance. At the birth age an infant is not ready for prolonged environmental impingement.

It is precisely by reason of its being significant to the infant that experience of the birth trauma is psychologically traumatic. The individual's personal 'going along' is interrupted by reactions to prolonged impingements. When birth trauma is significant every detail of impingement and reaction is, as it were, etched on the patient's memory in the way to which we become accustomed when patients relive traumatic experiences of later life (the sort of experiences that are sometimes successfully recovered by abreaction or by hypnosis). In collecting together examples of impingement I will not attempt to preserve any order because I have not yet decided how to do this; in the study of an analytic patient, however, one meets an order of detail which cannot fail to impress.

It may be pointed out that the most important thing is the trauma represented by the need to react. Reacting at this stage of human development means a temporary loss of identity. This gives an extreme sense of insecurity, and lays the basis for an expectation of further examples of loss of continuity of self, and even a congenital (but not inherited) hopelessness in respect of the attainment of a personal life.

The repeated phases of unconsciousness (here the word is used in the physical sense) either due to brain changes or to the anaesthetic administered to the mother, are unlikely to prove significant. When the patient gives a clear picture of having become unconscious once or several times in this situation it is likely that what is being re-enacted is the snapping of the thread of continuity of the self due to the repeated phases of prolonged reaction to environmental impingements, such as pressure. Unconsciousness (as after concussion) is not remembered.

Among features typical of the true birth memory is the feeling of being in the grips of something external, so that one is helpless. You will note that I am not saying that the baby feels that the mother is gripping. This would not be talking in terms of a baby at this stage. The point is that the external impingements require the baby to adapt to them, whereas at the birth age the baby requires an active adaptation from the environment. The infant can stand having to react to impingement over a limited period of time. There is a very clear relation here between what the baby experiences and what the mother experiences in being confined, as it is called. There comes a state in the labour in which, in health, a mother has to be able to resign herself to a process almost exactly comparable to the infant's experience at the same time.[1]

Belonging to this feeling of helplessness is the intolerable nature of experiencing something without any knowledge whatever of when it will end. A prisoner-of-war may say that the worst part of the experience is that there is no knowing when the imprisonment will end; this makes three years worse at the time than a twenty years' sentence. It is for this reason fundamentally that form in music is so important. Through form, the end is in sight from the beginning. One could say that many babies could be helped if one could only convey to them during prolonged birth that the birth process would last only a certain limited length of time. However, the baby is unable to understand our language; moreover there is no precedent for the baby to use, no yardstick for measurement. The birth-age baby has a rudimentary knowledge of impingements which produce reaction, so that the ordinary birth process can be accepted by the infant as a further example of what has already happened; but a difficult birth goes far beyond any prenatal experience of impingement that produces reaction.

In the case of one patient in whose analysis there was a particularly good opportunity to watch the birth process, since it was relived repeatedly, I

[1] I now call this special state of sensitivity in the mother 'Primary maternal preoccupation', 1957. (See Chapter XXIV.)

became able to detect each ego nucleus as it appeared in reaction appropriate to the type of impingement. To mention a few: urinary-tract nucleus, flatus nucleus, anal nucleus, faecal nucleus, skin nucleus, saliva nucleus, forehead nucleus, breathing nucleus, etc. Perhaps these considerations throw light on the difficulty we have in describing the weak ego of the immature individual knowing as we do how tremendously strong each ego nucleus is. What is weak is the integration of a total ego organization.

In the present context there is a great deal that can be said about what happens when, with extremely immature ego organization, an infant has to cope with an environment which insists on being important. There can be a false integration which involves some kind of abstract thinking which is unnatural. Here again there are two alternatives; in the one case there is a precocious intellectual development; in the other case there is a failure of intellectual development. Anything in between these two extremes is of no use. This intellectual development is a nuisance because it is derived from too early a stage in the history of the individual, so that it is pathologically unrelated to the body with its functions, and to the feelings and instincts and sensations of the total ego.[1]

Here it may be observed that the infant that is disturbed by being forced to react is disturbed out of a state of 'being'. This state of 'being' can obtain only under certain conditions. When reacting, an infant is not 'being'. The environment that impinges cannot yet be felt by the infant to be a projection of personal aggression, since the stage has not yet been reached at which this means anything. In my opinion a severe birth trauma (psychological) can cause a condition which I will call congenital, but not inherited, paranoia. Observation of many infants in my clinic gives me the impression that a severe paranoid basis can be present immediately after birth. I cannot better illustrate my meaning than by giving you a dream which a patient (woman, age 28, diagnosis: schizophrenia with paranoid features) dreamed in reaction to reading Rank's *Trauma of Birth*.

She dreamed that she was under a pile of gravel. Her whole body at the surface was extremely sensitive to a degree which it is hardly possible to imagine. Her skin was burned, which seemed to her to be her way of saying that it was extremely sensitive and vulnerable. She was burned all over. She knew that if anyone came and did anything at all to her, the pain would be just impossible to bear, both physical and mental pain. She knew of the danger that people would come and take the gravel off and do things to her in order to cure her, and the situation was intolerable. She emphasized that with this were intolerable feelings comparable to those which belonged to her suicide attempt. 'You just can't bear anything any longer. It's the awfulness of having a body at all, and the mind that's just had too much. It was the

[1] Idea developed further in 'Mind and its Relation to the Psyche-Soma', Chapter XIX.

185

entirety of it, the completeness of the job that made it so impossible. If only people would leave me alone. If only people wouldn't keep getting at me.' However, what happened in the dream was that someone came and poured oil over the gravel with her inside it. The oil came through and came on to her skin, and covered her. Then she was left without any interference whatever for three weeks, at the end of which time the gravel could be removed without her suffering pain, and when it was taken away her skin had almost entirely healed. There was, however, a little sore patch between her breasts, a triangular area which the oil had not reached, from which there came something like a little penis or a cord. This had to be attended to, and of course it was slightly painful but quite bearable. This simply didn't matter, someone just pulled it off.

Here is much less of the sophisticated overlay than there was in the dreams of the patient Miss H. (page 178), since the patient was not an hysteric, but was psychotic. Hence the true affect is evident. The person who understood, and who poured oil over the patient was I, the analyst, and the dream indicated a degree of confidence gained through my handling of her case. However, the dream itself is a reaction to an impingement (the reading of Rank's book) and the analysis suffered a temporary set-back.

The Head. In the ordinary birth the head of the infant is the forward point and does the work of dilating the maternal soft parts. There are several ways in which this is remembered. There may be retained as important a mode of progression which can be described by the word 'reptation'. This word appears in a book by Casteret called *My Caves.* The author is describing the way he gets through holes in deep cave exploration. The point about reptation is that the arms are not of any use, nor the hands. In fact the reason why there is any forward movement is not clearly known to the author. I suppose that in the memory trace of a normal birth there would be no sense of helplessness. The infant would feel that the swimming movements of which we know a foetus is capable, and the movements that I have referred to under the word reptation, produce the forward movement. The actual birth can easily be felt by the infant, in the normal case, to be a successful outcome of personal effort owing to the more or less accurate timing. I do not believe that the facts justify the theory that in the birth process itself there is *essentially* a condition in which the infant feels helpless. Very frequently, however, delay produces this very thing, helplessness, or sense of infinite delay.

There can very easily be delay at a time when there is constriction round the head, and it is my definite view that the type of headache which is clearly described as a band round the head is sometimes a direct derivative of birth sensations remembered in somatic form. In analytic work this band round the head can be found to be related to the experience of being caught up in an environmental impingement that has no predictable end. It is possible to conceive that there are all sorts of sensations not quite so clearly delineated, such as noises, blood rushing to the head, a feeling of congestion at the top, and the feeling 'that something gives way, as if blood is escaping'. These and other common head-symptoms in the psychosomatic field are related to the psychotic delusions in which there is a discharge through the top of the head, and I have known helmets and hoods to be important as providing reassurance that the self will not escape through the top of the head. Scalping has primary significance, and is not merely a castration displacement. Associated with this are all the variations on the theme of horns and unicorns which may derive an important root from the extension forward of the personality in this birth process whereby the body propels itself.

There is a basis here for a fantasy of re-entry into the mother head-first. This was brought out clearly in one analytic experience. The patient, the second of twins, had been unexpected and had been left for a long time after birth unattended. In the analysis there was a time when the patient's dilemma was whether to retain the relationship that was known or to become a separate entity with no external object presenting itself. The former alternative provided a false object relationship and was represented in the analysis at that time by a compulsion to have the hand over the forehead, the hand representing the mother's body. This easily got woven into a kind of false homosexuality in which the patient went into the woman head first. In this case the arms were notably useless. In the first dream she brought to me she was attempting to have intercourse without use of arms and she had developed rheumatoid arthritis confined at first to the elbows and wrists so that arms for which she had no fundamental use had virtually become eliminated. Needless to say, oral erotism was severely inhibited as part of the same complex, and she had already had all her teeth removed.

The identification of the whole body with the male genital often appears in psycho-analytic work. It should not be forgotten that there can be a basis for this in the birth experience in which the body acts as a whole, and without the arms and without oral or any other erotism (except that of the muscles employed in swimming or reptation movements). The body simply proceeds through a narrowed environment.

The Chest. The next in importance to the experiences of the head are those of the chest. This part of my description can be divided into three parts: first there is the memory of actual constricting bands at various levels around the chest. These constrictions can be desired, and we meet this especially in certain perversions, but also in the ordinary details of clothing. One could say that the individual with the strong memory trace of such a thing as a constriction round the chest would rather feel a constriction which is known and under control than continue to suffer from a delusion of a constriction based on memory traces of birth.

The second part of this description is in terms of function. I have found that the memory trace of restriction of chest expansion during traumatic birth process can be very strong, and an important thing about this is the contrast between reactive chest activity and the chest activity of true anger. During the birth process, in reaction to the construction of the maternal tissues, the infant has to make what would be (if there were any air available) an *inspiratory* movement. After birth, if all goes well, the cry establishes the expression of liveliness by *expiration*. This is an example in terms of physical function of the difference between reacting and simply going on 'being'. When there is delay and exceptional difficulty the changeover to normal crying is not definite enough and the individual is always left with some confusion about anger and its expression. Reactive anger detracts from ego establishment. Yet in the form of the cry anger can be ego-syntonic from very early, an expulsive function with clear aim, to live one's own way and not reactively.

The third thing about the chest and birth is the simple feeling of a lack of something, a lack which could be relieved if breathing could be freed. In a case with history of placenta praevia with very much delayed birth and marked asphyxiation, the patient when only six years old complained of a constant feeling of 'lack of oxygen'. She had known before then that the air seemed to lack something, and when she heard of oxygen she used the idea of it immediately. This feeling persisted as a very important symptom. The actual experience of breathing difficulty in the birth process must not be forgotten, in my opinion, when one is tracing out the various roots of breathing disturbances and the perversions that include breathing obstruction. The desire to be suffocated can be extremely strong and turns up as a masturbation fantasy, in the acting out of which many who had no suicidal intention have died. It is present in inverted suicide which is commonly called murder. By a reversal of roles, active suffocating can be a perverted kindness, the active person feeling that the passive one must be longing to be suffocated. There is something of all this, as of everything else, in the healthy passionate sexual relationship.

Study of the need to be able to do without breathing, a need that can be found in the mystical practices of various religions of the East, cannot be complete unless the individual's body-memory of his birth can be taken into consideration. There are of course other equally important things entering into the mystic's denial of the necessity to breathe, particularly his attempt to deny the difference between internal reality and external reality.

Conclusions

In order to preserve the personal way of life at the very beginning the individual needs a minimum of environmental impingements producing reaction. All individuals are really trying to find a new birth in which the line of their own life will not be disturbed by a quantity of reacting greater than that which can be experienced without a loss of the sense of continuity of personal existence. The mental health of the individual is laid down by the mother who, because she is devoted to her infant, is able to make active adaptation. This presupposes a basic state of relaxation in the mother, and also an understanding of the individual infant's way of life, which again arises out of her capacity for identification with her infant. This relationship between the mother and the infant starts before the infant is born and is continued in some cases through the birth process and after. As I see it, the trauma of birth is the break in the continuity of the infant's going on being, and when this break is significant the details of the way in which the impingements are sensed, and also of the infant's reaction to them, become in turn significant factors adverse to ego development. In the majority of cases the birth trauma is therefore mildly important and determines a good deal of the general urge towards rebirth. In some cases this adverse factor is so great that the individual has no chance (apart from rebirth in the course of analysis) of making a natural progress in emotional development, even if subsequent external factors are extremely good.

In consideration of the theoretical point of the origin of anxiety it would be a false step to link such a universal phenomenon as anxiety with a special case of birth, birth that is traumatic. It would be logical, however, to attempt to relate anxiety with the *normal* birth experience, but the suggestion is made in this paper that not enough is known yet about the normal birth experiences from the infant's point of view for us to be able to say that there is an intimate relationship between anxiety and normal untraumatic birth. Traumatic birth experience seems to me to determine not so much the pattern of subsequent anxiety as to determine the pattern of subsequent persecution.

RECAPITULATION

The study of birth trauma is an important study in its own right.

The clues to the understanding of infant psychology, including birth trauma, must come through psycho-analytic experience where regression is a feature. This takes priority over intuitive understanding and even over the objective study of infants and the infant-mother relationship in its early stages.

When birth material turns up in an analysis in a significant way the patient is certainly showing other signs of being in an extremely infantile state. A child may be playing games that contain birth symbolism, and in the same way an adult frequently reports fantasy related consciously or unconsciously to birth. This is *not* the same as the acting out of memory traces derived from birth experience, that which provides the material for study of birth trauma. It is psychotic patients who tend to relive such early infantile phenomena, bypassing fantasy which employs symbols.

I have postulated a *normal birth experience* which is non-traumatic. I have not been able to prove this. Nevertheless in order to clarify my ideas I have assumed the existence of a normal birth experience and have invented two grades of traumatic birth, the one being common, and largely annulled as to its effects by subsequent good management, and the other being definitely traumatic, difficult to counteract even by most careful nursing, and leaving its permanent mark on the individual.

If these assumptions should be found to be justified, there would seem to follow certain theoretical considerations.

Since anxiety is a universal phenomenon it cannot be directly correlated with a special case of birth, namely a traumatic birth.

Perhaps the clue to the well-known fact that there is a relation clinically between anxiety manifestations and the details of birth trauma may be that birth trauma determines the pattern of subsequent persecutions; in this way birth trauma determines *by indirect method* the way in which anxiety manifests itself in certain cases.

A by-product of this theory is that it provides a way of looking at the fairly common congenital, though not inherited, paranoia. The point that I am making is contained in the title of Greenacre's two articles as well as in her text. She writes of a predisposition to anxiety. She does not, however, exactly state that the traumatic birth experience determines the *pattern of expected persecution*. The suggestion is that a traumatic birth experience can determine the existence as well as the pattern of a paranoid disposition. In other words, if one accepts Melanie Klein's theory of paranoid anxiety, in which relief in analysis only comes from a full acceptance on the part of the patient of oral sadism and ambivalence towards the good object, one has to consider what one thinks about the fairly common cases in which the paranoid history dates from birth. My suggestion, which is based on psychoanalytic work, is that in certain cases in which the history goes back to birth, there is so strong a predisposition to ideas of persecution (as well as a set pattern for persecution) that probably the paranoia in such a case is not consequent on oral sadism. In other words, in my opinion there are certain cases of latent paranoia in which the analysis of the paranoia along the lines of recovering the full extent of the oral sadism does not bring about the complete resolution because there is needed in addition a reliving of the traumatic birth experience in the analytic setting. An environmental factor needs to be displaced.

May I be clearly understood? No paranoid case can be analysed by enabling the patient simply to relive the birth trauma. I am only suggesting that in a percentage of paranoid cases there is this additional fact that birth was traumatic, and placed a pattern on the infant of expected interference with basic 'being'. Probably with more experience one could sort these cases out from other paranoid cases according to their clinical picture as well as by very careful history-taking.

In another way I find a link between birth trauma and the psychosomatic disorders, notably certain headaches, and breathing disturbances of various kinds. In this case one could say that the birth trauma can influence the pattern of the hypochondria.

A positive statement can now be made. Freud recognizes a continuity between intra-uterine and extra-uterine life. I think we do not know how much Freud was able to support this intuitive flash from his analytic work. In the very close and detailed observation of one case I have been able to satisfy myself that *the patient was able to bring to the analytic hour, under certain very specialized conditions, a regression of part of the self to an intra-uterine state.* In such a case the to and fro from extra-uterine to intra-uterine existence and back involves experiences that belong to that individual's birth, and this has to be distinguished from the usually more important and more common movement *in fantasy* in and out of the mother's body and in and out of the patient's inner world.

One can certainly assume that from conception onwards the body and the psyche develop together, at first fused and gradually becoming distinguishable the one from the other. Certainly before birth it can be said of the psyche (apart from the soma) that there is a personal going-along, a continuity of experiencing. This continuity, which could be called the beginnings of the self, is periodically interrupted by phases of reaction to impingement. The self begins to include memories of limited phases in which reaction to impingement disturbs the continuity. By the time of birth the infant is prepared for such phases, and my suggestion is that *in the non-traumatic birth the reaction to impingement which birth entails does not exceed that for which the foetus is already prepared.*

It is generally assumed that the new experience of breathing must be traumatic. It is more likely that delay in breathing associated with prolonged birth provides the traumatic factor rather than the initiation of breathing. My psycho-analytic experience makes me think that it is not necessarily true in all cases that the initiation of breathing is significant.

It seems to me that *it is in relation to the border-line of intolerable reaction phases that the intellect begins to work as something distinct from the psyche.* It is as if the intellect collects together the impingements to which there had to be reaction, and holds them in exact detail and sequence, in this way protecting the psyche until there is a return of the continuing-to-exist state. In a rather more traumatic situation the intellect develops excessively and can even seem to become more important than the psyche, and subsequent to birth the intellect can continue to expect and even to go out to meet persecutions so as to collect them and hold them, still with the aim of preserving the psyche. The value of this defence is shown when the individual ultimately comes to analysis, for in the analytic setting we find that carefully collected primary persecutions can be remembered. Then, at long last, the patient can afford to forget them.

I am indebted to Dr Margaret Little for the observation that this may account for the way in which in paranoia scattered persecutions become integrated and organized as in the common clinical picture. The organizing is done by the intellect of the individual in defence of the psyche, and for this reason the organization of scattered persecutions itself is stoutly defended.

A corollary of this is that in some cases there is such a muddle of persecution that the intellect fails to bind and hold the sequence, and in that case instead of enhanced intellect one finds clinically an apparent mental defect, this in spite of the original normal brain tissue development.[1]

It would be possible to develop this subject by a description of the physical sensations belonging to birth trauma which appear in common psychosomatic symptomatology. The important thing, however, is that *for the individual patient the pattern is carefully set,* and also that in the reliving which can occur in the course of psycho-analytic work, a definite sequence in time is maintained. In any analysis of this kind of case one becomes familiar with the sensations and their sequence in so far as they belong to that particular patient.

An important practical point in this connection is the way in which *one thing at a time can be dealt with, whereas two or more factors spell confusion.* One of the main principles of the psycho-analytic technique is that a setting is provided in which the patient can deal with one thing at a time. There is nothing more important in our analytic work than that we try to see what the *one* thing is that the patient is bringing for interpretation or for reliving in any one particular hour. A good analyst confines his interpretations and his actions to the detail exactly presented by the patient. It is bad practice to interpret whatever one feels one understands, acting according to one's own needs, thus spoiling the patient's attempt to cope by dealing with one thing at a time. It seems that this is the more true the further back one gets. The integration of the immature psyche at the time of birth can be strengthened by one experience, even a reaction to impingement, provided it does not last too long. Two impingements, however, require two reactions, and these tear the psyche in half. The ego effort which I have described is an attempt to hold the impingements at bay by mental activity, so that the reactions to them can be allowed one at a time and without disruption of the psyche. All this can be very clearly demonstrated in psycho-analytic work provided one is able to follow

[1] See Chapter XIX.

the patient right back in emotional development as far as he needs to go, by regression to dependence, in order to get behind the period at which impingements became multiple and unmanageable.

Finally, I repeat that *there is no such thing as treatment by the analysis of birth trauma alone.* To arrive at these early stages one has to have shown to the patient one's competence in the whole range of the ordinary psycho-analytic understanding. Moreover, when the patient has been fully dependent and has started to come forward again, one will require a very sure understanding of the depressive position, and of the gradual development towards genital primacy, and of the dynamics of interpersonal relationships as well as of the urge to attain independence out of dependence.

Chapter XV

Hate in the Countertransference[1]
[1947]

IN THIS PAPER I wish to examine one aspect of the whole subject of ambivalence, namely, hate in the countertransference. I believe that the task of the analyst (call him a research analyst) who undertakes the analysis of a psychotic is seriously weighted by this phenomenon, and that analysis of psychotics becomes impossible unless the analyst's own hate is extremely well sorted-out and conscious. This is tantamount to saying that an analyst needs to be himself analysed, but it also asserts that the analysis of a psychotic is irksome as compared with that of a neurotic, and inherently so.

Apart from psycho-analytic treatment, the management of a psychotic is bound to be irksome. From time to time I have made acutely critical remarks about the modern trends in psychiatry, with the too easy electric shocks and the too drastic leucotomies. (Winnicott, 1947, 1949.) Because of these criticisms that I have expressed I would like to be foremost in recognition of the extreme difficulty inherent in the task of the psychiatrist, and of the mental nurse in particular. Insane patients must always be a heavy emotional burden on those who care for them. One can forgive those engaged in this work if they do awful things. This does not mean, however, that we have to accept whatever is done by psychiatrists and neuro-surgeons as sound according to principles of science.

Therefore although what follows is about psycho-analysis, it really has value to the psychiatrist, even to one whose work does not in any way take him into the analytic type of relationship to patients.

To help the general psychiatrist the psycho-analyst must not only study for him the primitive stages of the emotional development of the ill individual, but also must study the nature of the emotional burden which the psychiatrist

[1] Based on a paper read to the British Psycho-Analytical Society on 5th February, 1947. *Int. J. Psycho-Anal.*, Vol. XXX, 1949.

bears in doing his work. What we as analysts call the countertransference needs to be understood by the psychiatrist too. However much he loves his patients he cannot avoid hating them and fearing them, and the better he knows this the less will hate and fear be the motives determining what he does to his patients.

One could classify countertransference phenomena thus:

1. Abnormality in countertransference feelings, and set relationships and identifications that are under repression in the analyst. The comment on this is that the analyst needs more analysis, and we believe this is less of an issue among psycho-analysts than among psychotherapists in general.
2. The identifications and tendencies belonging to an analyst's personal experiences and personal development which provide the positive setting for his analytic work and make his work different in quality from that of any other analyst.
3. From these two I distinguish the truly objective countertransference, or if this is difficult, the analyst's love and hate in reaction to the actual personality and behaviour of the patient, based on objective observation.

I suggest that if an analyst is to analyse psychotics or antisocials he must be able to be so thoroughly aware of the countertransference that he can sort out and study his *objective* reactions to the patient. These will include hate. Countertransference phenomena will at times be the important things in the analysis.

I wish to suggest that the patient can only appreciate in the analyst what he himself is capable of feeling. In the matter of motive: the *obsessional* will tend to be thinking of the analyst as doing his work in a futile obsessional way. A *hypo-manic* patient who is incapable of being depressed, except in a severe mood swing, and in whose emotional development the depressive position has not been securely won, who cannot feel guilt in a deep way, or a sense of concern or responsibility, is unable to see the analyst's work as an attempt on the part of the analyst to make reparation in respect of his own (the analyst's) guilt feelings. A *neurotic* patient tends to see the analyst as ambivalent towards the patient, and to expect the analyst to show a splitting of love and hate; this patient, when in luck, gets the love, because someone else is getting the analyst's hate. Would it not follow that if a *psychotic* is in a 'coincident love-hate' state of feeling he experiences a deep conviction that the analyst is also only capable of the same crude and dangerous state of coincident love-hate relationship? Should the analyst show love, he will surely at the same moment kill the patient.

This coincidence of love and hate is something that characteristically recurs in the analysis of psychotics, giving rise to problems of management which can easily take the analyst beyond his resources. This coincidence of love and hate to which I am referring is something distinct from the aggressive component complicating the primitive love impulse, and implies that in the history of the patient there was an environmental failure at the time of the first object-finding instinctual impulses.

If the analyst is going to have crude feelings imputed to him he is best forewarned and so forearmed, for he must tolerate being placed in that position. Above all he must not deny hate that really exists in himself. Hate *that is justified* in the present setting has to be sorted out and kept in storage and available for eventual interpretation.

If we are to become able to be the analysts of psychotic patients we must have reached down to very primitive things in ourselves, and this is but another example of the fact that the answer to many obscure problems of psycho-analytic practice lies in further analysis of the analyst. (Psycho-analytic research is perhaps always to some extent an attempt on the part of an analyst to carry the work of his own analysis further than the point to which his own analyst could get him.)

A main task of the analyst of any patient is to maintain objectivity in regard to all that the patient brings, and a special case of this is the analyst's need to be able to hate the patient objectively.

Are there not many situations in our ordinary analytic work in which the analyst's hate is justified? A patient of mine, a very bad obsessional, was almost loathsome to me for some years. I felt bad about this until the analysis turned a corner and the patient became lovable, and then I realized that his unlikeableness had been an active symptom, unconsciously determined. It was indeed a wonderful day for me (much later on) when I could actually tell the patient that I and his friends had felt repelled by him, but that he had been too ill for us to let him know. This was also an important day for him, a tremendous advance in his adjustment to reality.

In the ordinary analysis the analyst has no difficulty with the management of his own hate. This hate remains latent. The main thing, of course, is that through his own analysis he has become free from vast reservoirs of unconscious hate belonging to the past and to inner conflicts. There are other reasons why hate remains unexpressed and even unfelt as such:

Analysis is my chosen job, the way I feel I will best deal with my own guilt, the way I can express myself in a constructive way.

I get paid, or I am in training to gain a place in society by psycho-analytic work.

I am discovering things.

I get immediate rewards through identification with the patient, who is making progress, and I can see still greater rewards some way ahead, after the end of the treatment.

Moreover, as an analyst I have ways of expressing hate. Hate is expressed by the existence of the end of the 'hour'.

I think this is true even when there is no difficulty whatever, and when the patient is pleased to go. In many analyses these things can be taken for granted, so that they are scarcely mentioned, and the analytic work is done through verbal interpretation of the patient's emerging unconscious transference. The analyst takes over the role of one or other of the helpful figures of the patient's childhood. He cashes in on the success of those who did the dirty work when the patient was an infant.

These things are part of the description of ordinary psycho-analytic work, which is mostly concerned with patients whose symptoms have a neurotic quality.

In the analysis of psychotics, however, quite a different type and degree of strain is taken by the analyst, and it is precisely this different strain that I am trying to describe.

Recently for a period of a few days I found I was doing bad work. I made mistakes in respect of each one of my patients. The difficulty was in myself and it was partly personal but chiefly associated with a climax that I had reached in my relation to one particular psychotic (research) patient. The difficulty cleared up when I had what is sometimes called a 'healing' dream. (Incidentally I would add that during my analysis and in the years since the end of my analysis I have had a long series of these healing dreams which, although in many cases unpleasant, have each one of them marked my arrival at a new stage in emotional development.)

On this particular occasion I was aware of the meaning of the dream as I woke or even before I woke. The dream had two phases. In the first I was in the 'gods' in a theatre and looking down on the people a long way below in the stalls. I felt severe anxiety as if I might lose a limb. This was associated with the feeling I have had at the top of the Eiffel Tower that if I put my hand over the edge it would fall off on to the ground below. This would be ordinary castration anxiety.

In the next phase of the dream I was aware that the people in the stalls were watching a play and I was now related through them to what was going on on the stage. A new kind of anxiety now developed. What I knew was that I had no right side of my body at all. This was not a castration dream. It was a sense of not having that part of the body.

As I woke I was aware of having understood at a very deep level what was my difficulty at that particular time. The first part of the dream represented the ordinary anxieties that might develop in respect of unconscious fantasies of my neurotic patients. I would be in danger of losing my hand or my fingers if these patients should become interested in them. With this kind of anxiety I was familiar, and it was comparatively tolerable.

The second part of the dream, however, referred to my relation to the psychotic patient. This patient was requiring of me that I should have no relation to her body at all, not even an imaginative one; there was no body that she recognized as hers and if she existed at all she could only feel herself to be a mind. Any reference to her body produced paranoid anxieties, because to claim that she had a body was to persecute her. What she needed of me was that I should have only a mind speaking to her mind. At the culmination of my difficulties on the evening before the dream I had become irritated and had said that what she was needing of me was little better than hair-splitting. This had had a disastrous effect and it took many weeks for the analysis to recover from my lapse. The essential thing, however, was that I should understand my own anxiety and this was represented in the dream by the absence of the right side of my body when I tried to get into relation to the play that the people in the stalls were watching. This right side of my body was the side related to this particular patient and was therefore affected by her need to deny absolutely even an imaginative relationship of our bodies. This denial was producing in me this psychotic type of anxiety, much less tolerable than ordinary castration anxiety. Whatever other interpretations might be made in respect of this dream the result of my having dreamed it and remembered it was that I was able to take up this analysis again and even to heal the harm done to it by my irritability which had its origin in a reactive anxiety of a quality that was appropriate to my contact with a patient with no body.

The analyst must be prepared to bear strain without expecting the patient to know anything about what he is doing, perhaps over a long period of time. To do this he must be easily aware of his own fear and hate. He is in the position of the mother of an infant unborn or newly born. Eventually, he ought to be able to tell his patient what he has been through on the patient's behalf, but an analysis may never get as far as this. There may be too little good experience in the patient's past to work on. What if there be no satisfactory relationship of early infancy for the analyst to exploit in the transference?

There is a vast difference between those patients who have had satisfactory early experiences which can be discovered in the transference, and those whose very early experiences have been so deficient or distorted that the analyst has to be the first in the patient's life to supply certain environmental essentials. In the treatment of a patient of the latter kind all sorts of things in analytic technique become vitally important, things that can be taken for granted in the treatment of patients of the former type.

I asked a colleague whether he does analysis in the dark, and he said:

'Why, no! Surely our job is to provide an ordinary environment: and the dark would be extraordinary.' He was surprised at my question. He was orientated towards analysis of neurotics. But this provision and maintenance of an ordinary environment can be in itself a vitally important thing in the analysis of a psychotic, in fact it can be, at times, even more important than the verbal interpretations which also have to be given. For the neurotic the couch and warmth and comfort can be *symbolical* of the mother's love; for the psychotic it would be more true to say that these things *are* the analyst's physical expression of love. The couch *is* the analyst's lap or womb, and the warmth *is* the live warmth of the analyst's body. And so on.

There is, I hope, a progression in my statement of my subject. The analyst's hate is ordinarily latent and is easily kept so. In analysis of psychotics the analyst is under greater strain to keep his hate latent, and he can only do this by being thoroughly aware of it. I want to add that in certain stages of certain analyses the analyst's hate is actually sought by the patient, and what is then needed is hate that is objective. If the patient seeks objective or justified hate he must be able to reach it, else he cannot feel he can reach objective love.

It is perhaps relevant here to cite the case of the child of the broken home, or the child without parents. Such a child spends his time unconsciously looking for his parents. It is notoriously inadequate to take such a child into one's home and to love him. What happens is that after a while a child so adopted gains hope, and then he starts to test out the environment he has found, and to seek proof of his guardians' ability to hate objectively. It seems that he can believe in being loved only after reaching being hated.

During the second World War a boy of nine came to a hostel for evacuated children, sent from London not because of bombs but because of truancy. I hoped to give him some treatment during his stay in the hostel, but his symptom won and he ran away as he had always done from everywhere since the age of six when he first ran away from home. However, I had established contact with him in one interview in which I could see and interpret through a drawing of his that in running away he was unconsciously saving the inside of his home and preserving his mother from assault, as well as trying to get away from his own inner world, which was full of persecutors.

I was not very surprised when he turned up in the police station very near my home. This was one of the few police stations that did not know him intimately. My wife very generously took him in and kept him for three months, three months of hell. He was the most lovable and most maddening of children, often stark staring mad. But fortunately we knew what to expect. We dealt with the first phase by giving him complete freedom and a shilling whenever he went out. He had only to ring up and we fetched him from whatever police station had taken charge of him.

Soon the expected change-over occurred, the truancy symptom turned round, and the boy started dramatizing the assault on the inside. It was really a whole-time job for the two of us together, and when I was out the worst episodes took place.

Interpretation had to be made at any minute of day or night, and often the only solution in a crisis was to make the correct interpretation, as if the boy were in analysis. It was the correct interpretation that he valued above everything.

The important thing for the purpose of this paper is the way in which the evolution of the boy's personality engendered hate in me, and what I did about it.

Did I hit him? The answer is no, I never hit. But I should have had to have done so if I had not known all about my hate and if I had not let him know about it too. At crises I would take him by bodily strength, without anger or blame, and put him outside the front door, whatever the weather or the time of day or night. There was a special bell he could ring, and he knew that if he rang it he would be readmitted and no word said about the past. He used this bell as soon as he had recovered from his maniacal attack.

The important thing is that each time, just as I put him outside the door, I told him something; I said that what had happened had made me hate him. This was easy because it was so true.

I think these words were important from the point of view of his progress, but they were mainly important in enabling me to tolerate the situation without letting out, without losing my temper and without every now and again murdering him.

This boy's full story cannot be told here. He went to an Approved School. His deeply rooted relation to us has remained one of the few stable things in his life. This episode from ordinary life can be used to illustrate the general topic of hate justified in the present; this is to be distinguished from hate that is only justified in another setting but which is tapped by some action of a patient.

Out of all the complexity of the problem of hate and its roots I want to rescue one thing, because I believe it has an importance for the analyst of psychotic patients. I suggest that the mother hates the baby before the baby hates the mother, and before the baby can know his mother hates him.

Before developing this theme I want to refer to Freud. In *Instincts and their Vicissitudes* (1915), where he says so much that is original and illuminating about hate, Freud says: 'We might at a pinch say of an instinct that it "loves" the objects after which it strives for purposes of satisfaction, but to say that it "hates" an object strikes us as odd, so we become aware that the attitudes of love and hate cannot be said to characterize the relation of instincts to their objects, but are reserved for the relations of the ego as a whole to objects. . . .' This I feel is true and important. Does this not mean that the personality must be integrated before an infant can be said to hate? However early integration may be achieved—perhaps integration occurs earliest at the height of excitement or rage—there is a theoretical earlier stage in which whatever the infant does that hurts is not done in hate. I have used the term 'ruthless love' in describing this stage. Is this acceptable? As the infant becomes able to feel to be a whole person, so does the word hate develop meaning as a description of a certain group of his feelings.

The mother, however, hates her infant from the word go. I believe Freud thought it possible that a mother may in certain circumstances have only love for her boy baby; but we may doubt this. We know about a mother's love and we appreciate its reality and power. Let me give some of the reasons why a mother hates her baby, even a boy:

The baby is not her own (mental) conception.

The baby is not the one of childhood play, father's child, brother's child, etc.

The baby is not magically produced.

The baby is a danger to her body in pregnancy and at birth.

The baby is an interference with her private life, a challenge to preoccupation.

To a greater or lesser extent a mother feels that her own mother demands a baby, so that her baby is produced to placate her mother.

The baby hurts her nipples even by suckling, which is at first a chewing activity.

He is ruthless, treats her as scum, an unpaid servant, a slave.

She has to love him, excretions and all, at any rate at the beginning, till he has doubts about himself.

He tries to hurt her, periodically bites her, all in love.

He shows disillusionment about her.

His excited love is cupboard love, so that having got what he wants he throws her away like orange peel.

The baby at first must dominate, he must be protected from coincidences, life must unfold at the baby's rate and all this needs his mother's continuous and detailed study. For instance, she must not be anxious when holding him, etc.

At first he does not know at all what she does or what she sacrifices for him. Especially he cannot allow for her hate.

He is suspicious, refuses her good food, and makes her doubt herself, but eats well with his aunt.

After an awful morning with him she goes out, and he smiles at a stranger, who says: 'Isn't he sweet?'

If she fails him at the start she knows he will pay her out for ever.

He excites her but frustrates—she mustn't eat him or trade in sex with him.

I think that in the analysis of psychotics, and in the ultimate stages of the analysis, even of a normal person, the analyst must find himself in a position comparable to that of the mother of a new-born baby. When deeply regressed the patient cannot identify with the analyst or appreciate his point of view any more than the foetus or newly born infant can sympathize with the mother.

A mother has to be able to tolerate hating her baby without doing anything about it. She cannot express it to him. If, for fear of what she may do, she cannot hate appropriately when hurt by her child she must fall back on masochism, and I think it is this that gives rise to the false theory of a natural masochism in women. The most remarkable thing about a mother is her ability to be hurt so much by her baby and to hate so much without paying the child out, and her ability to wait for rewards that may or may not come at a later date. Perhaps she is helped by some of the nursery rhymes she sings, which her baby enjoys but fortunately does not understand?

> 'Rockabye Baby, on the tree top,
> When the wind blows the cradle will rock,
> When the bough breaks the cradle will fall,
> Down will come baby, cradle and all.'

I think of a mother (or father) playing with a small infant; the infant enjoying the play and not knowing that the parent is expressing hate in the words, perhaps in terms of birth symbolism. This is not a sentimental rhyme. Sentimentality is useless for parents, as it contains a denial of hate, and sentimentality in a mother is no good at all from the infant's point of view.

It seems to me doubtful whether a human child as he develops is capable of tolerating the full extent of his own hate in a sentimental environment. He needs hate to hate.

If this is true, a psychotic patient in analysis cannot be expected to tolerate his hate of the analyst unless the analyst can hate him.

If all this is accepted there remains for discussion the question of the interpretation of the analyst's hate to the patient. This is obviously a matter fraught with danger, and it needs the most careful timing. But I believe an analysis is incomplete if even towards the end it has not been possible for the analyst to tell the patient what he, the analyst, did unbeknown for the patient whilst he was ill, in the early stages. Until this interpretation is made the patient is kept to some extent in the position of infant — one who cannot understand what he owes to his mother.

An analyst has to display all the patience and tolerance and reliability of a mother devoted to her infant; has to recognize the patient's wishes as needs;

has to put aside other interests in order to be available and to be punctual and objective; and has to seem to want to give what is really only given because of the patient's needs.

There may be a long initial period in which the analyst's point of view cannot be appreciated (even unconsciously) by the patient. Acknowledgement cannot be expected because, at the primitive root of the patient that is being looked for, there is no capacity for identification with the analyst; and certainly the patient cannot see that the analyst's hate is often engendered by the very things the patient does in his crude way of loving.

In the analysis (research analysis) or in ordinary management of the more psychotic type of patient, a great strain is put on the analyst (psychiatrist, mental nurse) and it is important to study the ways in which anxiety of psychotic quality and also hate are produced in those who work with severely ill psychiatric patients. Only in this way can there be any hope of the avoidance of therapy that is adapted to the needs of the therapist rather than to the needs of the patient.

Chapter XVI

Aggression in Relation to Emotional Development
[1950–5]

I

CONTRIBUTION TO SYMPOSIUM[1]

THE MAIN IDEA behind this study of aggression is that if society is in danger, it is not because of man's aggressiveness but because of the repression of personal aggressiveness in individuals.

In a study of the psychology of aggression a severe strain is imposed on the student, for the following reason. In a total psychology, being-stolen-from is the same as stealing, and is equally aggressive. Being weak is as aggressive as the attack of the strong on the weak. Murder and suicide are fundamentally the same thing. Perhaps most difficult of all, possession is as aggressive as is greedy acquisition; indeed acquisition and possession form a psychological unit, either is incomplete without the other. This is not saying that acquiring and possessing are good or bad.

These considerations are painful, because they draw attention to dissociations that are hidden in current social acceptance; they cannot be left out of a study of aggression. Also, the basis for a study of actual aggression must be a study of the roots of aggressive intention.

Prior to integration of the personality there is aggression.[2] A baby kicks in the womb; it cannot be assumed that he is trying to kick his way out. A baby of a few weeks thrashes away with his arms; it cannot be assumed that he means to hit. A baby chews the nipple with his gums; it cannot be assumed that he is meaning to destroy or to hurt. At origin aggressiveness is almost synonymous with activity; it is a matter of part-function.

[1] Symposium with Anna Freud, Royal Society of Medicine, Psychiatry Section, 16th January, 1950. For Anna Freud's contribution see *The Psychoanalytic Study of the Child*, Vol. III-IV, p. 37.

[2] I would now link this idea with that of motility (cf. Marty et Fain, 1955).

It is these part-functions that are organized by the child gradually, as he becomes a person, into aggression. In illness a patient may display activities and aggressiveness not fully meant. Integration of a personality does not arrive at a certain time on a certain day. It comes and goes, and even when well attained it can be lost through unfortunate environmental chance. Nevertheless, purposive behaviour is eventually arrived at if there is health. In so far as behaviour is purposive, aggression is meant. Here immediately comes the main source of aggression, instinctual experience. Aggression is part of the primitive expression of love. A description of this in oral terms is appropriate since I am studying the first love impulses.

Oral erotism gathers to itself aggressive components, and in health it is oral love that carries the basis of the greater part of actual aggressiveness — that is, aggression intended by the individual and felt as such by the people around.

All experience is both physical and non-physical. Ideas accompany and enrich bodily function, and bodily functioning accompanies and realizes[1] ideation. Also, of the sum of ideas and of memories it must be said that these gradually separate out into that which is available to consciousness, that which is available to consciousness only in certain circumstances, and that which is in the repressed unconscious, unavailable because of intolerable affect.

I am aware that I am mixing the theme of actual aggressiveness with that of aggressive impulse. I do feel, however, that the one cannot be studied without the other. No one act of aggression can be fully understood as an isolated phenomenon; and in fact the study of any one act of a child involves consideration of the following:

The child in his environment, with adults caring for him.

The child mature according to his chronological and emotional age.

The child who, although mature according to his age, contains within himself all degrees of immaturity reaching right back to the primary state.

The child as an ill person, having fixations at immature levels.

The child in a relatively unorganized emotional state, still liable with more or less ease to regression and to spontaneous recovery from regression.

Aggression at Various Stages

It would be helpful if we could start at the beginning of the individual's life, but here there is much that is not known with certainty. A complete study would trace aggressiveness as it appears at the various stages of ego development:

Early . . . . $\begin{cases} \text{Pre-integration} \\ \text{Purpose without concern} \end{cases}$

[1] cf. Sechehaye's term: 'symbolic realization'.

Intermediate . . $\begin{cases} \text{Integration} \\ \text{Purpose with concern} \\ \text{Guilt} \end{cases}$

Total personal . . $\begin{cases} \text{Inter-personal relationships} \\ \text{Triangular situations, etc.} \\ \text{Conflict, conscious and unconscious} \end{cases}$

What I attempt here is mainly a development of the second of these three themes, the intermediate.[1]

Pre-Concern

It is necessary to describe a theoretical stage of unconcern or ruthlessness in which the child can be said to exist as a person and to have purpose, yet to be unconcerned as to results. He does not yet appreciate the fact that what he destroys when excited is the same as that which he values in quiet intervals between excitements. His excited love includes an imaginative attack on the mother's body. Here is aggression as a part of love.[2]

One can see some degree of this appearing as a dissociation between quiet and excited aspects of the personality, so that children who are ordinarily nice and lovable will 'act out of character' and do aggressive things to people they love, not feeling fully responsible for their actions.

If aggression is lost at this stage of emotional development there is also some degree of loss of capacity to love, that is to say, to make relationships with objects.

Stage of Concern

Now comes the stage described by Melanie Klein as the 'depressive position' in emotional development. For my purpose I will call this the Stage of Concern. The individual's ego integration is sufficient for him to appreciate the personality of the mother figure, and this has the tremendously important result that he is concerned as to the results of his instinctual experience, physical and ideational.

The stage of concern brings with it the capacity to feel guilty. Henceforth some of the aggression appears clinically as grief or a feeling of guilt or some physical equivalent, such as vomiting. The guilt refers to the damage which is felt to be done to the loved person in the excited relationship. In health the infant can hold the guilt, and so with the help of a personal and live mother (who embodies a time factor) is able to discover his own personal urge to give and to construct and to mend. In this way much of the aggression is

[1] In Part II of this chapter, I attempt to deal with the theme of aggression relative to the early stages of ego development.

[2] This has been called 'pre-ambivalent', but this term avoids the issue of the integration of part-object and whole object, breast and mother who holds and cares.

transformed into the social functions, and appears as such. In times of helplessness (as when no person can be found to accept a gift or to acknowledge effort to repair) this transformation breaks down, and aggression reappears. *Social activity cannot be satisfactory* except it be based on a feeling of *personal* guilt in respect of aggression.

Anger

In my description there now comes a place for anger at frustration. Frustration, which is inevitable in some degree in all experience, encourages the dichotomy: 1. innocent aggressive impulses towards frustrating objects, and 2. guilt-productive aggressive impulses towards good objects. Frustration acts as a seduction away from guilt and fosters a defence mechanism, namely, the direction of love and hate along separate lines. If this splitting of objects into good and bad[1] takes place, there is an easing of guilt feeling; but in payment the love loses some of its valuable aggressive component, and the hate becomes the more disruptive.

Growth of Inner World

The psychology of the infant from now on becomes more complicated. The individual child becomes concerned not only with the effect on his mother of his impulses, but he also notes the results of his experiences in his own self. Instinctual satisfactions make him feel good, and he perceives intake and output in a psychological as well as in a physical sense. He becomes filled with what he feels to be good, and this initiates and maintains his confidence in himself and in what he feels he may expect from life. At the same time he has to reckon with his angry attacks, as a result of which he feels he becomes filled with what is bad or malign or persecuting. These evil things or forces, being inside him, as he feels, form a threat from within to his own person, and to the good which forms the basis of his trust in life.

He now starts a life-long task of management of his inner world, a task which, however, cannot be started until he is well lodged in his body and able to differentiate between what is inside himself and what is external, and between what is actual and what is his own fantasy. His management of the external world depends on his management of his inner world.

An extremely complex series of defence mechanisms develops, which should be examined in any attempt to understand aggression in a child who has reached this stage of emotional development. It will be impossible here to do more than enumerate some of the ways in which this part of human psychology is relevant to the present theme.

First I will describe the return from introversion, since this is an important and common source of actual aggression.

[1] I should now say 'idealized and bad' instead of 'good and bad' (1957).

In health the child's interest is directed both towards external reality and towards the inner world, and he has bridges between the one world and the other (dreams, play, etc.). In ill-health the child may re-arrange his relationships so that the good is concentrated within and the bad is projected. He now lives in his inner world. He may be said to have become introverted (or pathologically introverted).

A recovery from pathological introversion involves a new turning out into what is for such a child an external world full of persecutors, *and at this point in his recovery the child regularly becomes aggressive*. This is an important source of aggressive *behaviour*. If in a child's recovery from introversion the attack-in-defence is mishandled by those in charge, the child easily slips back into introversion. Apart from illness, some degree of this state of affairs is met daily in the life of any small child, and the concept is by no means a purely theoretical one. An individual is in a sensitive state on coming round after a period of concentration on a personal task.

It must be remembered that in childhood we are watching the human being only gradually becoming able to distinguish between the subjective and objective. A state of what looks like delusional madness easily appears through the child's projection of inner world experience. Even the healthy child of two or three commonly wakes in the night and feels he is in a world which (from our point of view) is his own inner world, not the external reality that we can share with him. In daytime small children become deluded in their play activities and, in fact, children can be found to be living chiefly in their inner world when apparently to us they are in our world. This need not be unhealthy, but in the management of such a child we cannot expect to meet with logic, which applies only to external or shared reality. A large proportion even of adults never achieve a reliable capacity for objectivity, and those who are most reliably objective are often comparatively out of touch with their own inner world's richness.

Three other examples will be given of the way in which the child's management of his own inner world explains aggressive behaviour.

In the child's fantasy the inner world is localized primarily in the belly or secondarily in the head or some other specific bodily area.

A child who has reached a certain degree of personality organization meets with an experience such that it is beyond his power to deal with it by identification. For instance, his parents quarrel in front of him at a time when he is fully occupied over some other problem. He manages only by taking the whole experience into himself in order to master it. It can then be said that a fixed state of parents quarrelling is living inside him, and a quantity of energy is thenceforth directed towards the control of the internalized bad relationship. Clinically he becomes tired, or depressed, or physically ill. At certain times the internalized bad relationship takes over, and then the child behaves as if 'possessed' by the quarrelling parents. We see him as compulsively aggressive, nasty, unreasonable, deluded.[1]

Alternatively the child with introjected quarrelling parents periodically engineers quarrelling in the people around him, then using the real external badness as a projection of what was 'bad' within. In such a case, there may easily be times of madness with true hallucination of quarrelling voices or people.

In the child's management of his inner world and in the attempt to preserve in it what is felt to be benign, there are moments when he feels that all would be well if a unit of malign influence could be eliminated. (This is equivalent to the scapegoat idea.)

Clinically there appears a dramatization of ejection of badness (kicking, passage of flatus, spitting, etc.). Alternatively the child is accident-prone, or there is a suicide attempt — with the aim to destroy the bad within the self; in the total fantasy of the suicide there is to be a survival, with the bad elements destroyed, but survival may not occur.

The management of inner world phenomena, felt by the child to be in the belly (or head, etc.), from time to time presents so great a difficulty that the child puts on a comprehensive control — with depressive mood as the clinical result. This leads to a state of inner deadness which is intolerable. The complementary state of mania is liable to occur. In this the inner world liveliness takes over and activates the child, who may clinically be violently aggressive, without obvious external stimulus for anger. These phases of mania are not the same as that which is called the manic defence, in which there is a denial of inner deadness by artificial activity (the so-called manic defence against depression, Klein). The clinical result of the manic defence is not an aggressive outburst, but a state of common anxious restlessness, hypomania, in which there is mild aggression in the form of untidiness, messiness, irritability with lack of constructive perseverance.

In health, the individual can store badness within for use in an attack on external forces that seem to threaten what is felt to be worth preserving. Aggression then has social value.

The value of this (as compared with maniacal or delusional aggression) lies in the fact that objectivity is preserved, and the enemy can be met with economy of effort. The enemy then does not need to be loved in order to be attacked.

Summary

The foregoing mainly describes the relation of aggression to what I have called the *intermediate* stage of emotional development. This stage precedes

[1] This state of affairs is related to that which Anna Freud has termed 'identification with the aggressor' (1937). The work of Melanie Klein introduced us to the concept of the omnipotent control of inner phenomena as a defence.

the *total personal*, with its interpersonal relationships and the triangular situations of the Oedipus complex, and it follows on after the *early* stages of ruthlessness, and of the era before purpose and before the integration of the personality.

Aggression that belongs to the stage that I have called *total personal* is already familiar to the present generation through the accepted work of Freud.

Important sources of aggression date from the *very early* stages of the development of the human being, and some of these will be traced in the next part of this chapter.

II

VERY EARLY ROOTS OF AGGRESSION[1]

In its simplest form the question that we ask is: does aggression come ultimately from anger aroused by frustration, or has it a root of its own?

The answer is necessarily highly complex unless a deliberate effort is made to cut through the great mass of clinical fact that goes to make up our daily analytic practice. If we do this, however, we run the risk of being accounted unaware of what we have in fact deliberately ignored.

We can say that in the primitive love impulse we shall always be able to detect reactive aggression, since in practice there is no such thing as a complete id satisfaction. Is it necessary therefore to attempt to dissect down? I think it is necessary because of the confusion that results from failure to do so. This is especially true in view of the fact that the primitive love impulse is operative at a stage when ego growth is only starting, when integration, for instance, is not an established fact. There is a primitive love that is operative when there is not yet a capacity for taking responsibility. In this era there is not even ruthlessness; it is a pre-ruth era, and if destruction be part of the aim in the id impulse, then destruction is only incidental to id satisfaction. Destruction only becomes an ego responsibility when there is ego integration and ego organization sufficient for the existence of anger, and therefore of fear of the talion. However early anger and fear can be detected, there is still room for recognition of those ego developments before which it is not sensible to talk of the individual's anger.

Hate is relatively sophisticated and cannot be said to exist in these early stages. It is necessary therefore to examine aggression apart altogether from the reactive aggression that inevitably follows the id impulse because of failure of id experience due to the operation of the reality principle.

It is convenient then to say that the primitive love impulse (id) has a

[1] Paper given to a private group, January 1955.

destructive quality, though it is not the infant's aim to destroy since the impulse is experienced in the pre-ruth era.

From this assumption it is possible to go into the matter of the root of the destructive element in the primitive love (id) impulse.

To simplify matters, the variable factor of birth trauma can be left out, and a normal or non-traumatic birth can be taken for granted. By normal here I mean that the birth is felt by the infant to be the result of his own effort. Neither delay nor precipitation interfered with this (see page 180).

The early id experiences bring into play a new element for the baby, instinctual crises, characterized by a preparatory period, a climax, and a period following some degree of satisfaction. Each of these three phases brings its own problems for the infant.

Our task is to examine the pre-history of the aggressive element (destructive by chance) in the earliest id experience. We have at hand certain elements which date from at least as early as the onset of foetal movements — namely motility. No doubt a corresponding element on the sensory side must eventually be added. Can this motility that dates from intra-uterine life, and that persists in infancy (and indeed throughout life), be linked up with the activity inherent in id experience proper? Indeed, is this activity to be classified as an id or an ego element? Or is it better to allow an undifferentiated ego-id phase (Hartmann, 1952) and to leave aside the attempt to classify motility on the ground that it appears before ego-id differentiation?

Each infant must be able to pour as much as possible of primitive motility into the id experiences. Here no doubt comes the truth of the need the infant has for the frustrations of reality — since id satisfaction if it could be complete and without hindrance would leave the infant with that which is derived from the motility root unsatisfied (Riviere, 1936).

In the pattern of id experience that belongs to any one infant there is x per cent of primitive motility included in the id experience. There is then $(100 - x)$ per cent left over for use in other ways — and here indeed is a reason for the vast difference in the experience of various individuals in regard to their aggressiveness. Here also is the origin of one kind of masochism (see later).

It is profitable to examine the patterns that evolve round this matter of motility (Marty et Fain, 1955).

In one pattern, the environment is constantly discovered and rediscovered because of motility. Here each experience within the framework of primary narcissism emphasizes the fact that it is in the centre that the new individual is developing, and contact with environment is *an experience of the individual* (in its undifferentiated ego-id state, at first). In the second pattern the environment impinges on the foetus (or baby) and instead of a series of individual experiences there is a series of *reactions to impingement*. Here then develops a withdrawal to rest which alone allows of individual existence. Motility is then only experienced as a reaction to impingement.

In a third pattern, which is extreme, this is exaggerated to such a degree that there is not even a resting place for individual experience, and the result is a failure in the primary narcissistic state to evolve an individual. The 'individual' then develops as an extension of the shell rather than of the core, and as an extension of the impinging environment. What there is left of a core is hidden away and is difficult to find even in the most far-reaching analysis. The individual then *exists by not being found*. The true self is hidden, and what we have to deal with clinically is the complex *false self* whose function is to keep this true self hidden. The false self may be conveniently society-syntonic, but the lack of true self gives an instability which becomes more evident the more society is deceived into thinking that the false self is the true self. The patient's complaint is of a sense of futility.

The first pattern is what we call healthy. It depends for its formation on good-enough mothering, with love expressed (as at first it can only be expressed) in physical terms. The mother holds the baby (in womb, or in arms) and through love (identification) knows how to adapt to ego needs. Under these conditions, and under these alone, the individual may start to exist, and starting to exist to have id experiences. The stage is set for the maximum of infusion of motility into id experiences. There is a fusion of the x per cent of motility potential with erotic potential (with x quantitatively high). Nevertheless even here there is $(100 - x)$ per cent of motility potential left out of the pattern of fusion, and available for pure motility use.

It must be remembered that the fusion allows of experience *apart from the action of opposition* (reaction to frustration). That which is fused with the erotic potential is satisfied in instinctual gratification. By contrast, the $(100 - x)$ per cent unfused motility potential *needs to find opposition*. Crudely, it needs something to push against, unless it is to remain unexperienced and a threat to well-being. In health, however, by definition, the individual can enjoy going around looking for appropriate opposition.

In the second and third patterns it is only through environmental impingement that the motility potential becomes a matter of experience. Here is ill-health. To a lesser or a greater degree, the individual *must* be opposed, and only if opposed does the individual tap the important motility source. This is satisfactory while environment consistently impinges, but:

Environmental impingement must continue.

Environmental impingement must have a pattern of its own, else chaos reigns since the individual cannot develop a personal pattern.

This means dependence, out of which the individual might not grow.

Withdrawal becomes an essential feature in the pattern. (Except in the extreme degree, with true self hidden; then even withdrawal is not available as a primitive defence.)

When the second and third patterns are operative there can be no health, and no treatment is of avail unless it changes the basic pattern in the direction of the pattern I have described first. Patients who have developed according to the second and third patterns do, however, come to analysis, and they may seem at first to be able to make especially good use of the analyst's work done on the false assumption that the patient really exists.

Here is a special comment on the positive value of the neurotic patient's resistances. The fact of these resistances, which can be analysed, gives a good prognosis. The absence of resistances leads to a diagnosis of disturbance in the early patterning of the kind I have described.

It would follow from these considerations that it is not possible to bring about a higher degree of fusion of motility and erotic potentials by analysis except in those who are normal by this method of classification. Where the first pattern is not established there cannot be a fusion except in a secondary way, through the 'erotization' of aggressive elements. Here is a root for compulsive sadistic trends, which can turn round into masochism. The individual feels real only when destructive and ruthless. He tries to bring about relationships through interplay with another individual by finding an erotic component to fuse with the aggression which is not in itself much more than pure motility. Here the erotic achieves fusion with motility, whereas in health it is more true to say that motility fuses with the erotic.

It is probable that in the perversions two kinds of masochism can be distinguished; one kind comes from a sadism which is an erotization of a crude motility urge, and the other kind is a more direct erotization of the passive of active motility; and it would appear that the development is directed one way or the other according to whether the first partner was masochistic or sadistic. The partnership produces a relationship which is valued the more because relationships were feeble when developed out of the erotic life, owing to relative lack of fusion of motility elements into the erotic life.

The sense of real comes especially from the motility (and corresponding sensory) roots, and erotic experiences with a weak infusion of the motility element do not strengthen the sense of reality or of existing. In fact such erotic experiences may be avoided precisely because they lead the subject to a sense of not existing, that is to say, in individuals whose early pattern is not of the variety that I have placed first in my description.

We are left with the conclusion that a great deal happens prior to the first feed, even if ego organization is immature. The summation of motility experiences contributes to the individual's ability to start to exist, and out of primary identification to repudiate the shell and to become the core. The good-enough environment makes this development possible. Only if the early environment is good enough does it make sense for us to discuss the early psychology of the human infant, since, *unless the environment has been good enough, the human being has not become differentiated, and has not come up as a subject for discussion in terms of normal psychology.* Where the individual does exist, however, we may say that one main way in which the ego and id, now differentiated, maintain a relationship, and keep a relationship in spite of the difficulties that belong to the operation of the reality principle, is through the fusion of a high proportion of primary motility potential in with erotic potential.

From these there follow other ideas that concern the problem of the external nature of objects. This subject is discussed in the third part of this chapter.

III

THE EXTERNAL NATURE OF OBJECTS[1]

In psycho-analytic practice, when an analysis has gone a long way, the analyst gets a privileged view of the early phenomena of emotional growth.

I have recently been struck by the following idea, derived from clinical work, that when a patient is engaged in discovering the aggressive root the analyst is more exhausted by the process, one way or another, than when the patient is discovering the erotic root of the instinctual life.

Immediately it will be observed that the material that concerns me here is that which is associated in our minds with the word 'de-fusion'. We assume a fusion of aggressive and erotic components in health, but we do not always give proper significance to the pre-fusion era, and to the task of fusion. We may easily take fusion too much for granted, and in this way we get into futile arguments as soon as we leave the consideration of an actual case.

It must be conceded that the task of fusion is a severe one, that even in health it is an uncompleted task, and that it is very common to find large quantities of unfused aggression complicating the psychopathology of an individual who is being analysed.

In analysis, if this be true, we have to deal with separate expressions of the aggressive and erotic components, and to hold each separately for the patient who, in the transference, cannot achieve a fusion of the two. In severe disorders that involve failure at the point of fusion, we find the patient's relationship to the analyst aggressive and erotic in turn. And it is here that I am claiming

[1] Paper given to a private group, November 1954.

that the analyst is more likely to be tired by the former than by the latter type of partial relationship.

The immediate conclusion to be drawn from this observation is that in the early stages, when the *Me* and the *Not-Me* are being established, it is the aggressive component that more surely drives the individual to a need for a *Not-Me* or an object that is felt to be *external*. The erotic experiences can be completed while the object is subjectively conceived or personally created, or while the individual is near to the narcissistic state of primary identification of earlier date.

The erotic experiences can be completed by anything that brings relief to the erotic instinctual drive, and that allows of forepleasure, rising tension of general and local excitement, climax and detumescence or its equivalent, followed by a period of lack of desire (which may itself produce anxiety because of the temporary annihilation of the subjective object created through desire). On the other hand, the aggressive impulses do not give any satisfactory experience unless there is opposition. The opposition must come from the environment, from the *Not-Me* which gradually comes to be distinguished from the *Me*. Erotic experience can be said to exist in the muscles and other tissues involved in effort, but this erotism is of a different order from that of the instinctual erotism associated with specific erotogenic zones.

Patients let us know that the aggressive experiences (more or less de-fused) feel real, much more real than do the erotic experiences (also de-fused). Both are real, but the former carry a feeling of real, which is greatly valued. The fusion of the aggression along with the erotic component of an experience enhances the feeling of the reality of the experience.

It is true that to some extent aggressive impulses can find their opposition without external opposition; this is displayed normally in the fish-movements of the spinal column that date from prenatal life, and abnormally in the to-and-fro (futile) movements of ill infants (rocking, or tension denoting a magical internal and invisible to-and-fro movement). In spite of those considerations can one not say that in normal development opposition from outside brings along the development of the aggressive impulse?

In normal birth the opposition encountered provides a type of experience which gives effort a head-first quality. Although birth is often not normal, so that it becomes a vast complication, and although birth may take place by breech instead of by head, there seems to be a general validity in the association between pure effort and a head-first relationship to opposition. This could be tested out by observation on infants who are making an effort to feed — according to my theory they can be helped by a degree of opposition to the top of the head.

This idea is usually expressed in the following terms: 'An infant does not thrive on perfect adaptation to need. A mother who fits in with a baby's desires too well is not a good mother. Frustration produces anger and this helps the infant to gain enhanced experience.' This is true and not true. In so far as it is untrue, it neglects two factors — one is that the infant does need perfect adaptation at the theoretical start, and then needs a carefully graduated failure of adaptation; the other is that this statement leaves out of consideration the lack of fusion of the aggressive and the erotic roots of experience, whereas in theory at least, the de-fused state (or the fore-fusion state) must be studied.

Those who make the statement more or less as quoted here only too easily assume that aggression is a reaction to frustration, that is to say, to frustration during erotic experience, during a phase of excitement with instinctual tension rising. That there is anger at frustration in such phases is only too obvious, but in our theory of the earliest feelings and states we need to be prepared for aggression that *precedes* the ego integration that makes anger at instinctual frustration possible, and that makes the erotic experience an experience.

It can be said that each baby has a potential of zonal erotic instinct, that this is biological, and that the potential is more or less the same for each baby. By contrast the *aggression component must be extremely variable*; by the time that we observe a baby's anger at frustration at a feeding delay a great deal has happened that has made the baby's aggressive potential great or little. To get to something in terms of aggression corresponding to the erotic potential it would be necessary to go back to the impulses of the foetus, to that which makes for movement rather than for stillness, to the aliveness of tissues and to the first evidence of muscular erotism. We need a term here such as life force.

No doubt the life-force potential of each individual foetus is more or less the same, just as is the erotic potential of each baby. The complication is that the amount of aggressive potential an infant carries depends on the amount of opposition that has been met with. In other words, opposition affects the conversion of life force into aggression potential. Moreover, excess of opposition introduces complications that make it impossible for the existence of an individual who, having aggressive potential, could achieve its fusion with the erotic.

It is not possible to go further with this argument without considering in detail the fate of the life force of the (prenatal) infant.

In health the foetal impulses bring about a discovery of environment, this latter being the opposition that is met through movement, and sensed during movement. The result here is an early recognition of a *Not-Me* world, and an early establishment of the *Me*. (It will be understood that in practice these things develop gradually, and repeatedly come and go, and are achieved and lost.)

In ill-health at this very early stage it is the environment that impinges, and the life force is taken up in reactions to impingement — the result being the opposite to the early firm establishment of the *Me*. In the extreme there is very little experience of impulses except as *reactions*, and the *Me* is not established. Instead we find a development based on the experience of reaction to impingement, and there comes into existence an individual that we call false because the personal impulsiveness is missing. In this case there is no fusion of the aggressive and erotic components, since the *Me* is not established when erotic experiences occur. The infant does indeed live, because of being seduced into erotic experience; but separately from the erotic life, which never feels real, is a purely aggressive reactive life, dependent on the experience of opposition.

It has been necessary, in this description, to discuss two extremes in the attempt to lead the way to a description of the common state in which *some degree of lack of fusion* has been a feature. The personality comprises three parts: a true self, with *Me* and *Not-Me* clearly established, and with some fusion of the aggressive and erotic elements; a self that is easily seduced along lines of erotic experience, but with the result of a loss of sense of real; a self that is entirely and ruthlessly given over to aggression. This aggression is not even organized to destruction, but it has value to the individual because it brings a sense of real and a sense of relating, but it is only brought into being by active opposition, or (later) persecution. It has no root in personal impulse, motivated in ego spontaneity.

The individual may achieve a false fusion of the aggressive and erotic by converting this pure de-fused aggression into masochism, but for this to occur there must be a reliable persecutor, and the reliable persecutor is a sadistic lover. In this way masochism can be primary to sadism. However, in following the development of an emotionally *healthy* human being we see sadism as primary to masochism. In health sadism implies successful fusion, that which is absent in the conditions in which masochism develops straight out of the pattern of reactive aggression, unfused.

The main conclusion to be made out of these considerations is that confusion exists through our using the term aggression sometimes when we mean spontaneity. The impulsive gesture reaches out and becomes aggressive when opposition is reached. There is reality in this experience, and it very easily fuses into the erotic experiences that await the new-born infant. I am suggesting: *it is this impulsiveness, and the aggression that develops out of it, that makes the infant need an external object*, and not merely a satisfying object.

Many infants, however, have a massive aggressive potential that belongs to reaction to impingement, that becomes activated by persecution: in so far as this is true the infant welcomes persecution, and feels real in reacting to it. But this represents a false mode of development since the infant needs continued persecution. The quantity of this reactive potential is not dependent on biological factors (which determine motility and erotism) but is dependent

217

on the chance of early environmental impingement, and therefore, often, on the mother's psychiatric abnormalities, and the state of the mother's emotional environment.

In adult and mature sexual intercourse, it is perhaps true that it is not the purely erotic satisfactions that need a specific object. It is the aggressive or destructive element in the fused impulse that fixes the object and determines the need that is felt for the partner's actual presence, satisfaction, and survival.

Chapter XVII

Psychoses and Child Care[1]
[1952]

IN THIS PAPER I shall try to show that some degree of psychosis in childhood is common, but it is not noticed because of the way in which the symptoms are hidden in the ordinary difficulties inherent in child care. The diagnosis is made when the environment fails to hide or to cope with distortions of emotional development, so that the child needs to organize along a certain defensive line which becomes recognizable as a disease entity. This theory assumes that the basis of the mental health of the personality is laid down in earliest infancy by the techniques which come naturally to a mother who is preoccupied with the care of her own infant. I shall make a brief sketch of the tasks involved in the early stages of the emotional development of the infant, tasks which cannot be accomplished by the infant except in an emotional environment that is good enough.

There are two methods by which the subject of childhood psychosis can be attacked. By one method mental disease organizations that are well known in adult psychiatry can be described as occurring before puberty and in the years of early childhood. Creak (1952) takes one type of psychosis in which there is an organized introversion, with consequent bizarre behaviour patterns and secondary disturbances of physical functioning, and she clearly describes a type of child that must be well-known to all child psychiatrists and to paediatricians. In the same way it would be possible to take melancholic states, manic-depressive mood swings, hypomanic restlessness, various kinds of confusional states, and to trace their common occurrence in childhood; the material for such a study is abundant.

I have chosen another method, perhaps because I wish to speak as a paediatrician who is in the habit of thinking of the developing child and indeed of

[1] Based on a lecture given to the Psychiatry Section of the Royal Society of Medicine, March 1952. *Brit. J. Med. Psychol.*, Vol. XXVI, 1953.

the developing infant. For the paediatrician there is a continuity of development of the individual; this development starts with conception, goes on throughout infancy and early childhood, and leads to the adult state, the child being father to the man. The aim in child care is not only to produce a healthy child but also to allow of the ultimate development of a healthy adult. The reverse of this statement is what concerns me here, which is that the health of the adult is laid down at all stages of infancy and childhood. The paediatrician is all the time aware of care and nurture, of the dependence of infants, and of the gradual maturation of the environmental factors which need to have a continuity just like the continuity of the inner development of the child. For this reason the paediatrician has much to contribute to psychiatry.

If some paediatricians have concentrated on the physical side and have neglected the psyche, I cannot help it; this is a phase that is passing, and no one can deny that it has paid rich dividends on the physical side.

Here I shall be concerned with the psyche and only secondarily with the soma; but I remain a paediatrician, and from the paediatric angle mental health is something which cannot be except as a fruition of previous development. The mental health of each child is laid down by the mother during her preoccupation with the care of her infant. The word 'devotion' can be rid of its sentimentality and can be used to describe the essential feature without which the mother cannot make her contribution, a sensitive and active adaptation to her infant's needs—needs which at the beginning are absolute. This word, devotion, also reminds us that in order to succeed in her task the mother need not be clever.

Mental health, then, is a product of the continuous care that enables a continuity of personal emotional growth. It is already an accepted view that neurosis has its origin in the early interpersonal relationships that arise when the child is beginning to take a place as a whole human being in the family. In other words, the health of an individual in terms of socialization and of absence of neurosis is laid down by the parents when the child is at the toddler age; but this statement assumes normal growth during infancy. It is not so well known (and indeed it is still a matter for proof) that disturbances which can be recognized and labelled as psychotic have their origin in distortions in emotional development arising before the child has clearly become a whole person capable of total relationships with whole persons.

This theory is accepted more readily for some types of psychotics than for others. Those who specialize in the study of these matters are fairly clear that the capacity to become depressed (in the sense of showing a reactive depression or mood change) is achieved in health by the infant who has reached the age at which weaning is meaningful. Depression is allied to concern, remorse, guilt, but in the depressed mood a relatively large proportion of unconscious affect is involved. The capacity to feel concerned, to feel grief, and to react to loss in an organized way so that recovery may take place in the course of time, is a developmental stage of great importance in healthy growth; and this capacity is laid down by the careful management of weaning, using weaning in the very broad sense of the management of infants of roughly speaking 9–18 months. It is not possible to do more in this paper than to refer to the very careful work done on this subject, work which is certainly relevant to the study of psychosis in so far as the term implies depression of various kinds and the manic-depressive types of disorder. Understanding of this started with Freud's paper 'Mourning and Melancholia' (1917) and the theme has been developed by others, notably Abraham (1924), Klein (1934), Rickman (1928). Also there is the extension of Klein's theory to cover the origins of certain types of paranoid organization. The concept of the healthy attainment of 'the depressive position in emotional development' (Klein) in its turn presupposes healthy previous development, and I wish in this paper to refer to the earliest and most primitive stages.

Just behind weaning is the wider subject of disillusionment. Weaning implies successful feeding and disillusionment implies the successful provision of opportunity for illusion.

PRIMITIVE STAGES OF EMOTIONAL DEVELOPMENT

This is a very difficult subject and I realize that much that I shall say is controversial. Nevertheless, it is necessary to explore the possibility that mental health in terms of lessened liability to schizoid states and to schizophrenia is laid down in the very earliest stages, when the infant is being introduced gradually to external reality. I say nothing in this lecture that is not fully substantiated *from my point of view* in my own analytic and other clinical work.

Elucidation of the earliest stages of emotional development must come chiefly in the psycho-analytic treatment room, psycho-analysis being by far the most precise instrument, whether it be used in the analysis of small children or of regressed adults or of psychotics of all ages or of relatively normal people who make temporary or even momentary regressions. Within the psycho-analytic framework there is opportunity for an infinite variety of experience, and if from various analyses certain common factors emerge, then we can make definite claims. At the same time there are the types of work in the field of direct observation. Here we have such published records as Freud & Burlingham (1942), Bowlby (1951), Spitz (1945, 1950). Also, careful history-taking is invaluable.

At first the individual is not the unit. As perceived from outside the unit is an environment-individual set-up. The outsider knows that the individual psyche can only start in a certain setting. In this setting the individual can gradually come to create a personal environment.[1] If all goes well the environment created by the individual becomes something that is like enough to the environment that can be generally perceived, and in such a case there arrives a stage in the process of development through which the individual passes from dependence to independence. This is an extremely tricky developmental era and it is in success here that mental health in respect of psychosis is principally laid down. It is this very difficult area that I am attempting to study in this lecture. I am far away therefore from the crude question: 'Is psychosis common or rare in infancy and childhood?' Rather am I trying to make a statement of the way in which emotional development in its primitive or earliest stages concerns exactly the same phenomena that appear in the study of adult schizophrenia, and of the schizoid states in general and of the organized defences against confusion and un-integration. The intimate study of a schizoid individual of whatever age becomes an intimate study of that individual's very early development, development within and emerging from the stage of the environment-individual set-up.

I have given myself the task therefore of studying the whole procedure of the early development of psyche-soma including the delays and distortions. I shall need to be dogmatic, and I hope to make my meaning clear by using diagrams.

Figs. 9 and 10 represent the way in which the individual is affected by environmental tendencies, especially at a very early stage. *Fig.* 9 shows how, by active adaptation to the child's needs, the environment enables him to be in undisturbed isolation. The infant does not know. In this state he makes a spontaneous movement and the environment is discovered without loss of sense of self. *Fig.* 10 shows faulty adaptation to the child, resulting in impingement of the environment so that the individual must become a reactor to this impingement. The sense of self is lost in this situation and is only regained by a return to isolation. (Note the introduction of the time factor which means that a *process* is involved.)

This simple statement can be used for clarification of extremely complex issues. The second type of experience, with failure of good-enough active environmental adaptation, produces a psychotic distortion of the environment-individual set-up. Relationships produce loss of the sense of self, and the latter is only regained by return to isolation. Being isolated, however, becomes less and less pure the further the child is from the beginning, involving more and more defensive organization in repudiation of environmental impingement. Therapy in respect of such a disorder must provide active

[1] According to my view the concept of the body-scheme as put forward by Scott (1949) concerns only the individual, and not the unit named here the environment-individual set-up.

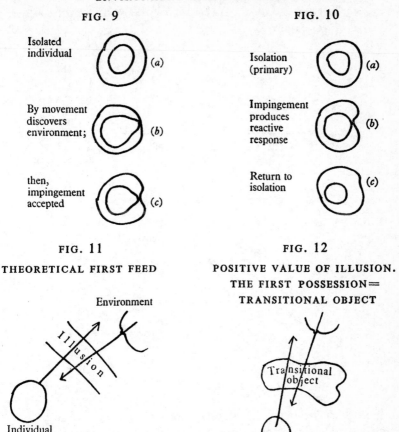

FIG. 9

Isolated individual *(a)*

By movement discovers environment; *(b)*

then, impingement accepted *(c)*

FIG. 10

Isolation (primary) *(a)*

Impingement produces reactive response *(b)*

Return to isolation *(c)*

FIG. 11

THEORETICAL FIRST FEED

Environment

Illusion

Individual

FIG. 12

POSITIVE VALUE OF ILLUSION.
THE FIRST POSSESSION =
TRANSITIONAL OBJECT

Transitional object

adaptation to the child and must gradually build up a respect for processes.

Fig. 11 illustrates a theoretical first feed. The creative potential of the individual arising out of need produces readiness for an hallucination. The mother's love and her close identification with her infant make her aware of the infant's needs to the extent that she provides something more or less in the right place and at the right time. This, much repeated, starts off the infant's ability to use *illusion*, without which no contact is possible between the psyche and the environment. If in the place of the word illusion we put the thumb, or that bit of blanket or that soft rag doll (fetish-object, Wulff (1946)) that some infants employ at 8–10–12 months for giving consolation or comfort, then one sees what I have tried to describe elsewhere under the term *transitional object* (*Fig.* 12). (See Chapter XVIII.)

By such a diagram as *Fig.* 13 one can again sort out this intermediate area of

223

FIG. 13
INTERMEDIATE AREA OF PRIMARY MADNESS

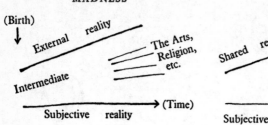

FIG. 14
AN ELABORATION OF FIG. 13

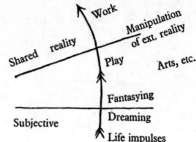

FIG. 15
BASIC SPLIT IN PERSONALITY

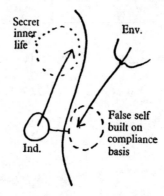

illusion which in infancy is an agreed area, unchallenged in respect of its being created by the infant or accepted as a bit of perceived reality. We allow the infant this madness, and only gradually ask for a clear distinguishing between the subjective and that which is capable of objective or scientific proof. We adults use the arts and religion for the off-moments which we all need in the course of reality-testing and reality-acceptance.

If an individual claims special indulgence in respect of this intermediate area we recognize psychosis; if the individual is an adult we use the epithet 'mad'. In observation of children we see here again the natural gradation from the ordinary predicaments of human nature to the psychotic illnesses. These psychotic illnesses only represent exaggerations here or there and do not imply any essential difference between sanity and insanity.

Fig. 14 shows one of the ways one can usefully elaborate the previous diagram.

In *Fig.* 15 I try to show how a tendency for a basic split in the environment-individual set-up can start through failure of active adaptation on the part of the environment at the beginning.

In the extreme case of splitting the secret inner life has very little in it derived from external reality. It is truly incommunicable.

Where there is a high degree of the tendency to a split at this early stage, the individual is in danger of being seduced into a false life, and the instincts then come in on the side of the seducing environment. Paediatrics at its worst (i.e. accent on physical health, denial of psyche-claims) can be said to be the organized exploitation of the betrayal of human nature by instincts. A successful seduction of this kind may produce a false self that seems satisfactory to the unwary observer, although the schizophrenia is latent and will claim attention in the end. The false self, developed on a compliance basis, cannot attain to the independence of maturity, except perhaps a pseudo-maturity in a psychotic environment.

It can certainly be claimed that adaptation to need is never complete, even at the beginning when the mother is biologically orientated to this highly specialized function. The gap between complete and incomplete adaptation is dealt with by the individual's intellectual processes, by which, gradually, the failures of the environment become allowed for, understood, tolerated, and even predicted. Intellectual understanding converts the not-good-enough environmental adaptation to the good-enough adaptation. Naturally, in the operation of this mechanism, the individual is in a much better condition if the environment behaves steadily. Variable adaptation because of its unpredictability is traumatic and annuls the good effect of occasional bouts of extremely sensitive adaptation.

Where there is restricted intellectual capacity (based on poor brain-tissue endowment) the infant's capacity to convert not-quite-good-enough environmental adaptation into good-enough environmental adaptation is lowered, with the result that certain psychoses are more common in defectives than in the normal population. Exceptional brain-tissue endowment may enable an infant to allow for a severe failure of adaptation to need, but in such a case there can be a prostitution of mental activity so that one finds clinically a hypertrophy of intellectual processes related to a potential schizophrenic breakdown.

I am not claiming that this is all that there is to be said about the origins of intellectual activity or of the psychoses of defectives, but it is useful to look at the problem of mental activity in this way as it shows how mental activity can be exploited and can become the enemy of the psyche.

Figs. 16 and 17 draw attention to the fact that the personality does not start off as a completed whole thing if we think of the infant's point of view. By various means the unity of the individual psyche becomes a fact, at first at moments (16b), and later over long and variable periods of time (16c) (see Glover, 1932).

No diagram is needed to illustrate another important development, which

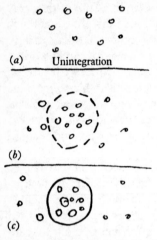

(a)   Unintegration

(b)

(c)

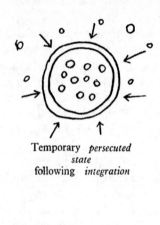

Temporary *persecuted*
state
following *integration*

is the way in which the individual psyche becomes lodged in the body. This process happens quite early at certain moments and gradually becomes more permanently established. Nevertheless, it can be lost in association with fatigue or lack of sleep or anxieties belonging to other stages of emotional development.

I can cite Humpty Dumpty at this juncture. He has just achieved integration into one whole thing, and has emerged from the environment-individual set-up so that he is perched on a wall, no longer devotedly held. He is notoriously in a precarious position in his emotional development, especially liable to irreversible disintegration.

Fig. 17 depicts the moments of the gathering together of the bits — dangerous moments for the individual. In respect of the total environment-individual set-up the integration activity produces an individual in a raw state, a potential paranoiac. The persecutors in the new phenomenon, the outside, become neutralized in ordinary healthy development by the fact of the mother's loving care, which physically (as in holding) and psychologically (as in understanding or empathy, enabling sensitive adaptation), makes the individual's primary isolation a fact. Environmental failure just here starts the individual off with a paranoid potential. This shows clinically so early and so clearly that one can forgive those who (not knowing about infant psychology) explain it in terms of heredity.[1]

In defence against the terrible anxieties of the paranoid state in very early life there is not infrequently organized a state which has been given various

---

[1] Melanie Klein has postulated a paranoid position in emotional development. I have described what I have found and I believe it to be related to that which Klein describes.

names (defensive pathological introversion, etc.). The infant lives permanently in his or her own inner world which is not, however, firmly organized.
The external persecution complication is kept at bay by non-achievement of
unit-status. In a relation with this kind of child one floats in and out of the
inner world in which the child lives, and while one is in it one is subjected to
more or less of omnipotent control, but not control from a strong central
point. It is a world of magic, and one feels mad to be in it. All of us who
have treated psychotic children of this kind know how mad we have to be to
inhabit this world, and yet we must be there, and must be able to stay there
for long periods in order to do any therapeusis.

It is difficult to make a satisfactory simple diagram of so complex a state of
affairs (see *Fig.* 18). This is a gross exaggeration of the healthy child's ordinary
preoccupation during play, but is distinguished from healthy play by the lack
of a beginning and end to the game, by the degree of magical control, by the
lack of organization of play material according to any one pattern, and by the
inexhaustibility of the child.

FIG. 18
A SCHIZOID STATE

P. = persecutors
T. = psycho-therapist

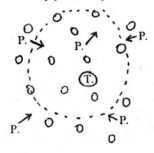

CONCLUSION

The subjects discussed in this chapter are common ground for infant care
and ordinary adult psychiatry. To go further I should have to give attention
to the depressive position and to the origins of sense of concern, and of the
ability to feel guilt, and to the building up in the individual of an inner
world of strains and stresses, and so on. All this I must leave out.

I have tried to show that a study of the theory of infant care brings us to
the theory of mental health and of psychiatric disorder (see Chapter XIII).

The basis for mental health is being laid down by the mother from conception onwards through the ordinary care that she gives her infant because of
her special orientation to that task. Mental ill-health of psychotic quality

arises out of delays and distortions, regressions and muddles, in the early stages of growth of the environment-individual set-up. Mental ill-health emerges imperceptibly out of the ordinary difficulties that are inherent in human nature and that give colour to the task of child care, whether it be done by parent, nurse, or school teacher. Prophylaxis against psychosis is therefore the responsibility of the paediatricians, did they but know it.

Chapter XVIII

Transitional Objects and Transitional Phenomena[1]
[1951]

A STUDY OF THE FIRST *NOT-ME* POSSESSION[2]

Introduction

IT IS WELL KNOWN that infants as soon as they are born tend to use fist, fingers, thumbs in stimulation of the oral erotogenic zone, in satisfaction of the instincts at that zone, and also in quiet union. It is also well known that after a few months infants of either sex become fond of playing with dolls, and that most mothers allow their infants some special object and expect them to become, as it were, addicted to such objects.

There is a relationship between these two sets of phenomena that are separated by a time interval, and a study of the development from the earlier into the later can be profitable, and can make use of important clinical material that has been somewhat neglected.

The First Possession

Those who happen to be in close touch with mothers' interests and problems will be already aware of the very rich patterns ordinarily displayed by babies in their use of the first *Not-Me* possession. These patterns, being displayed, can be subjected to direct observation.

There is a wide variation to be found in a sequence of events which starts with the new-born infant's fist-in-mouth activities, and that leads eventually on to an attachment to a teddy, a doll or soft toy, or to a hard toy.

[1] Based on a paper read before the British Psycho-Analytical Society on 30th May, 1951. *Int. J. Psycho-Anal.*, Vol. XXXIV, 1953.

[2] It is necessary to stress that the word used here is 'possession' and not 'object'. In the typed version distributed to members I did in fact use the word 'object' (instead of 'possession') in one place by mistake, and this led to confusion in the discussion. It was pointed out that the first *Not-Me object* is usually taken to be the breast. The reader's attention is drawn to the use of the word 'transitional' in many places by Fairbairn (1952, p. 35.).

It is clear that something is important here other than oral excitement and satisfaction, although this may be the basis of everything else. Many other important things can be studied, and they include:

The nature of the object.
The infant's capacity to recognize the object as *Not-Me*.
The place of the object — outside, inside, at the border.
The infant's capacity to create, think up, devise, originate, produce an object.
The initiation of an affectionate type of object relationship.

I have introduced the terms 'transitional object' and 'transitional phenomena' for designation of the intermediate area of experience, between the thumb and the teddy bear, between the oral erotism and true object relationship, between primary creative activity and projection of what has already been introjected, between primary unawareness of indebtedness and the acknowledgement of indebtedness ('Say: ta!').

By this definition an infant's babbling or the way an older child goes over a repertoire of songs and tunes while preparing for sleep come within the intermediate area as transitional phenomena, along with the use made of objects that are not part of the infant's body yet are not fully recognized as belonging to external reality.

It is generally acknowledged that a statement of human nature is inadequate when given in terms of interpersonal relationships, even when the imaginative elaboration of function, the whole of fantasy both conscious and unconscious, including the repressed unconscious, is allowed for. There is another way of describing persons that comes out of the researches of the past two decades, that suggests that of every individual who has reached to the stage of being a unit (with a limiting membrane and an outside and an inside) it can be said that there is an *inner reality* to that individual, an inner world which can be rich or poor and can be at peace or in a state of war.

My claim is that if there is a need for this double statement, there is need for a triple one; there is the third part of the life of a human being, a part that we cannot ignore, an intermediate area of *experiencing*, to which inner reality and external life both contribute. It is an area which is not challenged, because no claim is made on its behalf except that it shall exist as a resting-place for the individual engaged in the perpetual human task of keeping inner and outer reality separate yet inter-related.

It is usual to refer to 'reality-testing', and to make a clear distinction between apperception and perception. I am here staking a claim for an intermediate state between a baby's inability and growing ability to recognize and accept reality. I am therefore studying the substance of *illusion*, that which is allowed to the infant, and which in adult life is inherent in art and religion.

We can share a respect for *illusory experience,* and if we wish we may collect together and form a group on the basis of the similarity of our illusory experiences. This is a natural root of grouping among human beings. Yet it is a hall-mark of madness when an adult puts too powerful a claim on the credulity of others, forcing them to acknowledge a sharing of illusion that is not their own.

I hope it will be understood that I am not referring exactly to the little child's teddy bear nor to the infant's first use of the fist (thumb, fingers). I am not specifically studying the first object of object relationships. I am concerned with the first possession, and with the intermediate area between the subjective and that which is objectively perceived.

Development of a Personal Pattern

There is plenty of reference in psycho-analytic literature to the progress from 'hand to mouth' to 'hand to genital', but perhaps less to progress leading to the handling of truly '*Not-Me*' objects. Sooner or later in an infant's development there comes a tendency on the part of the infant to weave other-than-me objects into the personal pattern. To some extent these objects stand for the breast, but it is not especially this point that is under discussion.

In the case of some infants the thumb is placed in the mouth while fingers are made to caress the face by pronation and supination movements of the forearm. The mouth is then active in relation to the thumb, but not in relation to the fingers. The fingers caressing the upper lip, or some other part, may be or may become more important than the thumb engaging the mouth. Moreover this caressing activity may be found alone, without the more direct thumb-mouth union. (Freud, 1905. Hoffer, 1949.)

In common experience one of the following occurs, complicating an auto-erotic experience such as thumb-sucking:

1. with the other hand the baby takes an external object, say a part of a sheet or blanket, into the mouth along with the fingers; or
2. somehow or other the bit of cloth[1] is held and sucked, or not actually sucked. The objects used naturally include napkins and (later) handkerchiefs, and this depends on what is readily and reliably available; or
3. the baby starts from early months to pluck wool and to collect it and to use it for the caressing part of the activity.[2] Less commonly, the wool is swallowed, even causing trouble; or

[1] A recent example is the blanket-doll of the child in the film *A Two-year-old Goes to Hospital* by James Robertson (Tavistock Clinic). cf. also Robertson *et al.* (1952).

[2] Here there could possibly be an explanation for the use of the term 'wool-gathering', which means: inhabiting the transitional or intermediate area.

4. mouthing, accompanied by sounds of 'mum-mum', babbling,[1] anal noises, the first musical notes and so on.

One may suppose that thinking, or fantasying, gets linked up with these functional experiences.

All these things I am calling *transitional phenomena*. Also, out of all this (if we study any one infant) there may emerge some thing or some phenomenon — perhaps a bundle of wool or the corner of a blanket or eiderdown, or a word or tune, or a mannerism, which becomes vitally important to the infant for use at the time of going to sleep, and is a defence against anxiety, especially anxiety of depressive type. (Illingworth, 1951.) Perhaps some soft object or cot cover has been found and used by the infant, and this then becomes what I am calling a *transitional object*. This object goes on being important. The parents get to know its value and carry it round when travelling. The mother lets it get dirty and even smelly, knowing that by washing it she introduces a break in continuity in the infant's experience, a break that may destroy the meaning and value of the object to the infant.

I suggest that the pattern of transitional phenomena begins to show at about 4–6–8–12 months. Purposely I leave room for wide variations.

Patterns set in infancy may persist into childhood, so that the original soft object continues to be absolutely necessary at bed-time or at time of loneliness or when a depressed mood threatens. In health, however, there is a gradual extension of range of interest, and eventually the extended range is maintained, even when depressive anxiety is near. A need for a specific object or a behaviour pattern that started at a very early date may reappear at a later age when deprivation threatens.

This first possession is used in conjunction with special techniques derived from very early infancy, which can include or exist apart from the more direct autoerotic activities. Gradually in the life of an infant teddies and dolls and hard toys are acquired. Boys to some extent tend to go over to use hard objects, whereas girls tend to proceed right ahead to the acquisition of a family. It is important to note, however, that *there is no noticeable difference between boy and girl in their use of the original Not-Me possession*, which I am calling the transitional object.

As the infant starts to use organized sounds (mum, ta, da) there may appear a 'word' for the transitional object. The name given by the infant to these earliest objects is often significant, and it usually has a word used by the adults partly incorporated in it. For instance, 'baa' may be the name, and the 'b' may have come from the adult's use of the word 'baby' or 'bear'.

I should mention that sometimes there is no transitional object except the mother herself. Or an infant may be so disturbed in emotional development

[1] cf. Scott (1955).

that the transition state cannot be enjoyed, or the sequence of objects used is broken. The sequence may nevertheless be maintained in a hidden way.

Summary of Special Qualities in the Relationship

1. The infant assumes rights over the object, and we agree to this assumption. Nevertheless some abrogation of omnipotence is a feature from the start.
2. The object is affectionately cuddled as well as excitedly loved and mutilated.
3. It must never change, unless changed by the infant.
4. It must survive instinctual loving, and also hating, and, if it be a feature, pure aggression.
5. Yet it must seem to the infant to give warmth, or to move, or to have texture, or to do something that seems to show it has vitality or reality of its own.
6. It comes from without from our point of view, but not so from the point of view of the baby. Neither does it come from within; it is not an hallucination.
7. Its fate is to be gradually allowed to be decathected, so that in the course of years it becomes not so much forgotten as relegated to limbo. By this I mean that in health the transitional object does not 'go inside' nor does the feeling about it necessarily undergo repression. It is not forgotten and it is not mourned. It loses meaning, and this is because the transitional phenomena have become diffused, have become spread out over the whole intermediate territory between 'inner psychic reality' and 'the external world as perceived by two persons in common', that is to say, over the whole cultural field.

At this point my subject widens out into that of play, and of artistic creativity and appreciation, and of religious feeling, and of dreaming, and also of fetishism, lying and stealing, the origin and loss of affectionate feeling, drug addiction, the talisman of obsessional rituals, etc.

Relationship of the Transitional Object to Symbolism

It is true that the piece of blanket (or whatever it is) is symbolical of some part-object, such as the breast. Nevertheless the point of it is not its symbolic value so much as its actuality. Its not being the breast (or the mother) is as important as the fact that it stands for the breast (or mother).

When symbolism is employed the infant is already clearly distinguishing between fantasy and fact, between inner objects and external objects, between primary creativity and perception. But the term transitional object, according to my suggestion, gives room for the process of becoming able to accept difference and similarity. I think there is use for a term for the root of symbolism in time, a term that describes the infant's journey from the purely subjective to objectivity; and it seems to me that the transitional object (piece of blanket, etc.) is what we see of this journey of progress towards experiencing.

It would be possible to understand the transitional object while not fully understanding the nature of symbolism. It seems that symbolism can only be properly studied in the process of the growth of an individual, and that it has at the very best a variable meaning. For instance, if we consider the wafer of the Blessed Sacrament, which is symbolic of the body of Christ, I think I am right in saying that for the Roman Catholic community it *is* the body, and for the Protestant community it is a *substitute*, a reminder, and is essentially not, in fact, actually the body itself. Yet in both cases it is a symbol.

A schizoid patient asked me, after Christmas, had I enjoyed eating her at the feast. And then, *had I really eaten her or only in fantasy*. I knew that she could not be satisfied with either alternative. Her split needed the double answer.

CLINICAL DESCRIPTION OF A TRANSITIONAL OBJECT

For anyone in touch with parents and children, there is an infinite quantity and variety of illustrative clinical material.[1] The following illustrations are given merely to remind readers of similar material in their own experiences.

Two Brothers: Contrast in early Use of Possessions

Distortion in use of transitional object. X, now a healthy man, has had to fight his way towards maturity. The mother 'learned how to be a mother' in her management of X when he was an infant and she was able to avoid certain mistakes with the other children because of what she learned with him. There were also external reasons why she was anxious at the time of her rather lonely management of X when he was born. She took her job as a mother very seriously and she breast-fed X for seven months. She feels that in his case this was too long and he was very difficult to wean. He never sucked his thumb or his fingers and when she weaned him 'he had nothing to fall back on'. He had never had the bottle or a dummy or any other form of feeding. He had a very strong and early *attachment to the mother herself*, as a person, and it was her actual person that he needed.

From twelve months he adopted a rabbit which he would cuddle and his

[1] There are excellent examples in the one article I have found on this same subject. Wulff ('Fetishism and Object Choice in Early Childhood', *Psychoanal. Quart.*, 1946, 15, p. 450) is clearly studying this same phenomenon, but he calls the objects 'fetish objects'. It is not clear to me that this term is correct, and I discuss this below. I did not actually know of Wulff's paper until I had written my own, but it gave me great pleasure and support to find the subject had already been considered worthy of discussion by a colleague. See also Abraham (1916) and Lindner (1879).

affectionate regard for the rabbit eventually transferred to real rabbits. This particular rabbit lasted till he was five or six years old. It could be described as a *comforter*, but it never had the true quality of a transitional object. It was never, as a true transitional object would have been, more important than the mother, an almost inseparable part of the infant. In the case of this particular boy the kind of anxieties which were brought to a head by the weaning at seven months later produced asthma, and only gradually did he conquer this. It was important for him that he found employment far away from the home town. His attachment to his mother is still very powerful. He comes within the wide definition of the term normal, or healthy. This man has not married.

Typical use of transitional object. X's younger brother, Y, has developed in quite a straightforward way throughout. He now has three healthy children of his own. He was fed at the breast for four months and then weaned without difficulty.[1] Y sucked his thumb in the early weeks and this again 'made weaning easier for him than for his older brother'. Soon after weaning at five to six months he adopted the end of the blanket where the stitching finished. He was pleased if a little bit of the wool stuck out at the corner and with this he would tickle his nose. This very early became his 'Baa'; he invented this word for it himself as soon as he could use organized sounds. From the time when he was about a year old he was able to substitute for the end of the blanket a soft green jersey with a red tie. This was not a 'comforter' as in the case of the depressive older brother. but a 'soother'. It was a sedative which always worked. This is a typical example of what I am calling a *Transitional Object*. When Y was a little boy it was always certain that if anyone gave him his 'Baa' he would immediately suck it and lose anxiety, and in fact he would go to sleep within a few minutes if the time for sleep were at all near. The thumb-sucking continued at the same time, lasting until he was three or four years old, and he remembers thumb-sucking and a hard place on one thumb which resulted from it. He is now interested (as a father) in the thumb-sucking of his own children and their use of 'Baas'.

The story of seven ordinary children in this family brings out the points, arranged for comparison in the table on page 236.

In consultation with a parent it is often valuable to get information about the early techniques and possessions of all the children of the family. This starts the mother on a comparison of her children one with another, and enables her to remember and compare their characteristics at an early age.

Information can often be obtained from a child in regard to transitional objects; for instance, Angus (11 years 9 months) told me that his brother 'has tons of teddies and things' and 'before that he had little bears', and he fol-

[1] The mother had 'learned from her first child that it was a good idea to give one bottle feed while breast feeding', that is, to allow for the positive value of substitutes for herself, and by this means she achieved easier weaning than with X.

lowed this up with a talk about his own history. He said he never had teddies. There was a bell rope which hung down, a tag end of which he would go on hitting, and so go off to sleep. Probably in the end it fell, and that was the end of it. There was, however, something else. He was very shy about this. It was a purple rabbit with red eyes. 'I wasn't fond of it. I used to throw it around. Jeremy has it now. I gave it to him. I gave it to Jeremy because it was naughty. It *would* fall off the chest of drawers. *It still visits me. I like it to visit me.*' He surprised himself when he drew the purple rabbit. It will be noted that

		Thumb	*Transitional Object*		*Type of Child*
X	Boy	O	Mother	Rabbit (comforter)	Mother-fixated
Y	Boy	+	'Baa'	Jersey (soother)	Free
Twins {	Girl	O	Dummy	Donkey (friend)	Late maturity
	Boy	O	'Ee'	Ee (protective)	Latent psychopathic
Chil- {	Girl	O	'Baa'	Blanket (reassurance)	Developing well
dren {	Girl	+	Thumb	Thumb (satisfaction)	,, ,,
of Y {	Boy	+	'Mimis'*	Objects (sorting)	,, ,,

* Innumerable similar soft objects distinguished by colour, length, width, and early subjected to sorting and classification.

this eleven-year-old boy with the ordinary good reality-sense of his age spoke as if lacking in reality-sense when describing the transitional object's qualities and activities. When I saw the mother later she expressed surprise that Angus remembered the purple rabbit. She easily recognized it from the coloured drawing.

I deliberately refrain from giving more case material here, particularly as I wish to avoid giving the impression that what I am reporting is rare. In practically every case history there is something to be found that is interesting in the transitional phenomena, or in their absence (cf. Stevenson, Olive, 1954).

THEORETICAL STUDY

There are certain comments that can be made on the basis of accepted psycho-analytic theory.

1. The transitional object stands for the breast, or the object of the first relationship.
2. The transitional object antedates established reality-testing.
3. In relation to the transitional object the infant passes from (magical) omnipotent control to control by manipulation (involving muscle erotism and coordination pleasure).
4. The transitional object may eventually develop into a fetish object and

so persist as a characteristic of the adult sexual life. (See Wulff's development of the theme.)

5. The transitional object may, because of anal-erotic organization, stand for faeces (but it is not for this reason that it may become smelly and remain unwashed).

Relationship to Internal Object (Klein)

It is interesting to compare the transitional object concept with Melanie Klein's concept of the internal object. The transitional object is *not an internal object* (which is a mental concept) — it is a possession. Yet it is not (for the infant) an external object either.

The following complex statement has to be made. The infant can employ a transitional object when the internal object is alive and real and good enough (not too persecutory). But this internal object depends for its qualities on the existence and aliveness and behaviour of the external object (breast, mother figure, general environmental care). Badness or failure of the latter indirectly leads to deadness or to a persecutory quality of internal object. After a persistence of failure of the external object the internal object fails to have meaning to the infant, and then, and then only, does the transitional object become meaningless too. The transitional object may therefore stand for the 'external' breast, but *indirectly* so, through standing for an 'internal' breast.

The transitional object is never under magical control like the internal object, nor is it outside control as the real mother is.

Illusion–Disillusionment

In order to prepare the ground for my own positive contribution to this subject I must put into words some of the things that I think are taken too easily for granted in many psycho-analytic writings on infantile emotional development, although they may be understood in practice.

There is no possibility whatever for an infant to proceed from the pleasure-principle to the reality principle or towards and beyond primary identification (see Freud, 1923, p. 14),[1] unless there is a good enough mother.[2] The good enough 'mother' (not necessarily the infant's own mother) is one who makes active adaptation to the infant's needs, an active adaptation that gradually

---

[1] See also Freud (1921), p. 65.

[2] One effect, and the main effect, of failure of the mother in this respect at the start of an infant's life, is discussed clearly (in my view) by Marion Milner (1952, p. 181). She shows that because of the mother's failure there is brought about a premature ego development, with precocious sorting out of a bad from a good object. The period of illusion (or my Transitional Phase) is disturbed. In analysis or in various activities in ordinary life an individual can be seen to be going on seeking the valuable resting-place of illusion. Illusion in this way has its positive value. See also Freud (1950).

lessens, according to the infant's growing ability to account for failure of adaptation and to tolerate the results of frustration. Naturally the infant's own mother is more likely to be good enough than some other person, since this active adaptation demands an easy and unresented preoccupation with the one infant; in fact, success in infant care depends on the fact of devotion, not on cleverness or intellectual enlightenment.

The good-enough mother, as I have stated, starts off with an almost complete adaptation to her infant's needs, and as time proceeds she adapts less and less completely, gradually, according to the infant's growing ability to deal with her failure.

The infant's means of dealing with this maternal failure include the following:

> The infant's experience, often repeated, that there is a time limit to frustration. At first, naturally, this time limit must be short.
> A growing sense of process.
> The beginnings of mental activity.
> The employment of auto-erotic satisfactions.
> Remembering, reliving, fantasying, dreaming; the integrating of past, present, and future.

If all goes well the infant can actually come to gain from the experience of frustration, since incomplete adaptation to need makes objects real, that is to say hated as well as loved. The consequence of this is that *if all goes well* the infant can be disturbed by a close adaptation to need that is continued too long, not allowed its natural decrease, since exact adaptation resembles magic and the object that behaves perfectly becomes no better than an hallucination. Nevertheless *at the start* adaptation needs to be almost exact, and unless this is so it is not possible for the infant to begin to develop a capacity to experience a relationship to external reality, or even to form a conception of external reality.

Illusion and the Value of Illusion

The mother, at the beginning, by an almost 100 per cent adaptation affords the infant the opportunity for the *illusion* that her breast is part of the infant. It is, as it were, under magical control. The same can be said in terms of infant care in general, in the quiet times between excitements. Omnipotence is nearly a fact of experience. The mother's eventual task is gradually to disillusion the infant, but she has no hope of success unless at first she has been able to give sufficient opportunity for illusion.

In another language, the breast is created by the infant over and over again out of the infant's capacity to love or (one can say) out of need. A subjective phenomenon develops in the baby which we call the mother's breast.[1] The mother places the actual breast just there where the infant is ready to create, and at the right moment.

From birth, therefore, the human being is concerned with the problem of the relationship between what is objectively perceived and what is subjectively conceived of, and in the solution of this problem there is no health for the human being who has not been started off well enough by the mother. *The intermediate area to which I am referring is the area that is allowed to the infant between primary creativity and objective perception based on reality-testing*. The transitional phenomena represent the early stages of the use of illusion, without which there is no meaning for the human being in the idea of a relationship with an object that is perceived by others as external to that being.

The idea illustrated in *Fig.* 19 is this: that at some theoretical point early in the development of every human individual an infant in a certain setting provided by the mother is capable of conceiving of the idea of something which would meet the growing need which arises out of instinctual tension. The infant cannot be said to know at first what is to be created. At this point in time the mother presents herself. In the ordinary way she gives her breast and her potential feeding urge. The mother's adaptation to the infant's needs, when good enough, gives the infant the *illusion* that there is an external reality that corresponds to the infant's own capacity to create. In other words, there is an overlap between what the mother supplies and what the child might conceive of. To the observer the child perceives what the mother actually presents, but this is not the whole truth. The infant perceives the breast only in so far as a breast could be created just there and then. There is no interchange between the mother and the infant. Psychologically the infant takes from a breast that is part of the infant, and the mother gives milk to an infant that is part of herself. In psychology, the idea of interchange is based on an illusion.

In *Fig.* 20 a shape is given to the area of illusion, to illustrate what I consider to be the main function of the transitional object and of transitional phenomena. The transitional object and the transitional phenomena start each human being off with what will always be important for them, i.e. a neutral area of experience which will not be challenged. *Of the transitional object it can be said that it is a matter of agreement between us and the baby that we will never ask the question 'Did you conceive of this or was it presented to you from*

[1] I include the whole technique of mothering. When it is said that the first object is the breast, the word 'breast' is used, I believe, to stand for the technique of mothering as well as for the actual flesh. It is not impossible for a mother to be a good-enough mother (in my way of putting it) with a bottle for the actual feeding. If this wide meaning of the word 'breast' is kept in mind, and maternal technique is seen to be included in the total meaning of the term, then there is a bridge forming between the wording of Melanie Klein's statement of early history and that of Anna Freud. The only difference left is one of dates, which is in fact an unimportant difference which will automatically disappear in the course of time.

FIG. 19   FIG. 20

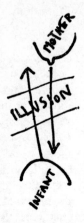

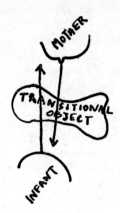

without?' The important point is that no decision on this point is expected. The question is not to be formulated.

This problem, which undoubtedly concerns the human infant in a hidden way at the beginning, gradually becomes an obvious problem on account of the fact that the mother's main task (next to providing opportunity for illusion) is disillusionment. This is preliminary to the task of weaning, and it also continues as one of the tasks of parents and educators. In other words, this matter of *illusion* is one which belongs inherently to human beings and which no individual finally solves for himself or herself, although a *theoretical* understanding of it may provide a *theoretical* solution. If things go well, in this gradual disillusionment process, the stage is set for the frustrations that we gather together under the word weaning; but it should be remembered that when we talk about the phenomena (which Klein has specifically illuminated) that cluster round weaning we are assuming the underlying process, the process by which opportunity for illusion and gradual disillusionment is provided. If illusion-disillusionment has gone astray the infant cannot attain to so normal a thing as weaning, nor to a reaction to weaning, and it is then absurd to refer to weaning at all. The mere termination of breast feeding is not a weaning.

We can see the tremendous significance of weaning in the case of the normal child. When we witness the complex reaction that is set going in a certain child by the weaning process we know that this is able to take place in that child because the illusion-disillusionment process is being carried through so well that we can ignore it while discussing actual weaning.

It is assumed here that the task of reality-acceptance is never completed, that no human being is free from the strain of relating inner and outer reality, and that relief from this strain is provided by an intermediate area of experience which is not challenged (arts, religion, etc.). (cf. Riviere, 1936). This intermediate area is in direct continuity with the play area of the small child who is 'lost' in play.

In infancy this intermediate area is necessary for the initiation of a relationship between the child and the world, and is made possible by good enough mothering at the early critical phase. Essential to all this is continuity (in time) of the external emotional environment and of particular elements in the physical environment such as the transitional object or objects.

The transitional phenomena are allowable to the infant because of the parents' intuitive recognition of the strain inherent in objective perception, and we do not challenge the infant in regard to subjectivity or objectivity just here where there is the transitional object.

Should an adult make claims on us for our acceptance of the objectivity of his subjective phenomena we discern or diagnose madness. If, however, the adult can manage to enjoy the personal intermediate area without making claims, then we can acknowledge our own corresponding intermediate areas, and are pleased to find examples of overlapping, that is to say common experience between members of a group in art or religion or philosophy.

I wish to draw particular attention to the paper by Wulff, referred to above, in which clinical material is given illustrating exactly that which I am referring to under the heading of transitional objects and transitional phenomena. There is a difference between my point of view and that of Wulff which is reflected in my use of this special term and his use of the term 'fetish object'. A study of Wulff's paper seems to show that in using the word fetish he has taken back to infancy something that belongs in ordinary theory to the sexual perversions. I am not able to find in his article sufficient room for the consideration of the child's transitional object as a healthy early experience. Yet I do consider that transitional phenomena are healthy and universal. Moreover if we extend the use of the word fetish to cover normal phenomena we shall perhaps be losing some of the value of the term.

I would prefer to retain the word fetish to describe the object that is employed on account of a *delusion* of a maternal phallus. I would then go further and say that we must keep a place for the *illusion* of a maternal phallus, that is to say, an idea that is universal and not pathological. If we shift the accent now from the object on to the word illusion we get near to the infant's transitional object; the importance lies in the concept of illusion, a universal in the field of experience.

Following this, we can allow the transitional object to be potentially a maternal phallus but originally the breast, that is to say, the thing created by the infant and at the same time provided from the environment. In this way I think that a study of the infant's use of the transitional object and of transitional phenomena in general may throw light on the origin of the fetish object and of fetishism. There is something to be lost, however, in working backwards from the psychopathology of fetishism to the transitional phenomena which belong to the beginnings of experience and which are inherent in healthy emotional development.

SUMMARY

Attention is drawn to the rich field for observation provided by the earliest experiences of the healthy infant as expressed principally in the relationship to the first possession.

This first possession is related backwards in time to auto-erotic phenomena and fist- and thumb-sucking, and also forwards to the first soft animal or doll and to hard toys. It is related both to the external object (mother's breast) and to internal objects (magically introjected breast), but is distinct from each.

The transitional objects and transitional phenomena belong to the realm of illusion which is at the basis of initiation of experience. This early stage in development is made possible by the mother's special capacity for making adaptation to the needs of her infant, thus allowing the infant the illusion that what the infant creates really exists.

This intermediate area of experience, unchallenged in respect of its belonging to inner or external (shared) reality, constitutes the greater part of the infant's experience and throughout life is retained in the intense experiencing that belongs to the arts and to religion and to imaginative living, and to creative scientific work.

A positive value of illusion can therefore be stated.

An infant's transitional object ordinarily becomes gradually decathected, especially as cultural interests develop.

In psychopathology:

Addiction can be stated in terms of regression to the early stage at which the transitional phenomena are unchallenged.

Fetishism can be described in terms of a persistence of a specific object or type of object dating from infantile experience in the transitional field, linked with the delusion of a maternal phallus.

Pseudologia fantastica and thieving can be described in terms of an individual's unconscious urge to bridge a gap in continuity of experience in respect of a transitional object.

Chapter XIX

Mind and its Relation to the Psyche-Soma[1]
[1949]

'TO ASCERTAIN what exactly comprises the irreducible mental elements, particularly those of a dynamic nature, constitutes in my opinion one of our most fascinating final aims. These elements would necessarily have a somatic and probably a neurological equivalent, and in that way we should by scientific method have closely narrowed the age-old gap between mind and body. I venture to predict that then the antithesis which has baffled all the philosophers will be found to be based on an illusion. In other words, *I do not think that the mind really exists as an entity* — possibly a startling thing for a psychologist to say [my italics]. When we talk of the mind influencing the body or the body influencing the mind we are merely using a convenient shorthand for a more cumbrous phrase . . .' (Jones, 1946).

This quotation by Scott (1949) stimulated me to try to sort out my own ideas on this vast and difficult subject. The body scheme with its temporal and spatial aspects provides a valuable statement of the individual's diagram of himself, and in it I believe there is no obvious place for the mind. Yet in clinical practice we do meet with the mind as an entity localized somewhere by the patient; a further study of the paradox that 'mind does not really exist as an entity' is therefore necessary.

MIND AS A FUNCTION OF PSYCHE-SOMA

To study the concept of mind one must always be studying an individual, a total individual, and including the development of that individual from the very beginning of psychosomatic existence. If one accepts this discipline then

[1] A paper read before the Medical Section of the British Psychological Society, 14th December, 1949, and revised October 1953. *Brit. J. Med. Psychol.*, Vol. XXVII, 1954.

one can study the mind of an individual as it specializes out from the psyche part of the psyche-soma.

The mind does not exist as an entity in the individual's scheme of things provided the individual psyche-soma or body scheme has come satisfactorily through the very early developmental stages; mind is then no more than a special case of the functioning of the psyche-soma.

In the study of a developing individual the mind will often be found to be developing a *false entity*, and a *false localization*. A study of these abnormal tendencies must precede the more direct examination of the mind-specialization of the healthy or normal psyche.

We are quite used to seeing the two words mental and physical opposed and would not quarrel with their being opposed in daily conversation. It is quite another matter, however, if the concepts are opposed in scientific discussion.

The use of these two words physical and mental in describing disease leads us into trouble immediately. The psychosomatic disorders, half-way between the mental and the physical, are in a rather precarious position. Research into psychosomatics is being held up, to some extent, by the muddle to which I am referring (MacAlpine, 1952). Also, neuro-surgeons are doing things to the normal or healthy brain in an attempt to alter or even improve mental states. These 'physical' therapists are completely at sea in their theory; curiously enough they seem to be leaving out the importance of the physical body, of which the brain is an integral part.

Let us attempt, therefore, to think of the developing individual, starting at the beginning. Here is a body, and the psyche and the soma are not to be distinguished except according to the direction from which one is looking. One can look at the developing body or at the developing psyche. I suppose the word psyche here means the *imaginative elaboration of somatic parts, feelings, and functions*, that is, of physical aliveness. We know that this imaginative elaboration is dependent on the existence and the healthy functioning of the brain, especially certain parts of it. The psyche is not, however, felt by the individual to be localized in the brain, or indeed to be localized anywhere.

Gradually the psyche and the soma aspects of the growing person become involved in a process of mutual interrelation. This interrelating of the psyche with the soma constitutes an early phase of individual development (see Chapter XII). At a later stage the live body, with its limits, and with an inside and an outside, is *felt by the individual* to form the core for the imaginative self. The development to this stage is extremely complex, and although this development may possibly be fairly complete by the time a baby has been born a few days, there is a vast opportunity for distortion of the natural course of development in these respects. Moreover, whatever applies to very early stages also applies to some extent to all stages, even to the stage that we call adult maturity.

THEORY OF MIND

On the basis of these preliminary considerations I find myself putting forward a theory of mind. This theory is based on work with analytic patients who have needed to regress to an extremely early level of development in the transference. In this paper I shall only give one piece of illustrative clinical material, but the theory can, I believe, be found to be valuable in our daily analytic work.

Let us assume that health in the early development of the individual entails *continuity of being*. The early psyche-soma proceeds along a certain line of development provided its *continuity of being is not disturbed*; in other words, for the healthy development of the early psyche-soma there is a need for a *perfect* environment. At first the need is absolute.

The perfect environment is one which *actively adapts* to the needs of the newly formed psyche-soma, that which we as observers know to be the infant at the start. A bad environment is bad because by failure to adapt it becomes an *impingement* to which the psyche-soma (i.e. the infant) must *react*. This reacting disturbs the continuity of the going-on-being of the new individual. In its beginnings the good (psychological) environment is a physical one, with the child in the womb or being held and generally tended; only in the course of time does the environment develop a new characteristic which necessitates a new descriptive term, such as emotional or psychological or social. Out of this emerges the ordinary good mother with her ability to make active adaptation to her infant's needs arising out of her devotion, made possible by her narcissism, her imagination, and her memories, which enable her to know through identification what are her baby's needs.

The need for a good environment, which is absolute at first, rapidly becomes relative. *The ordinary good mother is good enough.* If she is *good enough* the infant becomes able to allow for her deficiencies by mental activity. This applies to meeting not only instinctual impulses but also all the most primitive types of ego need, even including the need for negative care or an alive neglect. The mental activity of the infant turns a *good-enough* environment into a perfect environment, that is to say, turns relative failure of adaptation into adaptive success. What releases the mother from her need to be near-perfect is the infant's understanding. In the ordinary course of events the mother tries not to introduce complications beyond those which the infant can understand and allow for; in particular she tries to insulate her baby from coincidences and from other phenomena that must be beyond the infant's ability to comprehend. In a general way she keeps the world of the infant as simple as possible.

The mind, then, has as one of its roots a variable functioning of the psyche-soma, one concerned with the threat to continuity of being that follows any failure of (active) environmental adaptation, It follows that mind-development is very much influenced by factors not specifically personal to the individual, including chance events.

In infant care it is vitally important that mothers, at first physically, and soon also imaginatively, can start off by supplying this active adaptation, but also it is a characteristic maternal function to provide *graduated failure of adaptation*, according to the growing ability of the individual infant to allow for relative failure by mental activity, or by understanding. Thus there appears in the infant a tolerance in respect of both ego need and instinctual tension.

It could perhaps be shown that mothers are released slowly by infants who eventually are found to have a low I.Q. On the other hand, an infant with an exceptionally good brain, eventually giving a high I.Q., releases the mother earlier.

According to this theory then, in the development of every individual, the mind has a root, perhaps its most important root, in the need of the individual, at the core of the self, for a perfect environment. In this connection, I might refer to my view of psychosis as an environmental deficiency disease (see chapter XVII). There are certain developments of this theory which seem to me to be important. Certain kinds of failure on the part of the mother, especially erratic behaviour, produce over-activity of the mental functioning. Here, in the overgrowth of the mental function reactive to erratic mothering, we see that there can develop an opposition between the mind and the psyche-soma, since in reaction to this abnormal environmental state the thinking of the individual begins to take over and organize the caring for the psyche-soma, whereas in health it is the function of the environment to do this. In health the mind does not usurp the environment's function, but makes possible an understanding and eventually a making use of its relative failure.

The gradual process whereby the individual becomes able to care for the self belongs to later stages in individual emotional development, stages that must be reached in due course, at the pace that is set by natural developmental forces.

To go a stage further, one might ask what happens if the strain that is put on mental functioning organized in defence against a tantalizing early environment is greater and greater? One would expect confusional states, and (in the extreme) mental defect of the kind that is not dependent on brain-tissue deficiency. As a more common result of the lesser degrees of tantalizing infant care in the earliest stages we find *mental functioning becoming a thing in itself*, practically replacing the good mother and making her unnecessary. Clinically, this can go along with dependence on the actual mother and a false personal growth on a compliance basis. This is a most uncomfortable state of affairs, especially because the psyche of the individual gets 'seduced' away into this mind from the intimate relationship which the psyche originally had with the soma. The result is a mind-psyche, which is pathological.

A person who is developing in this way displays a distorted pattern affecting all later stages of development. For instance, one can observe a tendency for easy identification with the environmental aspect of all relationships that involve dependence, and a difficulty in identification with the dependent individual. Clinically one may see such a person develop into one who is a *marvellously good mother to others* for a limited period; in fact a person who has developed along these lines may have almost magical *healing properties* because of an extreme capacity to make active adaptation to primitive needs. The falsity of these patterns for expression of the personality, however, becomes evident in practice. Breakdown threatens or occurs, because what the individual is all the time needing is *to find someone else* who will make real this 'good environment' concept, so that the individual may return to the dependent psyche-soma which forms the only place to live from. In this case, 'without mind' becomes a desired state.

There cannot of course be a direct partnership between the mind-psyche and the body of the individual. But the *mind*-psyche is localized by the individual, and is placed either inside the head or outside it in some special relation to the head, and this provides an important source for headache as a symptom.

The question has to be asked why the head should be the place inside which the mind tends to become localized by the individual, and I do not know the answer. I feel that an important point is the individual's need to localize the mind because it is an enemy, that is to say, for control of it. A schizoid patient tells me that the head is the place to put the mind because, *as the head cannot be seen by oneself*, it does not obviously exist as part of oneself. Another point is that the head has special experiences during the birth process, but in order to make full use of this latter fact I must go on to consider another type of mental functioning which can be specially activated during the birth process. This is associated with the word 'memorizing'.

As I have said, the continuity of being of the developing psyche-soma (internal and external relationships) is disturbed by reactions to environmental impingements, in other words by the results of failures of the environment to make active adaptation. By my theory a rapidly increasing amount of reaction to impingement disturbing continuity of psyche-soma becomes expected and allowed for according to mental capacity. Impingements demanding *excessive* reactions (according to the next part of my theory) cannot be allowed for. All that can happen apart from confusion is that the reactions can be *catalogued*.[1] Typically at birth there is apt to be an excessive

[1] Cf. Freud's theory of obsessional neurosis (1909).

disturbance of continuity because of reactions to impingements, and the mental activity which I am describing at the moment is that which is concerned with exact memorizing during the birth process. In my psycho-analytic work I sometimes meet with regressions fully under control and yet going back to prenatal life. Patients regressed in an ordered way go over the birth process again and again, and I have been astonished by the convincing proof that I have had that an infant during the birth process not only memorizes every reaction disturbing the continuity of being, but also appears to memorize these in the correct order. I have not used hypnosis, but I am aware of the comparable discoveries, less convincing to me, that are achieved through use of hypnosis. Mental functioning of the type that I am describing, which might be called memorizing or cataloguing, can be extremely active and accurate at the time of a baby's birth. I shall illustrate this by details from a case, but first I want to make clear my point that *this type of mental functioning is an encumbrance to the psyche-soma,* or to the individual human being's continuity of being which constitutes the self. The individual may be able to make use of it to relive the birth process in play or in a carefully controlled analysis. But this cataloguing type of mental functioning acts like a foreign body if it is associated with environmental adaptive failure that is beyond understanding or prediction.

No doubt in health it may happen that the environmental factors are held fixed by this method until the individual is able to make them his own after having experienced libidinous and especially aggressive drives, which can be projected. In this way, and it is essentially a false way, the individual gets to feel responsible for the bad environment for which in fact he was not responsible and which he could (if he knew) justly blame on the world because it disturbed the continuity of his innate developmental processes before the psyche-soma had become sufficiently well organized to hate or to love. Instead of hating these environmental failures the individual became disorganized by them because the process existed prior to hating.

CLINICAL ILLUSTRATION

The following fragment of a case history is given to illustrate my thesis. Out of several years' intensive work it is notoriously difficult to choose a detail; nevertheless, I include this fragment in order to show that what I am putting forward is very much a part of daily practice with patients.

A woman[1] who is now 47 years old had made what seemed to others but not to herself to be a good relationship to the world and had always been able to earn her own living. She had achieved a good education and was generally liked; in fact I think she was never actively disliked. She herself, however,

[1] Case referred to again in another paper (see Chapter XXII pp. 279-80).

felt completely dissatisfied, as if always aiming to find herself and never succeeding. Suicidal ideas were certainly not absent but they were kept at bay by her belief which dated from childhood that she would ultimately solve her problem and find herself. She had had a so-called 'classical' analysis for several years but somehow the core of her illness had been unchanged. With me it soon became apparent that this patient must make a very severe regression or else give up the struggle. I therefore followed the regressive tendency, letting it take the patient wherever it led; eventually the regression reached the limit of the patient's need, and since then there has been a natural progression with the true self instead of a false self in action.

For the purpose of this paper I choose for description one thing out of an enormous amount of material. In the patient's previous analysis there had been incidents in which the patient had thrown herself off the couch in an hysterical way. These episodes had been interpreted along ordinary lines for hysterical phenomena of this kind. In the deeper regression of this new analysis light was thrown on the meaning of these falls. In the course of the two years of analysis with me the patient has repeatedly regressed to an early stage which was certainly prenatal. The birth process had to be relived, and eventually I recognized how this patient's unconscious need to relive the birth process underlay what had previously been an hysterical falling off the couch.

A great deal could be said about all this, but the important thing from my point of view here is that evidently every detail of the birth experience had been retained, and not only that, but the details had been retained in the exact sequence of the original experience. A dozen or more times the birth process was relived and each time the reaction to one of the major external features of the original birth process was singled out for re-experiencing.

Incidentally, these relivings illustrated one of the main functions of acting out; by acting out the patient informed herself of the bit of psychic reality which was difficult to get at at the moment, but of which the patient so acutely needed to become aware. I will enumerate some of the acting-out patterns, but unfortunately I cannot give the sequence which nevertheless I am quite sure was significant.

The breathing changes to be gone over in most elaborate detail.
The constrictions passing down the body to be relived and so remembered.
The birth from the fantasy inside of the belly of the mother, who was a depressive, unrelaxed person.
The changeover from not feeding to feeding from the breast, and then from the bottle.
The same with the addition that the patient had sucked her thumb in the womb and on coming out had to have the fist in relation to the breast

or bottle, thus making continuity between object relationships within and without.

The severe experience of pressure on the head, and also the extreme of awfulness of the release of pressure on the head; during which phase, unless her head were held, she could not have endured the re-enactment. There is much which is not yet understood in this analysis about the bladder functions affected by the birth process.

The changeover from pressure all round (which belongs to the intra-uterine state) to pressure from underneath (which belongs to the extra-uterine state). Pressure if not excessive means love. After birth therefore she was loved on the under side only, and unless turned round periodically became confused.

Here I must leave out perhaps a dozen other factors of comparable significance.

> Gradually the re-enactment reached the worst part. When we were nearly there, there was the anxiety of having the head crushed. This was first got under control by the patient's identification with the crushing mechanism. This was a dangerous phase because if acted out outside the transference situation it meant suicide. In this acting-out phase the patient existed in the crushing boulders or whatever might present, and the gratification came to her then from *destruction* of the head (including mind and false psyche) which had lost significance for the patient as part of the self.
>
> Ultimately the patient had to accept annihilation. We had already had many indications of a period of blackout or unconsciousness, and convulsive movements made it likely that there was at some time in infancy a minor fit. It appears that in the actual experience there was a loss of consciousness which could not be assimilated to the patient's self until accepted as a death. When this had become real the word death became wrong and the patient began to substitute 'a giving-in', and eventually the appropriate word was 'a not-knowing'.

In a full description of the case I should want to continue along these lines for some time, but development of this and other themes must be made in future publications. Acceptance of not-knowing produced tremendous relief. 'Knowing' became transformed into 'the analyst knows', that is to say, 'behaves reliably in active adaptation to the patient's needs'. The patient's whole life had been built up around mental functioning which had become falsely the place (in the head) from which she lived, and her life which had rightly seemed to her false had been developed out of this mental functioning.

Perhaps this clinical example illustrates what I mean when I say that I got from this analysis a feeling that the cataloguing of reactions to environmental impingements belonging to the time around about birth had been exact and complete; in fact I felt that the only alternative to the success of this cataloguing was absolute failure, hopeless confusion and mental defect.

But the case illustrates my theme in detail as well as generally.

I quote again from Scott (1949):

> Similarly when a patient in analysis loses his mind in the sense that he loses the illusion of needing a psychic apparatus which is separate from all that which he has called his body, his world, etc., etc., this loss is equivalent to the gain of all that conscious access to and control of the connections between the superficies and the depths, the boundaries and solidity of his Body Scheme — its memories, its perceptions, its images, etc., etc., which he had given up at an earlier period in his life when the duality soma-psyche began.

> Not infrequently in a patient whose first complaint is of fear of 'losing his mind' — the desire to lose such a belief and obtain a better one soon becomes apparent.

At this point of not-knowing in this analysis there appeared the memory of a bird that was seen as 'quite still except for the movements of the belly which indicated breathing'. In other words, the patient had reached, at 47 years, the state in which physiological functioning in general constitutes living. The psychical elaboration of this could follow. This psychical elaboration of physiological functioning is quite different from the intellectual work which so easily becomes artificially a thing in itself and falsely a place where the psyche can lodge.

Naturally only a glimpse of this patient can be given, and even if one chooses a small part, only a bit of this part can be described. I would like, however, to pursue a little the matter of the gap in consciousness. I need not describe the gap as it appeared in more 'forward' terms, the bottom of a pit, for instance, in which in the dark were all sorts of dead and dying bodies. Just now I am concerned only with the most primitive of the ways in which the gap was found, by the patient, by the reliving processes belonging to the transference situation. The gap in continuity, which throughout the patient's life had been actively denied, now became something urgently sought. We found a need to have the head broken into, and violent head-banging appeared as part of an attempt to produce a blackout. At times there was an urgent need for the destruction of the mental processes located by the patient in the head. A series of defences against full recognition of the desire to reach the gap in continuity of consciousness had to be dealt with before there could be acceptance of the not-knowing state. It happened that on the day on which this work reached its climax the patient stopped writing her diary.[1] This diary had been kept throughout the analysis, and it would be possible to reconstruct the whole of her analysis up to this time from it. There is little that the patient could perceive that has not been at least indicated in this diary. The meaning of the diary now became clear — it was a projection of her mental apparatus, and not a picture of the true self, which, in fact, had never lived till, at the bottom of the regression, there came a new chance for the true self to start.

The results of this bit of work led to a temporary phase in which there was no mind and no mental functioning. There had to be a temporary phase in which the breathing of her body was all. In this way the patient became able to accept the not-knowing condition because I was holding her and keeping a continuity by my own breathing, while she let go, gave in, knew nothing; it could not be any good, however, if I held her and maintained my own continuity of life if she were dead. What made my part operative was that I could see and hear her belly moving as she breathed (like the bird) and therefore I knew that she was alive.

Now for the first time she was able to have a psyche, an entity of her own, a body that breathes and in addition the beginning of fantasy belonging to the breathing and other physiological functions.

We as observers know, of course, that the mental functioning which enables the psyche to be there enriching the soma is dependent on the intact brain. But we do not place the psyche anywhere, not even in the brain on which it depends. For this patient, regressed in this way, these things were at last not important. I suppose she would now be prepared to locate the psyche wherever the soma is alive.

This patient has made considerable progress since this paper was read. Now in 1953 we are able to look back on the period of the stage I have chosen for description, and to see it in perspective. I do not need to modify what I have written. Except for the violent complication of the birth process body-memories, there has been no major disturbance of the patient's regression to a certain very early stage and subsequent forward movement towards a new existence as a real individual who feels real.

MIND LOCALIZED IN THE HEAD

I now leave my illustration and return to the subject of the localizing of the mind in the head. I have said that the imaginative elaboration of body parts and functions is not localized. There may, however, be localizations which are quite logical in the sense that they belong to the way in which the body functions. For instance, the body takes in and gives out substances. An inner world of personal imaginative experience therefore comes into the scheme of things,

[1] The diary was resumed at a later date, for a time, with a looser function, and a more positive aim including the idea of one day using her experiences profitably.

and shared reality is on the whole thought of as outside the personality. Although babies cannot draw pictures, I think that they are capable (except through lack of skill) of depicting themselves by a circle at certain moments in their first months. Perhaps if all is going well, they can achieve this soon after birth; at any rate we have good evidence that at six months a baby is at times using the circle or sphere as a diagram of the self. It is at this point that Scott's body scheme is so illuminating and especially his reminder that we are referring to time as well as to space. In the body scheme as I understand it there seems to me to be no place for the mind, and this is not a criticism of the body scheme as a diagram; it is a comment on the falsity of the concept of the mind as a localized phenomenon.

In trying to think out why the head is the place where either the mind is localized, or else outside which it is localized, I cannot help thinking of the way in which the head of the human baby is affected during birth, the time at which the mind is furiously active cataloguing reactions to a specific environmental persecution.

Cerebral functioning tends to be localized by people in the head in popular thought, and one of the consequences of this deserves special study. Until quite recently surgeons could be persuaded to open the skulls of mentally defective infants to make possible further development of their brains which were supposed to be constricted by the bones of the skull. I suppose the early trephining of the skull was for relief of *mind* disorders, i.e. for cure of persons whose mental functioning was their enemy and who had falsely localized their mental functioning in their heads. At the present time the curious thing is that once again in medical scientific thought the brain has got equated with the mind, which is felt by a certain kind of ill person to be an enemy, and a thing in the skull. The surgeon who does a leucotomy would *at first* seem to be doing what the patient asks for, that is, to be relieving the patient of mind activity, the mind having become the enemy of the psyche-soma. Nevertheless, we can see that the surgeon is caught up in the mental patient's false localization of the mind in the head, with its sequel, the equating of mind and brain. When he has done his work he has failed in the second half of his job. The patient wants to be relieved of the *mind activity* which has become a threat to the psyche-soma, but the patient next needs the full-functioning brain tissue *in order to be able to have psyche-soma existence.* By the operation of leucotomy with its irreversible brain changes the surgeon has made this impossible. The procedure has been of no use except through what the operation means to the patient. But the imaginative elaboration of somatic experience, the psyche, and for those who use the term, the soul, depend on the intact brain, as we know. We do not expect the *unconscious* of anyone to know such things, but we feel the neuro-surgeon ought to be *to some extent* affected by intellectual considerations.

In these terms we can see that one of the aims of *psychosomatic illness* is to draw the psyche from the mind back to the original intimate association with the soma. It is not sufficient to analyse the hypochondria of the psychosomatic patient, although this is an essential part of the treatment. One has also to be able to see the *positive value of the somatic disturbance* in its work of counteracting a 'seduction' of the psyche into the mind. Similarly, the aim of physiotherapists and the relaxationists can be understood in these terms. They do not have to know what they are doing to be successful psychotherapists. In one example of the application of these principles, if one tries to teach a pregnant woman how to do all the right things one not only makes her anxious, but one feeds the tendency of the psyche to lodge in the mental processes. *Per contra*, the relaxation methods at their best enable the mother to become body-conscious, and (if she is not a mental case) these methods help her to a continuity of being, and enable her to live as a psyche-soma. This is essential if she is to experience child-birth and the first stages of mothering in a natural way.

SUMMARY

1. The true self, a continuity of being, is in health based on psyche-soma growth.

2. Mental activity is a special case of the functioning of the psyche-soma.

3. Intact brain functioning is the basis for psyche-being as well as for mental activity.

4. There is no localization of a mind self, and there is no thing that can be called mind.

5. Two distinct bases for normal mental functioning can already be given, viz.: (*a*) conversion of good enough environment into perfect (adapted) environment, enabling minimum of reaction to impingement, and maximum of natural (continuous) self-development; and (*b*) cataloguing of impingements (birth trauma, etc.) for assimilation at later stages of development.

6. It is to be noted that psyche-soma growth is universal and its complexities are inherent, whereas mental development is somewhat dependent on variable factors such as the quality of early environmental factors, the chance phenomena of birth and of management immediately after birth, etc.

7. It is logical to oppose psyche and soma and therefore to oppose the emotional development and the bodily development of an individual. It is not logical, however, to oppose the mental and the physical as these are not of the same stuff. Mental phenomena are complications of variable importance in psyche-soma continuity of being, in that which adds up to the individual's 'self'.

Chapter XX

Withdrawal and Regression[1]
[1954]

IN THE COURSE of the last decade I have had forced on me the experience of several adult patients who made a regression in the transference in the course of analysis.

I wish to communicate an incident in the analysis of a patient who did not actually become clinically regressed but whose regressions were localized in momentary withdrawal states which occurred in the analytic sessions. My management of these withdrawal states was greatly influenced by my experience with regressed patients.

(By withdrawal in this paper I mean momentary detachment from a waking relationship with external reality, this detachment being sometimes of the nature of brief sleep. By regression I mean regression to dependence and not specifically regression in terms of erotogenic zones.)

I am choosing to give a series of six significant episodes chosen out of all the material belonging to the analysis of a schizoid-depressive patient. The patient is a married man with a family. At the onset of the present illness he had a breakdown, in which he felt unreal and lost what little capacity he had had for spontaneity. He was unable to work until some months after the analysis started, and at first he came to me as a patient from a mental hospital. (This patient had had a short period of analysis with me during the war, as a result of which he had made a clinical recovery from an acute disturbance of adolescence, but without gaining insight.)

The main thing that keeps this patient consciously seeking analysis is his inability to be impulsive and to make original remarks, although he can join very intelligently in serious conversation originated by other people. He is

[1] Read at the XVIIème Conférence des Psychanalystes de Langues Romanes, Paris, November 1954, and to the British Psycho-Analytical Society, 29th June, 1955. *Revue Française de Psychanalyse*, tome XIX, nos. 1–2, Jan-Juin 1955; *Psyche*, heft X, 1956–7.

almost friendless because his friendships are spoiled by his lack of ability to originate anything, which makes him a boring companion. (He reported having laughed once at the cinema, and this small evidence of improvement made him feel hopeful about the outcome of the analysis.)

Over a long period his free associations were in the form of a rhetorical report of a conversation that was going on all the time inside, his free associations being carefully arranged and presented in a way that he felt would make the material interesting to the analyst.

Like many other patients in analysis, this patient at times sinks deep into the analytic situation; on important but rare occasions he becomes withdrawn; during these moments of withdrawal unexpected things happen which he is sometimes able to report. I shall pick out these rare happenings for the purpose of this paper from the vast mass of ordinary psycho-analytic material which I must ask my reader to take for granted.

Episodes 1 and 2

The first of these happenings (the fantasy of which he was only just able to capture and to report) was that, in a momentary withdrawn state on the couch, he had *curled up and rolled over the back of the couch*. This was the first direct evidence in the analysis of a spontaneous self. The next withdrawn moment occurred a few weeks later. He had just made an attempt to use me as a substitute for his father (who had died when the patient was 18) and had asked me my advice about a detail in his work. I had first of all discussed this detail with him, pointing out, however, that he needed me as an analyst and not as a father-substitute. He had said it would be a waste of time to go on talking in his ordinary way, and then said that he had become withdrawn and felt this as a flight from something. He could not remember any dream belonging to this moment of sleep. I pointed out to him that his withdrawal was at that time a flight from the painful experience of being exactly between waking and sleeping, or between talking to me rationally and being withdrawn. It was at this point that he just managed to tell me that he had again had the idea of being *curled up*, although in actual fact he was lying on his back as usual, with his hands together across his chest.

It is here that I made the first of the interpretations which I know I would not have made twenty years ago. This interpretation turned out to be highly significant. When he spoke of being curled up, he made movements with his hands to show that his curled-up position was somewhere in front of his face and that he was moving around in the curled-up position. I immediately said to him: 'In speaking of yourself as curled up and moving round, you are at the same time implying something which naturally you are not describing since you are not aware of it; you imply the *existence of a medium*.' After a while I asked him if he understood what I meant and I found that he had

256

immediately understood; he said, 'Like the oil in which wheels move.' Having now received the idea of the medium holding him, he went on to describe in words what he had shown with his hands, which was that he had been twirling round forwards, and he contrasted this with the twirling round backwards over the couch which he had reported a few weeks previously.

From this interpretation of the medium I was able to go on to develop the theme of the analytic situation and together we worked out a rather clear statement of the specialized conditions provided by the analyst, and of the limits of the analyst's capacity for adaptation to the patient's needs. Following this the patient had a very important dream, and the analysis of this showed that he had been able to discard a shield which was now no longer necessary since I had proved myself capable of supplying a suitable medium at the moment of his withdrawal. It appears that *through my immediately putting a medium around his withdrawn self I had converted his withdrawal into a regression*, and so had enabled him to use this experience constructively. I would have missed this opportunity in the early days of my analytic career. The patient described this analytic session as 'momentous'.

There was a very big result from this detail of analysis: a clearer understanding of the part I could play as analyst; a recognition of the dependence which must at times be very great even although painful to bear; and also a coming to grips with his reality situation both at work and at home in a completely new way. Incidentally he was able to tell me that his wife had become pregnant and this made it very easy for him to link his curled-up state in the medium with the idea of a foetus in the womb. He had in fact identified with his own child and at the same time had made an acknowledgement of his own original dependence on his mother.

The next time he met his mother after this session he was able for the first time to ask her how much the analysis was costing her, and to allow himself to feel concerned about this. In the next session he was able to get at his criticisms of me and to express his suspicion that I was a swindler.

Episode 3

The next detail came some months later, after a very rich period of analysis. It came at a time when the material was of an anal quality and the homosexual aspect of the transference situation, an aspect of analysis which especially frightened him, had been reintroduced. He reported that in childhood he had had a constant fear of being chased by a man. I made certain interpretations and he reported that while I had been talking he had been *far away, at a factory*. In ordinary language his 'thoughts had wandered'. This wandering off was very real to him, and he had felt as if he was actually working at the factory to which he had gone when he ended the earlier phase of his analysis with me (which had had to be terminated because of the war). Immediately

I made the interpretation that he had gone away *from my lap*. The word lap was appropriate because in his withdrawn state and in terms of emotional development he had been at a stage of infancy, so that the couch had automatically become the analyst's lap. It will readily be seen that there is a relationship between my supplying the lap for him to come back to, and my supplying the medium on which depended his capacity to move round in a curled-up position in space.

Episode 4

The fourth episode that I wish to pick out is not so clear. It came in a session in which he said that he was unable to make love. The general material enabled me to interpret the dissociation in his relation to the world; on the one hand spontaneity from the *true* self which has no hope of finding an object except in imagination; and, on the other hand, response to stimulus from a self that is somewhat *false* or unreal. In the interpretation I pointed out that he was hoping to be able to join up this split in himself in his relation to me. At this point he sank into a withdrawn state for a brief period, and then was able to tell me what had happened when he was withdrawn; *it had become dark, clouds had gathered and it had started to rain; the rain had beaten down on his naked body*. On this occasion I was able to put into this cruel, ruthless environment himself, a newborn baby, and to point out to him what kind of environment he might expect should he become integrated and independent. Here was the 'medium' interpretation in reversed form.

Episode 5

The fifth detail comes from the material presented after a break of nine weeks which included my summer holiday.

The patient came back after the long break saying that he was not sure why he had come back; and that he found it difficult to start again. The main thing he reported was a continued difficulty in making a spontaneous remark of any kind either at home or among friends. He could only join in a conversation, and this was easiest when there were two others present who were taking the responsibility by talking to each other. If he made a remark he felt he was usurping the function of one of the parents (that is to say in the primal scene) whereas what he needed was to be recognized by the parents as an infant. He told me enough about himself to keep me in touch with current affairs.

This fifth episode was reached through consideration of an ordinary dream.

The night after this first session he had a dream which he reported the following day. It was unusually vivid. He went on a weekend trip abroad, *going on the Saturday and returning on the Monday.* The main thing about the trip was that he would meet a patient who had gone abroad from a hospital for treatment. (This turned out to be a patient who has had a limb amputated. There were other important details that do not specifically concern the subject of this communication.)

My first interpretation was the comment that in the dream *he goes and comes back.* It is this comment that I wish to report, since it joins up with my comments on the first two episodes in which I had provided a medium and a lap, and with that on the fourth episode in which I put an individual in the bad environment that had been hallucinated. I followed with a fuller interpretation, namely that the dream expresses the two aspects of his relationship to analysis; in one he goes away and comes back, and in the other he goes abroad, the patient from hospital standing for this part of himself; he goes and keeps in touch with the patient, which means that he is trying to break down the dissociation between these two aspects of himself. My patient followed this up by saying that in the dream he was particularly keen to make contact with the patient, implying that he was becoming aware of dissociation or splitting in himself, and wishing to become integrated.

This episode could be in the form of a dream dreamed away from analysis because it contained both elements together, the withdrawn self and the environmental provision. The medium aspect of the analyst had become introjected.

I further interpreted: the dream showed how the patient dealt with the holiday; he had been able to enjoy the experience of escaping from the treatment while at the same time he knew that although he had gone away he would come back. In this way the particularly long break which might have been serious in this type of patient was not a great disturbance. The patient made a particular point that this matter of going off and away was closely associated in his mind with the idea of making an original remark or doing anything spontaneous. He then told me that he had had, on the very day of the dream, a return of a special fear of his, that he would find that he had suddenly kissed a person; it would be anyone who happened to be next him; this might turn out to be a man. He would not make such a fool of himself if he found he had unexpectedly kissed a woman.

He now began to sink more deeply into the analytic situation. He felt he was a little child at home, and if he spoke it would be wrong; because he would then be in the parents' place. There was a feeling of hopelessness about having a spontaneous gesture met (and this fits in with what is known of the home situation). Much deeper material now emerged and he felt that there were people going in and out of the doors; my interpretation that this was associated with breathing was supported by further associations on his part. Ideas are like breath; also they are like children, and if I do nothing to them he feels they are abandoned. His great fear is of the abandoned child or the abandoned idea or remark, or the wasted gesture of a child.

Episode 6

A week later the patient (unexpectedly from his point of view), came up against the fact that he had never accepted his father's death. This followed a dream in which his father had been present and had been able to discuss current sexual problems with him in a sensible and free way. Two days later he came and reported that he had been seriously disturbed because he had had a *headache*, quite different from any that he had ever had before. It dated more or less from the time of the previous session two days earlier. This headache was temporal and sometimes frontal and *it was as if it were situated just outside the head.* It was constant and made him feel ill and if he could have got sympathy from his wife he would not have come to analysis but would have gone to bed. He was bothered because as a doctor he could see that this was certainly a functional disorder and yet it could not be explained in terms of physiology. (It was therefore like a madness.)

In the course of the hour I was able to see what interpretation was applicable and I said: 'The pain being just *outside* the head represents your *need to have your head held* as you would naturally have it held if you were in a state of deep emotional distress as a child.' At first this did not mean very much to him but gradually it became clear. That the person who was more likely to have held his head at the right moment and in the right way when he was a child was not his mother but his father. In other words, after his father's death there was no one to hold his head should he break down into experiencing grief.

I linked up my interpretation with the key interpretation of the medium, and gradually he felt that my idea about the hands was right. He reported a momentary withdrawal with a feeling that I had a machine which I could activate and which would supply the trappings of sympathetic management. This meant to him that it was important that I did not hold his head actually and in fact, as this would have been a mechanical application of technical principles. *The important thing was that I understood immediately what he needed.*

At the end of the hour he surprised himself by remembering that he had spent the afternoon holding a child's head. The child had been having a minor operation under local anaesthetic and this had taken more than an hour. He had done all he could to help the child but without much success. What he had felt the child must need was that his head should be held.

He now felt in rather a deep way that my interpretation had been the thing for which he had come to analysis on that day, and he was therefore almost grateful to his wife that she had offered no sympathy whatever and had not held his head as she might have done.

SUMMARY

The idea behind this communication is that if we know about regression in the analytic hour, we can meet it immediately and in this way enable certain patients who are not too ill to make the necessary regressions in short phases, perhaps even almost momentarily. I would say that *in the withdrawn state a patient is holding the self* and that if immediately the withdrawn state appears *the analyst can hold the patient*, then what would otherwise have been a withdrawal state becomes a regression. The advantage of a *regression* is that it carries with it the opportunity for correction of inadequate adaptation-to-need in the past history of the patient, that is to say, in the patient's infancy management. By contrast the *withdrawn* state is not profitable and when the patient recovers from a withdrawn state he or she is not changed.

Whenever we understand a patient in a deep way and show that we do so by a correct and well-timed interpretation we are in fact holding the patient, and taking part in a relationship in which the patient is in some degree regressed and dependent.

It is commonly thought that there is some danger in the regression of a patient during psycho-analysis. The danger does not lie in the regression but in the analyst's unreadiness to meet the regression and the dependence which belongs to it. When an analyst has had experience that makes him confident in his management of regression, then it is probably true to say that the more quickly the analyst accepts the regression and meets it fully the less likely is it that the patient will need to enter into an illness with regressive qualities.

Chapter XXI

The Depressive Position in Normal Emotional Development[1]

[1954-5]

THIS IS AN ATTEMPT to give a personal account of Melanie Klein's concept of the Depressive Position. To be fair to her I ought to state that I was not in analysis with her, nor with anyone analysed by her. I was drawn to study her contribution by its value for me in my own work with children, and I received instruction from her between 1935 and 1940 in case supervision. Klein's own account is to be found in her writings (1935, 1940).

The word 'normal' in the title is important. The Oedipus complex characterizes normal or healthy development of children, and the Depressive Position is a normal stage in the development of healthy infants (and so also is absolute dependence, or primary narcissism, a normal stage of the healthy infant at or near the start).

What I shall stress is the depressive position in emotional development *as an achievement*.

A feature of the depressive position is that it applies to an area of clinical psychiatry that is half-way between the places of origin of psychoneurosis and of psychosis respectively.

The child (or adult) who has reached that capacity for interpersonal relationships which characterizes the toddler stage in health, and for whom ordinary analysis of the infinite variations of triangular human relationships is feasible, has passed *through and beyond* the depressive position. On the other hand, the child (or adult) who is chiefly concerned with the innate problems of personality integration and with the initiation of a relationship with environment is not yet at the depressive position in personal development.

In terms of environment: the toddler is in a family situation, working out an instinctual life in interpersonal relationships, and the baby is being held by

[1] Paper read before the British Psychological Society, Medical Section, February 1954. *Brit. J. Med. Psychol.* Vol. XXVIII, 1955.

a mother who adapts to ego needs; in between the two is the infant or small child arriving at the depressive position, being held by the mother, but more than that, being held over a phase of living. It will be noted that *a time factor* has entered, and the mother *holds a situation* so that the infant has the chance to work through the consequences of instinctual experiences; as we shall see, the working through is quite comparable to the digestive process, and is comparably complex.

The mother holds the situation, and does so over and over again, and at a critical period in the baby's life. The consequence is that something can be done about something. The mother's technique enables the infant's co-existing love and hate to become sorted out and interrelated and gradually brought under control from within in a way that is healthy.[1]

Think of a baby at the weaning age. The actual time of weaning varies according to the cultural pattern, but for me the weaning age is that at which the infant becomes able to play at dropping things. The game of dropping things starts somewhere about five months and is a regular feature till, say, one year or eighteen months. So let us think in terms of any baby who has developed the dropping game to a fine art — say nine months old (see Freud, 1920. See also Chapter IV).

The depressive position is an achievement that belongs to the weaning age. If all goes well the depressive position is reached and established somewhere in the second half of the first year. Often it takes much longer to become established, even in more or less healthy development. We know also that in many children and adults who are in analysis the approach and reapproach to the depressive position is an important feature of the analysis, indicating progress and at the same time implying earlier failure at this developmental stage. An exact age need not be fixed. Perhaps some infants reach a moment of depressive position achievement earlier than at six months, perhaps even much earlier. Such an achievement would provide a favourable sign, but would not imply that the depressive position had become an established phenomenon. If I find an analyst claiming too much for the depressive position in the development that belongs to the first six months of life, I feel inclined to make the comment: what a pity to spoil a valuable concept by making it difficult to believe in.

My reason for not looking for this phase in the first months is not that I think early infancy is without incident. Far from it! A great deal happens from the very start, and indeed from before birth; but I doubt whether it is of the high order of complexity which the depressive position involves — such as

---

[1] It is here that is to be found the origin of the capacity for ambivalence. The term ambivalence has come to be used popularly with the implication that repressed hate has distorted the positive elements in a relationship. This, however, should not be allowed to obscure the concept of a capacity for ambivalence as an achievement in emotional pevelopment.

the holding of an anxiety and a hope over a period of time. Nevertheless, if it be eventually proved that a baby had a depressive position moment in the first week of life I shall not feel disturbed. Meanwhile, the depressive position is something placed at six to twelve months as a gradually strengthening evidence of personal growth, growth that is dependent on sensitive and continued environmental provision.

We can state the preconditions for the depressive position achievement. We have a great deal of practical experience to draw upon because of the number of times we have watched patients, patients of any age, reach this stage in emotional development under the clear conditions of an analysis that is going well. The earlier stages must have been successfully negotiated either in real life or in the analysis, or in both, if the depressive position is to be reached. To reach the depressive position a baby must have become established as a whole person, and to be related to whole persons as a whole person. Here I am counting the breast as a whole person, because, as the baby becomes a whole person, then the breast, the mother's body, whatever there is of her, any part, becomes perceived by the baby as a whole thing.

If we take for granted everything that has gone before, we can say, in talking of a whole baby related to a whole mother, that the stage is set in which the depressive position can be reached. If this wholeness cannot be taken for granted, then nothing I have to say about the depressive position is relevant. The infant just gets on without it; and many do. In fact in schizoid types there may be no significant depressive position achievement, and magical re-creation has to be exploited in default of what is described as reparation and restitution. I have known analysts looking for the depressive position in patients when the preconditions were absent. It is of course rather pathetic to witness failure, and the resulting conclusion that the depressive position is a false concept is not very convincing. *Per contra*, analysts try to demonstrate depressive position phenomena when these are not the main issue, in analyses of patients who have already achieved the depressive position on attainment of unit status in infancy.

If in a baby's development we can take it for granted that the sense of wholeness is a fact for that baby, we can also assume that the baby is living in the body. This detail is important, but I cannot develop the theme here.

So here we have a person, a whole human baby, and the mother holding the situation, enabling the child to work through certain processes which I shall eventually describe.

First, however, I must make some observations on the name 'depressive position'.

The term 'depressive position' is a bad name for a normal process, but no one has been able to find a better. My own suggestion was that it should be called '*the Stage of Concern*'. I believe this term easily introduces the concept. Melanie Klein includes the word 'concern' in her own descriptions. However, this descriptive term does not cover the whole of the concept. I fear the original term will remain.

It has often been pointed out that a term that implies illness ought not to be used where a normal process is being described. The term depressive position seems to imply that infants in health pass through a stage of depression, or mood illness. Actually this is not what is meant.

When Spitz (1946) discovers and describes depression in infants who are deprived of ordinary good care he is right in saying that this is not an example of the depressive position; it has in fact nothing to do with it. The babies Spitz describes are depersonalized and hopeless about external contacts and essentially lack the preconditions for depressive position achievement.

In the concept of the depressive position in normal development there is no implication that infants normally become depressed. Depression, however common, is an illness symptom, and indicates a mood, and implies unconscious complexes that could become unconscious. The unconscious processes have to do with guilt feelings, and the guilt feelings belong to the destructive element inherent in loving. Depression as an affective disorder is neither unanalysable nor a normal phenomenon.

What then is this so-called depressive position about?

There is a helpful approach to the problem which starts with the word 'ruthless'. At first the infant (from our point of view) is ruthless; there is no concern yet as to results of instinctual love.[1] This love is originally a form of impulse, gesture, contact, relationship, and it affords the infant the satisfaction of self-expression and release from instinct tension; more, it places the object outside the self.

It should be noted that the infant does not feel ruthless, but looking back (and this does occur in regressions) the individual can say: I was ruthless then! The stage is one that is pre-ruth.

At some time or other in the history of the development of every normal human being there comes the change over from pre-ruth to ruth. No one will question this. The only thing is, when does this happen, how, and under what conditions? The concept of the depressive position is an attempt to answer these three questions. According to this concept the change from ruthlessness to ruth occurs gradually, under certain definite conditions of mothering, during the period around five to twelve months, and its establishment is not necessarily final until a much later date; and it may be found, in an analysis, that it has never occurred at all.

The depressive position, then, is a complex matter, an inherent element in a

---

[1] Here please allow for a quite different thing, which I must omit: aggression that is non-inherent and that belongs to all sorts of chance adverse persecutions which are the lot of some babies but not of the majority.

non-controversial phenomenon, that of the emergence of every human individual from pre-ruth to ruth or concern.

FUNCTION OF ENVIRONMENT

We are examining the psychology of the stage immediately following the new human being's attainment of unit status. It will be understood that everything that precedes the attainment of unit status is being omitted deliberately. I do want to throw in the observation here, however, that the further back one goes the more one sees it is true that there is no sense in talking about the individual without all the time postulating a good-enough environmental adaptation to the individual's needs. At the earliest stage one even arrives at a position at which it is only the observer who can distinguish between the individual and the environment (primary narcissism); the individual cannot do so, and it is therefore convenient here to speak of an environment-individual set-up, rather than of an individual.

Further development after unit status is reached is still dependent on stability and reliable simplicity of environment.

The mother needs to be able to combine two functions, and to persist with these two functions in time, so that the infant may have the opportunity to use this specialized setting. She has been adapting to infant needs generally by her technique of infant care (see A. Freud, 1953), and the infant has come to know this technique as part of the mother, just like her face and her ear and the necklaces she wears, and her varying attitudes (affected by hurry, laziness, anxiety, worry, excitement, etc.). The mother has been loved by the infant as the one who has embodied all this. The term affection comes in here, and it is these qualities of the mother that are embodied in the object that so many infants handle and hug (see Chapter XVIII).

At the same time the mother has been the object of assault during phases of instinctual tension. It may be seen that I am distinguishing between the functions of the mother according to whether the baby is quiet or excited. The mother has two functions corresponding to the infant's quiet and excited states.

At last the stage is set for a coming together in the mind of the infant of these two functions of the mother. It is just here that very great difficulties can arise, and these are especially studied in Melanie Klein's pioneer work, which was never more rich or productive than in this field.

The human infant cannot accept the fact that this mother who is so valued in the quiet phases is the person who has been and will be ruthlessly attacked in the excited phases.

The infant, being a whole person, is able to identify with the mother, but there is no clear distinction yet for the baby between what is intended and what really happens. Functions and their imaginative elaborations are not yet clearly distinguished as fact and fantasy. It is astonishing what the baby has to accomplish at just about this time.

Let us see what happens if the 'quiet' mother holds the situation in time, so that the baby may experience 'excited' relationships and meet the consequences.

In simplest possible terms the excited baby, scarcely knowing what is happening, becomes carried away by crude instinct and with ideas of the powerful kind that belong to instinct. (We must assume a relatively satisfactory feed, or other instinctual experience.)

The time comes for the infant to see that here are two completely different uses of the same mother. A new kind of need has arisen based on impulse and on instinct tension that seeks relief, and this involves a climax or orgasm. Where there is an orgastic experience there is necessarily an increase in pain at frustration. Once the excitement has started and tension has risen, risk has entered in.

I think we must take it that a great deal has to be experienced before the implication of all this is fully felt.[1]

As I have said, two things are happening. One is the perception of the identity of the two objects, the mother of the quiet phases, and the mother used and even attacked at the instinctual climax. The other is the beginning of the recognition of the existence of ideas, fantasy, imaginative elaboration of function, the acceptance of ideas and of fantasy related to fact but not to be confused with fact.

Such complex progression in emotional development of the individual cannot be made without good-enough environmental help. The latter is here represented by the survival of the mother. Until the child has collected memory material there is no room for the mother's disappearance.[2]

It seems to me to be a postulate of Klein's theory that the human individual cannot accept the crude fact of the excited or instinctual relationship or assault on the 'quiet' mother. Integration in the child's mind of the split between the child-care environment and the exciting environment (the two aspects of mother) cannot be made except by good-enough mothering and the mother's survival over a period of time.

Let us now think in terms of a day, with the mother holding the situation, assuming that at some point early in the day the baby has an instinctual experience. For simplicity's sake I think of a feed, for this is really at the basis of the whole matter. There appears a cannibalistic ruthless attack, which partly

[1] It must be remembered that I am talking clinically, and am describing real infancy situations as well as analytic situations.

[2] No doubt there are other early roots of fantasy appreciation but I must leave them out here.

shows in the baby's physical behaviour, and which partly is a matter of the infant's own imaginative elaboration of the physical function. The baby puts one and one together and begins to see that the answer is one, and not two. The mother of the dependent relationship (anaclitic) is also the object of instinctual (biologically driven) love.

The baby is fobbed off by the feed itself; instinct tension disappears, and the baby is both satisfied and cheated. It is too easily assumed that a feed is followed by satisfaction and sleep. Often distress follows this fobbing off, especially if physical satisfaction too quickly robs the infant of zest. The infant is then left with: aggression undischarged — because not enough muscle erotism or primitive impulse (or motility), was used in the feeding process; or a sense of 'flop'—since a source of zest for life has gone suddenly, and the infant does not know it will return. All this appears clearly in clinical analytic experience, and is at least not contradicted by direct observation of infants.

But we cannot deal with too many complications at once. Let us take it for granted that the baby experienced instinctual discharge. The mother is holding the situation and the day proceeds, and the infant realizes that the 'quiet' mother was involved in the full tide of instinctual experience, and has survived. This is repeated day after day, and adds up eventually to the baby's dawning recognition of the difference between what is called fact and fantasy, or outer and inner reality.

DEPRESSIVE ANXIETY

A more complex matter now awaits description. Instinctual experience brings the baby two types of anxiety. The first is this that I have described: anxiety about the object of instinctual love. The mother is not the same after as before. If we like we can use words to describe what the infant feels and say: there is a hole, where previously there was a full body of richness. There are plenty of other ways of putting this, according to the way we allow the infant to get a few weeks older and to have more complex ideas.

The other anxiety is of the infant's own inside. The infant has had an experience and does not feel the same as before. It would be quite legitimate to compare this with the change for good or bad in an adult after sexual experience. Remember that all the time the mother is holding the situation. The infant's personal inner phenomena need now to be studied in detail.

Let us continue to use the feeding experience.[1] The infant takes in stuff. This stuff is felt to be good or bad according to whether it was taken in during

---

[1] I assume that the instinctual experience was in line with current ego processes, otherwise I would have to discuss the infant's reactions to the impingement from the environment represented by the instinct tension and by the reactive activity.

a satisfactory instinctual experience or during an experience complicated by excessive anger at frustration. Some anger at frustration is of course part and parcel even of satisfactory feeding.

I oversimplify the inside phenomenon here, but later I shall return to make a more true evaluation of the infant's fantasy of the inside of the self, with its contending forces, and its control systems.

We can talk of the infant's ideas about the inside because we have postulated the infant's attainment of unit status; the infant has already become a person with a limiting membrane, with an inside and an outside.

For our purposes here, this infant, after the feed, besides being apprehensive about the imagined hole in the body of the mother is also very much caught up in the struggle within the self, a struggle between what is felt to be good, that is to say self-supportive, and what is felt to be bad, that is to say persecutory to the self.

A complex state of affairs has been created within, and the child can only await the result, just exactly as the result of digestion must be awaited after a feed. A sorting out surely occurs, by silent process which has a speed of its own. Quite apart from intellectual control, and according to personal patterns that gradually develop, the supportive and the persecutory elements become interrelated until some sort of equilibrium is reached, as a result of which the infant retains or eliminates according to inner need. Along with the eliminating the infant once more gains some control, since elimination once more involves body functions.[1] But whereas in the physical process of digestion we see elimination only of useless material, in the imaginative process elimination has both good and bad potential.

I shall deliberately omit reference to anal and urethral experiences as types of instinctual satisfaction in themselves, since consideration of this belongs elsewhere; in this context anal and urethral experiences are the eliminative part of the whole ingestive and digestive process.

All the while the mother is holding the situation in time. Thus, the infant's day proceeds, physical digestion and also a corresponding working-through take place in the psyche. This working-through takes time and the infant can only await the outcome, passively surrendered to what is going on inside.[2] In health this personal inner world becomes the infinitely rich core of the self.

Towards the end of this day in the life of any healthy infant as a result of inner work done, the infant has good and bad to offer. The mother takes the good and the bad, and she is supposed to know what is offered as good and what is offered as bad. Here is the first giving, and without this giving there is no true receiving. All these are very practical everyday matters of infant care, and indeed of analysis.

[1] This is in line with a main trend in the work of Fairbairn (1952).

[2] This idea corresponds to ideas put forward by A. Freud (1952).

The infant that is blessed with a mother who survives, a mother who knows a gift gesture when it is made, is now in a position to do something about that hole, the hole in the breast or body, imaginatively made in the original instinctual moment. Here come in the words reparation and restitution, words which mean so much in the right setting, but which can easily become clichés if used loosely. The gift gesture may reach to the hole, if the mother plays her part.

You may see why I have insisted on the importance of the mother holding a situation in time.

There is now set up a benign circle. Among all the complications we can discern

A relationship between infant and mother complicated by instinctual experience.

A dim perception of the effect (hole).

An inner working-through, the results of experience being sorted out.

A capacity to give, because of the sorting out of the good and the bad within.

Reparation.

The result of a day-after-day reinforcement of the benign circle is that the infant becomes able to tolerate the hole (result of instinct love). Here then is the beginning of *guilt* feeling. This is the only true guilt, since implanted guilt is false to the self. Guilt starts through the bringing together of the two mothers, and of quiet and excited love, and of love and hate, and this feeling gradually grows to be a healthy and normal source of activity in relationships. Here is one source of potency and of social contribution, and of artistic performance (but not of art itself which has roots at a deeper level).

The very great importance of the depressive position is therefore evident, and Melanie Klein's contribution to psycho-analysis here is a true contribution to society, and to child care and education. *The healthy child has a personal source of sense of guilt*, and need not be taught to feel guilty or concerned. Of course a proportion of children are not healthy in this way, have not reached the depressive position, and do have to be taught a sense of right and wrong. This is a corollary of the first statement. But, theoretically at least, each child has the potential for a development of a guilt sense. Clinically we see children without sense of guilt, but there is no human child incapable of finding a personal sense of guilt if opportunity is given before it is too late for the attainment of the depressive position. In borderline cases we do actually see this development taking place apart from analysis, for instance, in observation of antisocial children being cared for in schools for the maladjusted, so-called.

In the operation of the benign circle, concern becomes tolerable to the infant through a dawning recognition that, given time, something can be done about the hole, and the various effects of id impulse on the mother's body.

Thus instinct becomes more free, and more risk can be taken. Greater guilt is generated, but there follows also an intensification of instinctual experience with its imaginative elaboration, so that a richer inner world results, followed in turn by bigger gift potential.

We see this over and over again in analysis, when the depressive position is reached in the transference. We see an expression of love followed by anxiety about the analyst and also by hypochondriacal fears. Or we see, more positively, a release of instinct, and a development towards richness in the personality, and an increase in potency or in general potential for social contribution.

It seems that after a time the individual can build up memories of experiences felt to be good, so that the experience of the mother holding the situation becomes part of the self, becomes assimilated into the ego. In this way the actual mother gradually becomes less and less necessary. The individual acquires an internal environment. The child thus becomes able to find new situation-holding experiences, and is able in time to take over the function of being the situation-holding person for someone else, without resentment.

Some very remarkable things come out of this concept of the benign circle of the depressive position:

1. When the benign circle is broken, and the situation-holding mother is no longer a fact, then an undoing of the process occurs, resulting first in instinct inhibition and general personal impoverishment, and then also in the loss of the capacity for sense of guilt. This guilt sense can be recovered, but only by the re-establishment of the situation-holding good-enough-mother fact. Without guilt sense the child can continue with instinctual sensual gratifications, but loses the capacity for affectionate feeling.

2. For a long while the small child needs someone who is not only loved but who will accept potency (whether it be boy or girl) in terms of reparative and restitutive giving. In other words the small child must go on having a chance to give in relation to guilt belonging to instinctual experience, because this is the way of growth. There is dependence here of a high order, but not the absolute dependence of the earliest phases.

This giving is expressed in play, but constructive play at first must have the loved person near, apparently involved if not actually appreciative of the true constructive attainment in the play. It is a sure sign of a lack of understanding of small children (or of deprived children who need regressive healing experiences) when an adult thinks to help by giving, failing to see the primary importance of being there to receive.

3. If the inner phenomena give trouble the child (or adult) wet-blankets the whole inner world and functions at a low level of vitality. The mood is depression. In my description this is the first time I have linked the term depression inherently with the depressive position concept.

The depressions that are encountered clinically in psychiatry are chiefly not of the type that is related to the 'depressive position'. They are more associated with depersonalization, or hopelessness in respect of object relationships; or with a sense of futility that results from the development of a false self. These phenomena belong to the era before that of the depressive position in the individual's development.

THE MANIC DEFENCE

In the individual's management of this depressed mood that is associated specifically with depressive position anxieties, there is the notorious holiday from depression: *the manic defence*. In the manic defence everything serious is negated. Death becomes exaggerated liveliness, silence becomes noise, there is neither grief nor concern, neither constructive work nor restful pleasure. This is the reaction formation relative to depression and it needs to be examined as a concept in its own right. Its presence clinically does imply that the depressive position has been reached, and that the depressive position is being held in abeyance and negated rather than lost.

The commonest diagnosis in a medical paediatric clinic is what I used to call (in 1930, before I met the Klein ideas) 'common anxious restlessness' (see p. 22) and this is a clinical state with negation of depression as its main feature. This illness in a child is sometimes missed since it gets hidden behind the quickness and restlessness that belong to young life. As an illness, common anxious restlessness corresponds to the hypomanic state of adults, that which brings in its train many and various psychosomatic disorders.

Manic restlessness has to be differentiated from persecutory restlessness and from elation and from mania.

INNER WORLD EXAMINED

Now, though too briefly, I come to a closer examination of the inner world phenomena. This is a very big subject indeed.

It will be remembered that I deliberately oversimplified by dealing with the depressive position in terms of feeding, and of the stuff taken in by the infant during a feed. But it is not just a matter of feeding and of milk or food. We are concerned with instinctual experiences of all kinds, and the good and bad objects turn out to be the good and bad feelings that result from the instinctual life of the individual, imaginatively elaborated. A more complex statement is due even in a short presentation such as this.

The inner world of the individual builds up in three main ways:

A. Instinctual experiences.
B. Stuffs incorporated, held, or eliminated.
C. Whole relationships or situations magically introjected.

Of these types the first is fundamental to all human beings everywhere, and always will be. The second is more or less similar among infants everywhere, though of course observers can see differences (breast, bottle, milk, banana, coconut juice, beer, etc.), according to the customs prevalent in the culture at the time. The third is essentially personal, belonging to the individual in the actual setting, including happenings with that actual mother, nurse, aunt, in that actual house, hut, tent, with the reality that actually presents itself. Included here should be the mother's anxiousness, moodiness, unreliability, as well as her ordinary good-enough mothering. Father comes in indirectly as husband and directly as mother-substitute.

In order to link up the inner world of the depressive position with the work of C. G. Jung and the analytical psychologists on archetypes we must confine ourselves to a study of the first group. What happens here belongs to mankind in general, and provides the basis for that which is *common* to the dreams, the arts and religions and myths of the world, regardless of time. This is the stuff of human nature, only, however, in so far as the individual has been brought to the depressive position achievement. This is not the whole of the inner world of the child, however, and we cannot neglect the other two groups in our clinical work.

Whatever we find of archetypal organizations in the inner world, we should remember that *permanent therapeutic changes can only be brought about by new instinctual experiences*, and these are only in hand when they occur in the transference neurosis of an analysis; we do not change archetypes by showing a patient that a fantasy is the same in the patient and in mythology.

When we look at the inner world of the individual who has achieved the depressive position we see:

Contending forces (group A).
Objects or object matter, good and bad (group B).
Good perceived matter, introjected for personal enrichment and stabilization (group C).
Bad perceived matter introjected in order to be controlled (group C).

When we say that in therapy *the real changes in respect of groups A and B come from the work in the transference*, we know that an orderly sequence is implied, though we acknowledge its infinite complexity in any actual case, even when the patient is a young child.

It is the analysis of the oral sadism in the transference that economically lessens the persecutory potential in the inner world of the patient.

TYPES OF DEFENCE

One defence against depressive anxiety is a relative inhibition of the instinct itself, which gives a quantitative diminution of all sequelae of instinctual experiences.

Other defence mechanisms are employed in the inner world, such as:

Overall control, gradually lifted (depressive mood).
Departmentalization.
Insulation of certain persecutory groupings.
Incapsulation.
Introjection of an idealized object.
Secret hiding of good things.
Magical projection of the good.
Magical projection of the bad.
Elimination.
Negation.

To go over this ground is like going over the whole range of a child's play; in fact it is precisely the same since everything appears in the playing. It is only too easy for the individual to get temporary relief from incapsulation of a persecutory grouping by a projection of it. The result, however, is a delusional state, and we call it madness, unless external reality happens to provide a perfect example of the material to be projected.

One more complication must be mentioned. It will already have been noted that this building up of the inner world through innumerable instinctual experiences has started long before the era that we are examining. Long before six months old the human baby is becoming made up out of the experiences that constitute the life of infancy, instinctual and non-instinctual, excited and quiet. On account of this it may be claimed that some of the things I am talking about start from birth or from the pre-birth era. This is not, however, to take the depressive position itself back to these early months and weeks and days, because the depressive position depends on the development of a sense of time, on an appreciation of the difference between fact and fantasy, and above all on the fact of the integration of the individual. It is very difficult to allow for all these things, to see the mother holding the situation and the baby really making use of this fact, except in the case of a baby who is old enough to play at dropping things.

(I watched a twelve-weeks-old baby put his finger into his mother's mouth whenever she fed him at the breast. He was beautifully cared for and is now about the most healthy boy of ten that I know. It is tempting to say that he perhaps was at the depressive position; but there are all the strange processes of identification to be considered, and, besides, it is not usual for this thing to occur as early as twelve weeks and very rare for it to occur earlier. We have also to allow for the apparent integration that comes from reliable handling rather than from the true attainment of integration in independence.)

If one begins to investigate not the depressive position but the origins of persecutors as well as of supportive forces within the ego, then one must go much further back than the second half of the first year. But then one must also go back to unintegration, to a lack of sense of living in the body, to a smudging of the line between fantasy and fact, and above all one must go back to dependence on the mother who is all the time holding the baby, and eventually to what may be called *double dependence*, where dependence is absolute because environment is not perceived.

But I can leave the extremely complex psychology of the early formation of benign and persecutory elements, and keep to my first intention, which is to start at the point at which the individual becomes a whole, a unit, and to deal with the important matters that inherently follow that stage in health.

REACTION TO LOSS

Melanie Klein's work has enriched the understanding Freud gave us of reaction to loss. If in an individual the depressive position has been achieved and fully established, then the reaction to loss is *grief*, or *sadness*. Where there is some degree of failure at the depressive position the result of loss is depression. Mourning means that the object lost has been magically introjected, and (as Freud showed) it is there subjected to hate. I suppose we mean that it is allowed contact with internal persecutory elements. Incidentally the inner world balance of forces is upset by this, so that the persecutory elements are increased and the benign or supportive forces are weakened. There is a danger situation, and the defensive mechanism of an overall deadening produces a mood of depression. The depression is a healing mechanism; it covers the battleground as with a mist, allowing for a sorting out at reduced rate, giving time for all possible defences to be brought into play, and for a working-through, so that eventually there can be a spontaneous recovery. Clinically, depression (of this sort) tends to lift, a well-known psychiatric observation.

In the subject whose depressive position is securely established there accrue what I have called the group C introjections, or memories of good experiences and of loved objects, and these enable the subject eventually to carry on even without environmental support. Love of the internal representation of an external object lost can lessen the hate of the introjected loved object which loss entails. In these and other ways mourning is experienced and worked through, and grief can be felt as such.

The child's play at throwing things away on which I have laid such stress is an indication of the child's growing ability to master loss, and it is therefore an indication for weaning.[1] This play indicates some degree of group C introjection.

[1] In speaking of weaning I must leave out reference here to the fact that behind weaning is disillusionment.

THE CONCEPT OF THE 'GOOD BREAST'

Finally, let us consider the term a 'good breast'.

Externally a good breast is one that having been eaten waits to be reconstructed. In other words, it turns out to be nothing more nor less than the mother holding the situation in time in the way I have described.

In so far as the good breast is an *inner* phenomenon (assuming the individual has achieved the depressive position) we must apply our principle of the three groupings in order to understand the concept.

Group A. There is no use for the term good breast in this grouping. Instead we refer to an archetypal experience, or a satisfactory instinctual experience.

Group B. There is no good breast recognizable here since, if good, it will have been eaten, and we hope enjoyed. There will be no breast material recognizable as such. The child grows out of this material and eliminates what is not needed or what is felt to be bad.

Group C. Here at last the term 'good internal breast' can be employed.

Memories of good situation-holding experiences help the child to tide over short periods in which the mother fails, and they provide the basis first for the 'transitional object' and then for the familiar succession of breast and mother substitutes.

I wish to add the reminder that a good breast introjection is sometimes highly pathological, a defence organization. The breast is then an idealized breast (mother) and this idealization indicates a hopelessness about inner chaos and the ruthlessness of instinct. A good breast based on selected memories, or on a mother's need to be good, provides reassurance. Such an introjected idealized breast dominates the scene; and all seems well for the patient. Not so for the patient's friends, however, since such an introjected good breast has to be advertised, and the patient becomes a 'good breast' advocate.

Analysts are faced with this difficult problem, shall we ourselves be recognizable in our patients? We always are. But we deplore it. We hate to become internalized good breasts in others, and to hear ourselves being advertised by those whose own inner chaos is being precariously held by the introjection of an idealized analyst.

What do we want? We want to be eaten, not magically introjected. There is no masochism in this. To be eaten is the wish and indeed the need of a mother at a very early stage in the care of an infant. This means that whoever is not cannibalistically attacked tends to feel outside the range of people's reparative and restitutive activities, and so outside society.

If and only if we have been eaten, worn down, stolen from, can we stand in a minor degree being also magically introjected, and being placed in the preserve department in someone's inner world.

To summarize, the depressive position which may be well on the way under favourable circumstances at six to nine months is quite commonly not reached till the subject comes into analysis. With regard to the more schizoid people, and the whole mental hospital population of persons who have never reached a true self-life or self-expression, the depressive position is not the thing that matters; it must remain for these like colour to the colour-blind. By contrast, for the whole manic-depressive group that comprises the majority of so-called normal people the subject of the depressive position in normal development is one that cannot be left aside; it is and it remains *the problem of life* except in so far as it is reached. With quite healthy people it becomes taken for granted, and incorporated in active living in society. The child, healthy in having reached the depressive position, can get on with the problem of the triangle in interpersonal relationships, the classical Oedipus complex.

Chapter XXII

Metapsychological and Clinical Aspects of Regression within the Psycho-Analytical Set-Up[1]
[1954]

THE STUDY of the place of regression in analytic work is one of the tasks Freud left us to carry out, and I think it is a subject for which this Society is ready. I base this idea on the fact that material relevant to the subject occurs frequently in papers read before the Society. Usually attention is not specifically drawn to this aspect of our work, or else it is referred to casually under the guise of the intuitive or 'art' aspect of psycho-analytic practice.

The subject of regression is one that has been forced on my attention by certain cases during the past dozen years of my clinical work. It is, of course, too vast for full presentation here and now. I shall choose therefore those aspects that seem to me to introduce the discussion in a fruitful way.

Analysis is not only a technical exercise. It is something that we become able to do when we have reached a stage in acquiring a basic technique. What we become able to do enables us to co-operate with the patient in following the *process*, that which in each patient has its own pace and which follows its own course; all the important features of this process derive from the patient and not from ourselves as analysts.

Let us therefore clearly keep before our minds the difference between technique and the carrying through of a treatment. It is possible to carry through a treatment with limited technique, and it is possible with highly developed technique to fail to carry through a treatment.

Let us also bear in mind that by the legitimate method of careful choice of case we may and usually do avoid meeting aspects of human nature that must take us beyond our technical equipment.

Choice of case implies classification. For my present purpose I group cases according to the technical equipment they require of the analyst. I divide

[1] Paper read before the British Psycho-Analytical Society on 17th March, 1954. *Int. J. Psycho-Anal.*, Vol. XXXVI, 1955.

cases into the following three categories. *First* there are those patients who operate as whole persons and whose difficulties are in the realm of inter-personal relationships. The technique for the treatment of these patients be-longs to psycho-analysis as it developed in the hands of Freud at the begin-ning of the century.

Then *secondly* there come the patients in whom the wholeness of the person-ality only just begins to be something that can be taken for granted; in fact one can say that analysis has to do with the first events that belong to and in-herently and immediately follow not only the achievement of wholeness but also the coming together of love and hate and the dawning recognition of dependence. This is the analysis of the stage of concern, or of what has come to be known as the 'depressive position'. These patients require the analysis of mood. The technique for this work is not different from that needed by patients in the first category; nevertheless some new management problems do arise on account of the increased range of clinical material tackled. Im-portant from our point of view here is the idea of the *survival of the analyst* as a dynamic factor.

In the *third* grouping I place all those patients whose analyses must deal with the early stages of emotional development before and up to the establish-ment of the personality as an entity, before the achievement of space-time unit status. The personal structure is not yet securely founded. In regard to this third grouping, the accent is more surely on management, and sometimes over long periods with these patients ordinary analytic work has to be in abeyance, management being the whole thing.

To recapitulate in terms of environment, one can say that in the first group-ing we are dealing with patients who develop difficulties in the ordinary course of their home life, assuming a home life in the pre-latency period, and assum-ing satisfactory development at the earlier infantile stages. In the second category, the analysis of the depressive position, we are dealing with the mother-child relationship especially around the time that weaning becomes a meaningful term. The mother holds a situation in time. In the third category there comes primitive emotional development, that which needs the mother actually holding the infant.

Into the last of these three categories falls one of my patients who has per-haps taught me most about regression. On another occasion I may be able to give a full account of this treatment, but at present I must do little more than point out that I have had the experience of allowing a regression absolutely full sway, and of watching the result.

Briefly, I have had a patient (a woman now in middle age) who had had an ordinary good analysis before coming to me but who obviously still needed help. This case had originally presented itself as one in the first category of my classification, but although the diagnosis of psychosis would never have been made by a psychiatrist, an analytical diagnosis needed to be made that took into account a very early development of a false self. For treatment to be effectual, there had to be a regression in search of the true self. Fortunately in this case I was able to manage the whole regression myself, that is to say, without the help of an institution. I decided at the start that the regression must be allowed its head, and no attempt, except once near the beginning, was made to interfere with the regressive process which followed its own course. (The one occasion was an interpretation I made, arising out of the material, of oral erotism and sadism in the transference. This was correct but about six years too early because I did not yet fully believe in the regression. For my own sake I had to test the effect of one ordinary interpretation. When the right time came for this interpretation it had become unnecessary.) It was a matter of about three or four years before the depth of the regression was reached, following which there started up a progress in emotional development. There has been no new regression. There has been an absence of chaos, though chaos has always threatened.

I have therefore had a unique experience even for an analyst. I cannot help being different from what I was before this analysis started. Non-analysts would not know the tremendous amount that this kind of experience of *one* patient can teach, but amongst analysts I can expect it to be fully understood that this one experience that I have had has tested psycho-analysis in a special way, and has taught me a great deal.

The treatment and management of this case has called on everything that I possess as a human being, as a psycho-analyst, and as a paediatrician. I have had to make personal growth in the course of this treatment which was painful and which I would gladly have avoided. In particular I have had to learn to examine my own technique whenever difficulties arose, and it has always turned out in the dozen or so resistance phases that the cause was in a counter-transference phenomenon which necessitated further self-analysis in the analyst. It is not my aim in this paper to give a description of this case, since one must choose whether to be clinical or theoretical in one's approach, and I have chosen to be theoretical. Nevertheless I have this case all the time in mind.[1]

The main thing is that in this case, as in many others that have led up to it in my practice, I have needed to re-examine my technique, even that adapted to the more usual case. Before I explain what I mean I must explain my use of the word regression.

For me, the word regression simply means the reverse of progress. This progress itself is the evolution of the individual, psyche-soma, personality, and mind with (eventually) character formation and socialization. Progress starts from a date certainly prior to birth. There is a biological drive behind progress.

[1] Case also referred to on p. 248.

It is one of the tenets of psycho-analysis that health implies continuity in regard to this evolutionary progress of the psyche and that health is maturity of emotional development appropriate to the age of the individual, maturity that is to say in regard to this evolutionary process.

On closer examination one observes immediately that *there cannot be a simple reversal of progress.* For this progress to be reversed there has to be in the individual an organization which enables regression to occur.

We see:

> A failure of adaptation on the part of the environment that results in the development of a false self.
> A belief in the possibility of a correction of the original failure represented by a latent capacity for regression which implies a complex ego organization.
> Specialized environmental provision, followed by actual regression.
> New forward emotional development, with complications that will be described later.

Incidentally I think it is not useful to use the word regression whenever infantile behaviour appears in a case history. The word regression has derived a popular meaning which we need not adopt. When we speak of regression in psycho-analysis we imply the existence of an ego organization and a threat of chaos. There is a great deal for study here in the way in which the individual stores up memories and ideas and potentialities. It is as if there is an expectation that favourable conditions may arise justifying regression and offering a new chance for forward development, that which was rendered impossible or difficult initially by environmental failure.

It will be seen that I am considering the idea of regression within a highly organized ego-defence mechanism, one which involves the existence of a false self. In the patient referred to above this false self gradually became a 'caretaker self', and only after some years could the caretaker self become handed over to the analyst, and the self surrender to the ego.

One has to include in one's theory of the development of a human being the idea that it is normal and healthy for the individual to be able to defend the self against specific environmental failure by a *freezing of the failure situation.* Along with this goes an unconscious assumption (which can become a conscious hope) that opportunity will occur at a later date for a renewed experience in which the failure situation will be able to be unfrozen and re-experienced, with the individual in a regressed state, in an environment that is making adequate adaptation. The theory is here being put forward of regression as part of a healing process, in fact, a normal phenomenon that can properly be studied in the healthy person. In the very ill person there is but little hope of new opportunity. In the extreme case the therapist would need to go to the patient and actively present good mothering, an experience that could not have been expected by the patient.

There are several ways in which the healthy individual deals with specific early environmental failures; but there is one of them that I am calling here the freezing of the failure situation. There must be a relation between this and the concept of the fixation point.

In psycho-analytic theory we often state that in the course of instinct development in the pregenital phases *unfavourable situations* can create fixation points in the emotional development of the individual. At a later stage, for instance at the stage of genital dominance, that is to say when the whole person is involved in interpersonal relationships (and when it is quite ordinarily Freudian to speak about the Oedipus complex and castration fears), anxiety may lead to a regression in terms of instinct quality to that operative at the fixation point, and the consequence is a reinforcement of the original failure situation. This theory has proved its value and is in daily use, and there is no need to abandon it while at the same time looking at it afresh.

A simple example would be that of a boy whose infancy had been normal, who at the time of tonsillectomy was given an enema, first by his mother, and then by a group of nurses who had to hold him down. He was then two. Following this he had bowel difficulty but at the age of nine (age at consultation) he appears clinically as a severe case of constipation. In the meantime there has been a serious interference with his emotional development in terms of genital fantasy. In this case there happens to be the complication that the boy has reacted to the giving of the enema as if it had been a revenge on the part of the mother on account of his homosexuality, and what went into repression was the homosexuality and along with it the anal-erotic potential. In the analysis of this boy one knows that there would be acting out to be dealt with, a repetition compulsion associated with the original trauma. One knows also that the changes in this boy would not follow a simple re-enactment of the trauma but would follow ordinary Oedipus complex interpretation in the transference neurosis.

I give this as an ordinary case illustrating a symptom which was a regression to a fixation point where a trauma was clearly present.

Analysts have found it necessary to postulate that more normally there are *good* pregenital situations to which the individual can return when in difficulties at a later stage. This is a health phenomenon. There has thus arisen the idea of two kinds of regression in respect of instinct development, the one being a going back to an early failure situation and the other to an early success situation.

I think that insufficient attention has been drawn to the difference between these two phenomena. In the case of the environmental failure situation what we see is evidence of *personal defences* organized by the individual and requiring analysis. In the case of the more normal early success situation what we see more obviously is the memory of *dependence*, and therefore we encounter an *environmental situation* rather than a personal defence organization. The personal organization is not so obvious because it has remained fluid, and less defensive. I should mention at this point that I am relying on an assumption which I have often made before and which is by no means always accepted, namely, that towards the theoretical beginning there is less and less of personal failure, eventually only failure of environmental adaptation.

We are concerned, therefore, not merely with regression to good and bad points in the instinct experiences of the individual, but also to good and bad points in the environmental adaptation to ego needs and id needs in the individual's history.

We can think in terms of genital and pregenital stages of the development of *instinct* quality, we can use the word regression simply as a reversal of progress, a voyage back from genital to phallic, phallic to excretory, excretory to ingestive. But however much we develop our thinking in this direction we have to admit that a great deal of clinical material cannot be fitted into the framework of this theory.

The alternative is to put the accent on ego development and on dependence, and in this case when we speak of regression we immediately speak of environmental adaptation in its successes and failures. One of the points that I am trying to make especially clear is that our thinking on this subject has been confused by an attempt to trace back the ego without ourselves evolving as we go an increasing interest in environment. We can build theories of *instinct* development and agree to leave out the environment, but there is no possibility of doing this in regard to formulation of *early ego* development. We must always remember, I suggest, that the end result of our thinking about ego development is primary narcissism. In primary narcissism the environment is holding the individual, and *at the same time* the individual knows of no environment and is at one with it.

If I had time I would point out the way in which an organized regression is sometimes confused with pathological withdrawal and defensive splittings of various kinds. These states are related to regression in the sense that they are defensive organizations. The organization that makes regression useful has this quality distinct from the other defence organizations in that it carries with it the hope of a new opportunity for an unfreezing of the frozen situation and a chance for the environment, that is to say, the present-day environment, to make adequate though belated adaptation.

From this is derived the fact, if it be a fact, that it is from psychosis that a patient can make spontaneous recovery, whereas psychoneurosis makes no spontaneous recovery and the psycho-analyst is truly needed. In other words, psychosis is closely related to health, in which innumerable environmental failure situations are frozen but are reached and unfrozen by the various healing phenomena of ordinary life, namely friendships, nursing during physical illness, poetry, etc., etc.

It seems to me that it is only lately in the literature that *regression to dependence* has taken its rightful place in clinical descriptions. The reason for this must be that it is only recently that we have felt strong enough in our understanding of individual psyche-soma and mental development to be able to allow ourselves to examine and allow for the part that environment plays.

I now want to go directly to Freud, and I want to make a somewhat artificial distinction between two aspects of Freud's work. We see Freud developing the psycho-analytic method out of the clinical situation in which it was logical to use hypnosis.

Let us look and see what Freud did in choosing his cases. We can say that out of the total psychiatric pool, which includes all the mad people in asylums as well as those outside, he took those cases which had been *adequately provided for in earliest infancy*, the psychoneurotics. It might not be possible to confirm this by a close examination of the early cases on which Freud did work, but of one thing we can be certain, and this is most important, that Freud's own early personal history was of such a kind that he came to the Oedipus or prelatency period in his life as a whole human being, ready to meet whole human beings, and ready to deal in interpersonal relationships. His own infancy experiences had been good enough, so that in his self-analysis he could take the mothering of the infant for granted.

Freud takes for granted the early mothering situation and my contention is that *it turned up in his provision of a setting for his work*, almost without his being aware of what he was doing. Freud was able to analyse himself as an independent and whole person, and he interested himself in the anxieties that belong to interpersonal relationships. Later of course he looked at infancy theoretically and postulated pregenital phases of instinct development, and he and others proceeded to work out details and to go further and further back in the history of the individual. This work on the pregenital phases could not come to full fruition because it was not based on the study of patients who needed to regress in the analytic situation.[1]

---

[1] You will observe that I am not saying that this theoretical work on pregenital instinct could not succeed on account of a lack in Freud of direct contact with infants, because I see no reason why Freud should not have had very good experience as an observer of the mother-infant situation within his own family and his work. Further I am reminded that Freud worked in a children's clinic and made detailed observation on infants when studying Little's disease. The point that I wish to make here is that *fortunately* for us Freud found his interest at the beginning not in the patient's need to regress in the analysis but in what

Now I wish to make clear in what way I artificially divide Freud's work into two parts. First, there is the technique of psycho-analysis as it has gradually developed, and which students learn. The material presented by the patient is to be *understood* and to be *interpreted*. And, second, there is the *setting* in which this work is carried through.

Let us now glance at Freud's clinical setting. I will enumerate some of the very obvious points in its description.

1. At a stated time daily, five or six times a week, Freud put himself at the service of the patient. (This time was arranged to suit the convenience of both the analyst and the patient.)
2. The analyst would be reliably there, on time, alive, breathing.
3. For the limited period of time prearranged (about an hour) the analyst would keep awake and become preoccupied with the patient.
4. The analyst expressed love by the positive interest taken, and hate in the strict start and finish and in the matter of fees. Love and hate were honestly expressed, that is to say not denied by the analyst.
5. The aim of the analysis would be to get into touch with the process of the patient, to understand the material presented, to communicate this understanding in words. Resistance implied suffering and could be allayed by interpretation.
6. The analyst's method was one of objective observation.
7. This work was to be done in a room, not a passage, a room that was quiet and not liable to sudden unpredictable sounds, yet not dead quiet and not free from ordinary house noises. This room would be lit properly, but not by a light staring in the face, and not by a variable light. The room would certainly not be dark and it would be comfortably warm. The patient would be lying on a couch, that is to say, comfortable, if able to be comfortable, and probably a rug and some water would be available.
8. The analyst (as is well known) keeps moral judgment out of the relationship, has no wish to intrude with details of the analyst's personal life and ideas, and the analyst does not wish to take sides in the persecutory systems even when these appear in the form of real shared situations, local, political, etc. Naturally if there is a war or an earthquake or if the king dies the analyst is not unaware.
9. In the analytic situation the analyst is much more reliable than people are in ordinary life; on the whole punctual, free from temper tantrums, free from compulsive falling in love, etc.

happens in the analytic situation when regression is *not* necessary and when it is possible to take for granted the work done by the mother and by the early environmental adaptation in the individual patient's past history.

10. There is a very clear distinction in the analysis between fact and fantasy, so that the analyst is not hurt by an aggressive dream.
11. An absence of the talion reaction can be counted on.
12. The analyst survives.

A good deal more could be said, but the whole thing adds up to the fact that the analyst *behaves* himself or herself, and behaves without too much cost simply because of being a relatively mature person. If Freud had not behaved well he could not have developed the psycho-analytic technique or the theory to which the use of his technique led him. This is true however clever he might at the same time have been. The main point is that almost any one detail can be found to be of extreme importance at a specific phase of an analysis involving some regression of the patient.

There is rich material here for study, and it will be noted that there is a very marked similarity between all these things and the ordinary task of parents, especially that of the mother with her infant or with the father playing a mother role, and in some respects with the task of the mother at the very beginning.

Let me add that for Freud there are three people, one of them excluded from the analytic room. If there are only two people involved then there has been a regression of the patient in the analytic setting, and the setting represents the mother with her technique, and the patient is an infant. There is a further state of regression in which there is only one present, namely the patient, and this is true even if in another sense, from the observer's angle, there are two.

My thesis up to this point can be stated thus:

Psychotic illness is related to environmental failure at an early stage of the emotional development of the individual. The sense of futility and unreality belongs to the development of a false self which develops in protection of the true self.

The setting of analysis reproduces the early and earliest mothering techniques. It invites regression by reason of its reliability.

The regression of a patient is an organized return to early dependence or double dependence. The patient and the setting merge into the original success situation of primary narcissism.

Progress from primary narcissism starts anew with the true self able to meet environmental failure situations without organization of the defences that involve a false self protecting the true self.

To this extent psychotic illness can only be relieved by specialized environmental provision interlocked with the patient's regression.

Progress from the new position, with the true self surrendered to the total ego, can now be studied in terms of the complex processes of individual growth.

In practice there is a sequence of events:

1. The provision of a setting that gives confidence.
2. Regression of the patient to dependence, with due sense of the risk involved.
3. The patient feeling a new sense of self, and the self hitherto hidden becoming surrendered to the total ego. A new progression of the individual processes which had stopped.
4. An unfreezing of an environmental failure situation.
5. From the new position of ego strength, anger related to the early environmental failure, felt in the present and expressed.
6. Return from regression to dependence, in orderly progress towards independence.
7. Instinctual needs and wishes becoming realizable with genuine vitality and vigour.

All this repeated again and again.

Here a comment must be made on the diagnosis of psychosis.

In consideration of a group of mad people there is a big distinction to be drawn between those whose defences are in a chaotic state, and those who have been able to organize an illness. It must surely be that when psychoanalysis comes to be applied to psychosis it will be more likely to succeed where there is a highly organized illness. My own personal horror of leucotomy and suspicion of E.C.T. derives from my view of psychotic illness as a defensive organization designed to protect the true self; and also, from my feeling that apparent health with a false self is of no value to the patient. Illness, with the true self well hidden away, however painful, is the only good state unless we can go back with the patient as therapists and displace the original environmental-failure situation.

Another consideration follows naturally here. In a group of psychotic patients there will be those who are clinically regressed and those who are not. It is by no means true that the clinically regressed are the more ill. From the psycho-analyst's point of view it may be easier to tackle the case of a patient who has had a breakdown than to tackle a comparable case in a state of flight to sanity.

It takes a great deal of courage to have a breakdown, but it may be that the alternative is a *flight to sanity*, a condition comparable to the manic defence against depression. Fortunately in most of our cases the breakdowns can be caught within the analytic hours, or they are limited and localized so that the social milieu of the patient can absorb them or cope with them.

To clarify the issue I wish to make a few comparisons:

The couch and the pillows are there for the patient's use. They will appear in ideas and dreams and then will stand for the analyst's body, breasts, arms, hands, etc., in an infinite variety of ways. In so far as the patient is regressed (for a moment or for an hour or over a long period of time) the couch *is* the analyst, the pillows *are* breasts, the analyst *is* the mother at a certain past era. In the extreme it is no longer true to say the couch stands for the analyst.

It is proper to speak of the patient's *wishes*, the wish (for instance) to be quiet. With the regressed patient the word wish is incorrect; instead we use the word *need*. If a regressed patient *needs* quiet, then without it nothing can be done at all. If the need is not met the result is not anger, only a reproduction of the environmental failure situation which stopped the processes of self growth. The individual's capacity to 'wish' has become interfered with, and we witness the reappearance of the original cause of a sense of futility.

The regressed patient is near to a reliving of dream and memory situations; an acting out of a dream may be the way the patient discovers what is urgent, and talking about what was acted out follows the action but cannot precede it.

Or take the detail of being on time. The analyst is not one who keeps patients waiting. Patients dream about being kept waiting and all the other variations on the theme, and they can be angry when the analyst is late. This is all part of the way the material goes. But patients who regress are different about the initial moment. There come phases when everything hangs on the punctuality of the analyst. If the analyst is there ready waiting, all is well — if not, well then both analyst and patient may as well pack up and go home, since no work can be done. Or, if one considers the patient's own unpunctuality, a neurotic patient who is late may perhaps be in a state of negative transference. A depressive patient is more likely by being late to be giving the analyst a little respite, a little longer for other activities and interests (protection from aggression, greed).

The psychotic (regressive) patient is probably late because there is not yet established any hope that the analyst will be on time. It is futile to be on time. So much hangs on this detail that the risk cannot be taken, so the patient is late; therefore no work gets done.

Again, neurotic patients like to have the third person always *excluded*, and the hate roused by sight of other patients may disturb the work in unpredictable ways. Depressive patients may be glad to see other patients till they reach the primitive or greedy love, which engenders their guilt. Regressive patients either have no objection to there being other patients or else they cannot conceive of there being another patient. Another patient is none other than a new version of the self.

A patient curls up on the couch and rests the head on the hand and seems warm and contented. The rug is right over the head. The patient is alone. Of course we are used to all varieties of angry withdrawal, but the analyst has to be able to recognize this *regressive* withdrawal in which he is not being insulted but is being used in a very primitive and positive way.

Another point is that regression to dependence is part and parcel of the analysis of early infancy phenomena, and if the couch gets wetted, or if the patient soils, or dribbles, we know that this is inherent, not a complication. Interpretation is not what is needed, and indeed speech or even movement can ruin the process and can be excessively painful to the patient.

An important element in this theory is the postulate of the observing ego. Two patients very similar in their immediate clinical aspect may be very different in regard to the degree of organization of the observer ego. At one extreme the observing ego is almost able to identify with the analyst and there can be a recovery from the regression at the end of the analytic hour. At the other extreme there is very little observing ego, and the patient is unable to recover from the regression in the analytic hour, and must be nursed.

Acting out has to be tolerated in this sort of work, and with the acting out in the analytic hour the analyst will find it necessary to play a part, although usually in token form. There is nothing more surprising both to the patient and to the analyst than the revelations that occur in these moments of acting out. The actual acting out in the analysis is only the beginning, however, and there must always follow a putting into words of the new bit of understanding. There is a sequence here:

1. A statement of what happened in the acting out.
2. A statement of what was needed of the analyst. From this can be deduced:
3. What went wrong in the original environmental failure situation.
   This produces some relief, but there follows:
4. Anger belonging to the original environmental failure situation. This anger is being felt perhaps for the first time, and the analyst may now have to take part by being used in respect of his failures rather than of his successes. This is disconcerting unless it is understood. The progress has been made through the analyst's very careful attempt at adaptation, and yet it is the *failure* that at this moment is singled out as important on account of its being a reproduction of the original failure or trauma. In favourable cases there follows at last:

5. A new sense of self in the patient and a sense of the progress that means true growth. It is this last that must be the analyst's reward through his identification with his patient. Not always will a further stage arrive in which the patient is able to understand the strain which the analyst has undergone and is able to say thank-you with real meaning.

This strain on the analyst is considerable, especially if lack of understanding and unconscious negative countertransference complicate the picture. On the other hand, I can say that in this kind of treatment I have not felt bewildered, and this is to some extent a compensation. The strain can be quite simple.

In one vitally important hour near the beginning of such a treatment I remained and knew I must remain absolutely still, only breathing. This I found very difficult indeed, especially as I did not yet know the special significance of the silence to my patient. At the end the patient came round from the regressed state and said: 'Now I know you can do my analysis.'

The idea is sometimes put forward: of course everyone wants to regress; regression is a picnic; we must stop our patients from regression; or, Winnicott likes or invites his patients to regress.

Let me make some basic observations on the subject of organized regression to dependence.

This is always extremely painful for the patient:

(*a*) at one extreme is the patient who is fairly normal; here pain is experienced almost all the time;

(*b*) midway we find all degrees of painful recognition of the precariousness of dependence and of double dependence;

(*c*) at the other extreme is the mental hospital case; here the patient presumably does not suffer at the time on account of dependence. Suffering results from sense of futility, unreality, etc.

This is not to deny that in a localized way extreme satisfaction can be derived from the regression experience. This satisfaction is not sensuous. It is due to the fact that regression reaches and provides a starting-place, what I would call a *place* from which to operate. The self is reached. The subject becomes in touch with the basic self-processes that constitute true development, and what happens from here is felt as real. The satisfaction belonging to this is so much more important than any sensuous element in the regression experience that the latter need not be more than mentioned.

There are no reasons why an analyst should *want* a patient to regress, except grossly pathological reasons. If an analyst likes patients to regress, this must eventually interfere with the management of the regressed situation. Further, psycho-analysis which involves clinical regression is very much more difficult all along than that in which no special adaptive environmental provision has to be made. In other words it would be pleasant if we were to be able to take for analysis only those patients whose mothers at the very start and also in the first months had been able to provide good-enough conditions. But this era of psycho-analysis is steadily drawing to a close.

But the question arises, what do analysts do when regression (even of minute quantity) turns up?

Some crudely say: Now sit up! Pull your socks up! Come round! Talk! But this is not psycho-analysis.

Some divide their work into two parts, though unfortunately they do not always fully acknowledge this:

(a) they are strictly analytic (free association in words; interpretation in words; no reassurances);

and also

(b) they act intuitively.

Here comes the idea of psycho-analysis as an *art*.

Some say: unanalysable, and throw up the sponge. A mental hospital takes over.

The idea of psycho-analysis as an art must gradually give way to a study of environmental adaptation relative to patients' regressions. But while the scientific study of environmental adaptation is undeveloped, then I suppose analysts must continue to be artists in their work. An analyst may be a good artist, but (as I have frequently asked): what patient wants to be someone else's poem or picture?

I know from experience that some will say: all this leads to a theory of development which ignores the early stages of the development of the individual, which ascribes early development to environmental factors. This is quite untrue.

In the early development of the human being the environment that behaves well enough (that makes good-enough active adaptation) *enables personal growth to take place*. The self processes then may continue active, in an unbroken line of living growth. If the environment behaves not well enough, then the individual is engaged in reactions to impingement, and the self processes are interrupted. If this state of affairs reaches a quantitative limit the core of the self begins to get protected; there is a hold-up, the self cannot make new progress unless and until the environment failure situation is corrected in the way I have described. With the true self protected there develops a false self built on a defence-compliance basis, the acceptance of reaction to impingement. The development of a false self is one of *the most successful defence organizations* designed for the protection of the true self's core, and its existence results in the sense of futility. I would like to repeat myself and to say that while the individual's operational centre is in the false self there is a sense of futility, and in practice we find the change to the feeling that life is worth while coming at the moment of shift of the operational centre from the false to the true self, even before full surrender of the self's core to the total ego.

From this one can formulate a fundamental principle of existence: that which proceeds from the true self feels real (later good) whatever its nature, however aggressive; that which happens in the individual as a reaction to environmental impingement feels unreal, futile (later bad), however sensually satisfactory.

Lastly, let us examine the concept of regression by putting up against it the concept of reassurance. This becomes necessary because of the fact that the adaptive technique that must meet a patient's regression is often classed (wrongly, I am sure) as reassurance.

We assume that reassurance is not part of the psycho-analytic technique. The patient comes into the analytic setting and goes out of it, and within that setting there is no more than interpretation, correct and penetrating and well-timed.

In teaching psycho-analysis we must continue to speak against reassurance.

As we look a little more carefully, however, we see that this is too simple a language. It is not just a question of reassurance and no reassurance.

In fact, the whole matter needs examination. What is a reassurance? What could be more reassuring than to find oneself being well analysed, to be in a reliable setting with a mature person in charge, capable of making penetrating and accurate interpretation, and to find one's personal process respected? It is foolish to deny that reassurance is present in the classical analytic situation.

The whole set-up of psycho-analysis is one big reassurance, especially the reliable objectivity and behaviour of the analyst, and the transference interpretations constructively using instead of wastefully exploiting the moment's passion.

This matter of reassurance is much better discussed in terms of *counter-transference*. Reaction formations in the behaviour of the analyst are harmful not because they appear in the form of reassurances and denials but because they represent repressed unconscious elements in the analyst, and these mean limitation of the analyst's work.

What would be said of an analyst's *inability* to reassure? If an analyst were suicidal? *A belief in human nature and in the developmental process exists in the analyst* if work is to be done at all, and this is quickly sensed by the patient.

There is no value to be got from describing regression to dependence, with its concomitant environmental adaptation, in terms of reassurance, just as there is a very real point in considering harmful reassurance in terms of countertransference.

What, if anything, am I asking analysts to do about these matters in their practical work?

1. I am *not* asking them to take on psychotic patients.
2. Nothing I have said affects the principles of ordinary practice in so far as
    (*a*) the analyst is in the first decade of his analytic career;
    (*b*) the case is a true neurotic (not psychotic).
3. I do suggest that while analysts are waiting to be in a position, through their increasing personal experience, to tackle a case in which regression must occur, there is much they can do to prepare themselves. They can:
    (*a*) watch the operation of setting factors;
    (*b*) watch the minor examples of regression with natural termination that appear in the course of analytic sessions, and
    (*c*) watch and use the regressive episodes that occur in the patient's life outside analysis, episodes, I may say, which are usually wasted, much to the impoverishment of the analysis.

The main result of the ideas I am putting forward, if they are accepted, will be a more accurate, rich, and profitable use of the setting phenomena in ordinary analyses of non-psychotics, resulting, I believe, in a new approach to the understanding of psychosis, and its treatment by psycho-analysts doing psycho-analysis.

SUMMARY

Attention is drawn to the subject of regression as it occurs in the psycho-analytic setting. Case reports of successful psychological treatments of adults and children show that techniques that allow of regression are increasingly being used. It is the psycho-analyst, familiar with the technique required in treatment of psychoneurosis, who can best understand regression and the theoretical implication of the patient's expectations that belong to the need to regress.

Regression can be of any degree, localized and momentary, or total and involving a patient's whole life over a phase. The less severe regressions provide fruitful material for research.

Emerging from such study comes a fresh understanding of the 'true self' and the 'false self', and of the 'observing ego', and also of the ego organization which enables regression to be a healing mechanism, one that remains potential unless there be provided a new and reliable environmental adaptation which can be used by the patient in correction of the original adaptive failure.

Here the therapeutic work in analysis links up with that done by child care, by friendship, by enjoyment of poetry, and cultural pursuits generally. But psycho-analysis can allow and use the hate and anger belonging to the original failure, important effects which are liable to destroy the value of therapeusis brought about by non-analytic methods.

On recovery from regression the patient, with the self now more fully surrendered to the ego, needs ordinary analysis as designed for the management of the depressive position and of the Oedipus complex in interpersonal relationships. For this reason, if for no other, the student should acquire proficiency in the analysis of the carefully-chosen non-psychotic before proceeding to the study of regression. Preliminary work can be done by a study of the setting in classical psycho-analysis.

Chapter XXIII

Clinical Varieties of Transference[1]
[1955-6]

MY CONTRIBUTION to this Symposium on Transference deals with one special aspect of the subject. It concerns the influence on analytical practice of the new understanding of infant care which has, in turn, derived from analytical theory.

In the history of psycho-analysis there has often been a delay in the direct application of analytical metapsychology. Freud was able to formulate a theory of the very early stages of the emotional development of the individual at a time when theory was being applied only in the treatment of the well-chosen neurotic case. (I refer to the period of Freud's work between 1905 and 1914.)

For instance the theory concerning the primary process, primary identification, and primary repression appeared in analytical practice only in the form of a greater respect that analysts had, as compared with others, for the dream and for psychic reality.

As we look back now we may say that cases were well-chosen as suitable for analysis if in the very early personal history of the patient there *had been good-enough infant care*. This good-enough adaptation to need at the beginning had enabled the individual's ego to come into being, with the result that the *earlier stages* of the establishment of the ego *could be taken for granted* by the analyst. In this way it was possible for analysts to talk and write as if the human infant's first experience was the first feed, and as if the object relationship between mother and infant that this implied was the first significant relationship. This was satisfactory for the practising analyst but it could not satisfy the direct observer of infants who are in the care of their mothers.

At that time theory was groping towards a deeper insight into this matter of

[1] Read before the 19th International Psycho-Analytical Congress, Geneva, 1955. *Int. J. Psycho-Anal.*, Vol. XXXVII, p. 386, 1956.

the mother with her infant, and indeed the term 'primary identification' implies an environment that is not yet differentiated from that which will be the individual. When we see a mother holding an infant soon after the birth, or an infant not yet born, at this same time we know that there is another point of view, that of the infant if the infant were already there; and from this point of view the infant is either not yet differentiated out, or else the process of differentiation has started and there is absolute dependence on the immediate environment and its behaviour. It has now become possible to study and use this vital part of old theory in a new and practical way in analytical work, work either with borderline cases or else with the psychotic phases or moments that occur in the course of the analyses of neurotic patients or normal people. This work widens the concept of transference since at the time of the analysis of these phases the ego of the patient cannot be assumed as an established entity, and there can be no transference neurosis for which, surely, there must be an ego, and indeed an intact ego, an ego that is able to maintain defences against anxiety arising out of instinct, the responsibility for which is accepted.

I have referred to the state of affairs that exists when a move is made in the direction of emergence from primary identification. Here at first is absolute dependence. There are two possible kinds of outcome: by the one, environmental adaptation to need is good enough, so that there comes into being an ego which, in time, can experience id impulses; by the other, environmental adaptation is not good enough, and so there is no true ego establishment, but instead there develops a *pseudo-self* which is a collection of innumerable reactions to a succession of failures of adaptation. I would like here to refer to Anna Freud's paper: 'The Widening Scope of Indications for Psycho-Analysis' (1954). The environment, when it successfully adapts at this early stage, is not recognized, or even recorded, so that in the original stage there is no feeling of dependence; whenever the environment fails in its task of making active adaptation, however, it automatically becomes recorded as an impingement, something that interrupts the continuity of being, that very thing which, if not broken up, would have formed itself into the ego of the differentiating human being.

There may be extreme cases in which there is no more than a collection of reactions to environmental failures of adaptation at the critical stage of emergence from primary identification. I am sure this condition is compatible with life, and with physical health. In the cases on which my work is based there has been what I call a true self hidden, protected by a false self. This false self is no doubt an aspect of the true self. It hides and protects it, and it reacts to the adaptation failures and develops a pattern corresponding to the pattern of environmental failure. In this way the true self is not involved in the reacting, and so preserves a continuity of being. However, this hidden true self suffers an impoverishment that derives from lack of experience.

The false self may achieve a deceptive false integrity, that is to say a false ego-strength, gathered from an environmental pattern, and from a good and reliable environment; for it by no means follows that early maternal failure must lead to a general failure of child care. The false self cannot, however, experience life or feel real.

In the favourable case the false self develops a fixed maternal attitude towards the true self, and is permanently in a state of holding the true self as a mother holds a baby at the very beginning of differentiation and of emergence from primary identification.

In the work that I am reporting the analyst follows the basic principle of psycho-analysis, that the patient's unconscious leads and is alone to be pursued. In dealing with a regressive tendency the analyst must be prepared to follow the patient's unconcious process if he is not to issue a directive and so step outside the analyst's role. I have found that it is not necessary to step outside the analyst's role and that it is possible to follow the patient's unconscious lead in this type of case as in the analysis of neurosis. There are differences, however, in the two types of work.

Where there is an intact ego and the analyst can take for granted these earliest details of infant care, then the setting of the analysis is unimportant relative to the interpretative work. (By setting, I mean the summation of all the details of management.) Even so there is a basic ration of management in ordinary analysis which is more or less accepted by all analysts.

In the work I am describing the setting becomes more important than the interpretation. The emphasis is changed from the one to the other.

The behaviour of the analyst, represented by what I have called the setting, by being good enough in the matter of adaptation to need, is gradually perceived by the patient as something that raises a hope that the true self may at last be able to take the risks involved in its starting to experience living.

Eventually the false self hands over to the analyst. This is a time of great dependence, and true risk, and the patient is naturally in a deeply regressed state. (By regression here I mean regression to dependence and to the early developmental processes.) This is also a highly painful state because the patient is aware, as the infant in the original situation is not aware, of the risks entailed. In some cases so much of the personality is involved that the patient must be in care at this stage. The processes are better studied, however, in those cases in which these matters are confined, more or less, to the time of the analytic sessions.

One characteristic of the transference at this stage is the way in which we must allow the patient's past to *be* the present. This idea is contained in Mme Sechehaye's book and in her title *Symbolic Realization*. Whereas in the transference neurosis the past comes into the consulting-room, in this work it is more true to say that the present goes back into the past, and *is* the past. Thus the analyst finds himself confronted with the patient's primary process in the setting in which it had its original validity.

Good enough adaptation by the analyst produces a result which is exactly that which is sought, namely, a shift in the patient of the main site of operation from a false to a true self. There is now for the first time in the patient's life an opportunity for the development of an ego, for its integration from ego nuclei, for its establishment as a body ego, and also for its repudiation of an external environment with the initiation of a relatedness to objects. For the first time the ego can experience id impulses, and can feel real in so doing, and also in resting from experiencing. And from here there can at last follow an ordinary analysis of the ego's defences against anxiety.

There builds up an ability of the patient to use the analyst's limited successes in adaptation, so that the ego of the patient becomes able to begin to recall the original failures, all of which were recorded, kept ready. These failures had a disruptive effect at the time, and a treatment of the kind I am describing has gone a long way when the patient is able to take an example of original failure and to be angry about it. Only when the patient reaches this point, however, can there be the beginning of reality-testing. It seems that something like primary repression overtakes these recorded traumata once they have been used in the treatment.

The way that this change comes about from the experience of being disrupted to the experience of anger is a matter that interests me in a special way, as it is at this point in my work that I found myself surprised. *The patient makes use of the analyst's failures.* Failures there must be, and indeed there is no attempt to give perfect adaptation; I would say that it is less harmful to make mistakes with these patients than with neurotic patients. Others may be surprised, as I was, to find that while a gross mistake may do but little harm, a very small error of judgment may produce a big effect. The clue is that the analyst's failure is being used and must be treated as a *past* failure, one that the patient can perceive and encompass, and be angry about now. The analyst needs to be able to make use of his failures in terms of their meaning for the patient, and he must if possible account for each failure even if this means a study of his unconscious countertransference.

In these phases of analytic work that which would be called resistance in work with neurotic patients always indicates that *the analyst has made a mistake*, or in some detail has behaved badly; in fact, the resistance remains until the analyst has found out the mistake and has tried to account for it, and has used it. If he defends himself, the patient misses the opportunity for being angry about a past failure just where anger was becoming possible for the first time. Here is a great contrast between this work and the analysis of neurotic patients with intact ego. It is here that we can see the sense in the dictum that every failed analysis is a failure not of the patient but of the analyst.

This work is exacting partly because the analyst has to have a sensitivity to the patient's needs and a wish to provide a setting that caters for these needs. The analyst is not, after all, the patient's natural mother.

It is exacting, also, because of the necessity for the analyst to look for his own mistakes whenever resistances appear. Yet it is only by using his own mistakes that he can do the most important part of the treatment in these phases, the part that enables the patient to become angry for the first time about the details of failure of adaptation that (at the time when they happened) produced disruption. It is this part of the work that frees the patient from dependence on the analyst.

In this way the negative transference of 'neurotic' analysis is replaced by objective anger about the analyst's failures, so there again is an important difference between the transference phenomena in the two types of work.

We must not look for an awareness of our adaptation successes, since these are not felt as such at a deep level. Although we cannot work without the theory that we build up in our discussions, this work inevitably finds us out if our understanding of our patient's need is a matter of the mind rather than of the psyche-soma.

In my clinical work I have proved, at least to myself, that one kind of analysis does not preclude the other. I find myself slipping over from one to the other and back again, according to the trend of the patient's unconscious process. When work of the special kind I have referred to is completed it leads naturally on to ordinary analytic work, the analysis of the depressive position and of the neurotic defences of a patient with an ego, an intact ego, an ego that is able to experience id impulses and to take the consequences. What needs to be done now is the study in detail of the criteria by which the analyst may know *when to work with the change of emphasis*, how to see that a need is arising which is of the kind that I have said must be met (at least in a token way) by active adaptation, the analyst keeping the concept of primary identification all the time in mind.

Chapter XXIV

Primary Maternal Preoccupation
[1956]

THIS CONTRIBUTION is stimulated by the discussion published in the *Psychoanalytic Study of the Child*, Volume IX, under the heading: 'Problems of Infantile Neurosis'. The various contributions from Miss Freud in this discussion add up to an important statement of present-day psycho-analytic theory as it relates to the very early stages of infant life, and of the establishment of personality.

I wish to develop the theme of the very early infant-mother relationship, a theme that is of maximal importance at the beginning, and that only gradually takes second place to that of the infant as an independent being.

It is necessary for me first to support what Miss Freud says under the heading, 'Current Misconceptions'. 'Disappointments and frustrations are inseparable from the mother-child relationship. . . . To put the blame for the infantile neurosis on the mother's shortcomings in the oral phase is no more than a facile and misleading generalization. Analysis has to probe further and deeper in its search for the causation of neurosis.' In these words Miss Freud expresses a view held by psycho-analysts generally.

In spite of this we may gain much by taking the mother's position into account. There is such a thing as an environment that is not good enough, and which distorts infant development, just as there can be a good-enough environment, one that enables the infant to reach, at each stage, the appropriate innate satisfactions and anxieties and conflicts.

Miss Freud has reminded us that we may think of pregenital patterning in terms of two people joined to achieve what for brevity's sake one might call 'homeostatic equilibrium' (Mahler, 1954). The same thing is referred to under the term 'symbiotic relationship'. It is often stated that the mother of an infant becomes biologically conditioned for her job of special orientation to the needs of her child. In more ordinary language there is found to be an identification — conscious but also deeply unconscious — which the mother makes with her infant.

I think that these various concepts need joining together and the study of the mother needs to be rescued from the purely biological. The term symbiosis takes us no further than to compare the relationship of the mother and the infant with other examples in animal and plant life — physical interdependence. The words homeostatic equilibrium again avoid some of the fine points which appear before our eyes if we look at this relationship with the care it deserves.

We are concerned with the very great *psychological* differences between, on the one hand, the mother's identification with the infant and, on the other, the infant's dependence on the mother; this latter does not involve identification, identification being a complex state of affairs inapplicable to the early stages of infancy.

Miss Freud shows that we have gone far beyond that awkward stage in psycho-analytic theory in which we spoke as if life started for the infant with oral instinctual experience. We are now engaged in the study of early development and of the early self which, if development has gone far enough, can be strengthened instead of disrupted by id experiences.

Miss Freud says, developing the theme of Freud's term 'anaclitic': 'The relationship to the mother, although the first to another human being, is not the infant's first relationship to the environment. What precedes it is an earlier phase in which not the object world but the body needs and their satisfaction or frustration play the decisive part.'

Incidentally I feel that the introduction of the word 'need' instead of 'desire' has been very important in our theorizing, but I wish Miss Freud had not used the words 'satisfaction' and 'frustration' here; a need is either met or not met, and the effect is not the same as that of satisfaction and frustration of id impulse.

I can bring in Greenacre's reference (1954) to what she names the 'lulling' type of rhythmic pleasures. Here we find an example of need that is met or not met, but it would be a distortion to say that the infant who is not lulled reacts as to a frustration. Certainly there is not anger so much as some kind of distortion of development at an early phase.

Be that as it may, a further study of the function of the mother *at the earliest phase* seems to me to be overdue, and I wish to gather together the various hints and put forward a proposition for discussion.

MATERNAL PREOCCUPATION

It is my thesis that in the earliest phase we are dealing with a very special state of the mother, a psychological condition which deserves a name, such as

Primary Maternal Preoccupation. I suggest that sufficient tribute has not yet been paid in our literature, or perhaps anywhere, to a very special psychiatric condition of the mother, of which I would say the following things:

It gradually develops and becomes a state of heightened sensitivity during, and especially towards the end of, the pregnancy.

It lasts for a few weeks after the birth of the child.

It is not easily remembered by mothers once they have recovered from it. I would go further and say that the memory mothers have of this state tends to become repressed.

This organized state (that would be an illness were it not for the fact of the pregnancy) could be compared with a withdrawn state, or a dissociated state, or a fugue, or even with a disturbance at a deeper level such as a schizoid episode in which some aspect of the personality takes over temporarily. I would like to find a good name for this condition and to put it forward as something to be taken into account in all references to the earliest phase of infant life. I do not believe that it is possible to understand the functioning of the mother at the very beginning of the infant's life without seeing that she must be able to reach this state of heightened sensitivity, almost an illness, and to recover from it. (I bring in the word 'illness' because a woman must be healthy in order both to develop this state and to recover from it as the infant releases her. If the infant should die, the mother's state suddenly shows up as illness. The mother takes this risk.)

I have implied this in the term 'devoted' in the words 'ordinary devoted mother' (Winnicott, 1949). There are certainly many women who are good mothers in every other way and who are capable of a rich and fruitful life but who are not able to achieve this' normal illness' which enables them to adapt delicately and sensitively to the infant's needs at the very beginning; or they achieve it with one child but not with another. Such women are not able to become preoccupied with their own infant to the exclusion of other interests, in the way that is normal and temporary. It may be supposed that there is a 'flight to sanity' in some of these people. Some of them certainly have very big alternative concerns which they do not readily abandon or they may not be able to allow this abandonment until they have had their first babies. When a woman has a strong male identification she finds this part of her mothering function most difficult to achieve, and repressed penis envy leaves but little room for primary maternal preoccupation.

In practice the result is that such women, having produced a child, but having missed the boat at the earliest stage, are faced with the task of making up for what has been missed. They have a long period in which they must closely adapt to their growing child's needs, and it is not certain that they can succeed in mending the early distortion. Instead of taking for granted the good effect of an early and temporary preoccupation they are caught up in the child's need for therapy, that is to say, for a prolonged period of adaptation to need, or spoiling. They do therapy instead of being parents.

The same phenomenon is referred to by Kanner (1943), Loretta Bender (1947) and others who have attempted to describe the type of mother who is liable to produce an 'autistic child' (Creak, 1951; Mahler, 1954).

It is possible to make a comparison here between the mother's task in making up for her past incapacity and that of society attempting (sometimes successfully) to bring round a deprived child from an antisocial state towards a social identification. This work of the mother (or of society) proves a great strain because it does not come naturally. The task in hand properly belongs to an earlier date, in this case to the time when the infant was only beginning to exist as an individual.

If this thesis of the normal mother's special state and her recovery from it be acceptable, then we can examine more closely the infant's corresponding state.

The infant has

A constitution.

Innate developmental tendencies ('conflict-free area in ego').

Motility and sensitivity.

Instincts, themselves involved in the developmental tendency, with changing zone-dominance.

The mother who develops this state that I have called 'primary maternal preoccupation' provides a setting for the infant's constitution to begin to make itself evident, for the developmental tendencies to start to unfold, and for the infant to experience spontaneous movement and become the owner of the sensations that are appropriate to this early phase of life. The instinctual life need not be referred to here because what I am discussing begins before the establishment of instinct patterns.

I have tried to describe this in my own language, saying that if the mother provides a good enough adaptation to need, the infant's own line of life is disturbed very little by reactions to impingement. (Naturally, it is the *reactions* to impingement that count, not the impingements themselves.) Maternal failures produce phases of reaction to impingement and these reactions interrupt the 'going on being' of the infant. An excess of this reacting produces not frustration but a *threat of annihilation*. This in my view is a very real primitive anxiety, long antedating any anxiety that includes the word death in its description.

In other words, the basis for ego establishment is the sufficiency of 'going on being', uncut by reactions to impingement. A sufficiency of 'going on being' is only possible at the beginning if the mother is in this state that (I suggest) is a very real thing when the healthy mother is near the end of her pregnancy, and over a period of a few weeks following the baby's birth.

Only if a mother is sensitized in the way I am describing can she feel herself into her infant's place, and so meet the infant's needs. These are at first body-needs, and they gradually become ego-needs as a psychology emerges out of the imaginative elaboration of physical experience.

There comes into existence an ego-relatedness between mother and baby, from which the mother recovers, and out of which the infant may eventually build the idea of a person in the mother. From this angle the recognition of the mother as a person comes in a positive way, normally, and not out of the experience of the mother as the symbol of frustration. The mother's failure to adapt in the earliest phase does not produce anything but an annihilation of the infant's self.

What the mother does well is not in any way apprehended by the infant at this stage. This is a fact according to my thesis. Her failures are not felt as maternal failures, but they act as threats to personal self-existence.

In the language of these considerations, the early building up of the ego is therefore silent. The first ego organization comes from the experience of threats of annihilation which do not lead to annihilation and from which, repeatedly, there is *recovery*. Out of such experiences confidence in recovery begins to be something which leads to an ego and to an ego capacity for coping with frustration.

It will, I hope, be felt that this thesis contributes to the subject of the infant's recognition of the mother as a frustrating mother. This is true later on but not at this very early stage. At the beginning the failing mother is not apprehended as such. Indeed a recognition of absolute dependence on the mother and of her capacity for primary maternal preoccupation, or whatever it is called, is something which belongs to *extreme sophistication*, and to a stage not always reached by adults. The general failure of recognition of absolute dependence at the start contributes to the fear of WOMAN that is the lot of both men and women (Winnicott, 1950, 1957a).

We can now say why we think the baby's mother is the most suitable person for the care of that baby; it is she who can reach this special state of primary maternal preoccupation without being ill. But an adoptive mother, or any woman who can be ill in the sense of 'primary maternal preoccupation', may be in a position to adapt well enough, on account of having some capacity for identification with the baby.

According to this thesis a good enough environmental provision in the earliest phase enables the infant to begin to exist, to have experience, to build a personal ego, to ride instincts, and to meet with all the difficulties inherent in life. All this feels real to the infant who becomes able to have a self that can eventually even afford to sacrifice spontaneity, even to die.

On the other hand, without the initial good-enough environmental provision, this self that can afford to die never develops. The feeling of real is absent and if there is not too much chaos the ultimate feeling is of futility. The inherent difficulties of life cannot be reached, let alone the satisfactions. If there is not chaos, there appears a false self that hides the true self, that complies with demands, that reacts to stimuli, that rids itself of instinctual experiences by having them, but that is only playing for time.

It will be seen that, by this thesis, constitutional factors are more likely to show up in the normal, where the environment in the first phase has been adaptive. By contrast, when there has been failure at this first phase, the infant is caught up in primitive defence mechanisms (false self, etc.) which belong to the threat of annihilation, and constitutional elements tend to become overridden (unless physically manifest).

It is necessary here to leave undeveloped the theme of the infant's introjection of illness patterns of the mother, though this subject is of great importance in consideration of the environmental factor in the next stages, after the first stage of absolute dependence.

In reconstructing the early development of an infant there is no point at all in talking of instincts, except on a basis of ego development.

There is a watershed:

Ego maturity — instinctual experiences strengthen ego.

Ego immaturity — instinctual experiences disrupt ego.

Ego here implies a summation of experience. The individual self starts as a summation of resting experience, spontaneous motility, and sensation, return from activity to rest, and the gradual establishment of a capacity to wait for recovery from annihilations; annihilations that result from reactions to environmental impingement. For this reason the individual needs to start in the specialized environment to which I have here referred under the heading: Primary Maternal Preoccupation.

Chapter XXV

The Antisocial Tendency[1]
[1956]

THE ANTISOCIAL tendency provides psycho-analysis with some awkward problems, problems of a practical as well as a theoretical nature. Freud, through his introduction to Aichhorn's *Wayward Youth*, showed that psycho-analysis not only contributes to the understanding of delinquency, but it is also enriched by an understanding of the work of those who cope with delinquents.

I have chosen to discuss the antisocial tendency, not delinquency. The reason is that the organized antisocial defence is overloaded with secondary gain and social reactions which make it difficult for the investigator to get to its core. By contrast the antisocial tendency can be studied as it appears in the normal or near-normal child, where it is related to the difficulties that are inherent in emotional development.

I will start with two simple references to clinical material:

For my first child analysis I chose a delinquent. This boy attended regularly for a year and the treatment stopped because of the disturbance that the boy caused in the clinic. I could say that the analysis was going well, and its cessation caused distress both to the boy and to myself in spite of the fact that on several occasions I got badly bitten on the buttocks. The boy got out on the roof and also he spilt so much water that the basement became flooded. He broke into my locked car and drove it away in bottom gear on the self-starter. The clinic ordered termination of the treatment for the sake of the other patients. He went to an approved school.

I may say that he is now 35, and he has been able to earn his living in a job that caters for his restlessness. He is married, with several children. Nevertheless I am afraid to follow up his case for fear that I should become

---

[1] Read before the British Psycho-Analytical Society, 20th June, 1956.

involved again with a psychopath, and I prefer that society should continue to take the burden of his management.

It can easily be seen that the treatment for this boy should have been not psycho-analysis but placement. Psycho-analysis only made sense if added after placement. Since this time I have watched analysts of all kinds fail in the psycho-analysis of antisocial children.

By contrast, the following story brings out the fact that an antisocial tendency may sometimes be treated very easily if the treatment be adjunctive to specialized environmental care.

I was asked by a friend to discuss the case of her son, the eldest of a family of four. She could not bring John to me in an open way because of her husband who objects to psychology on religious grounds. All she could do was to have a talk with me about the boy's compulsion to steal, which was developing into something quite serious; he was stealing in a big way from shops as well as at home. It was not possible for practical reasons to arrange for anything else but for the mother and myself to have a quick meal together in a restaurant, in the course of which she told me about the troubles and asked me for advice. There was nothing for me to do unless I could do it then and there. I therefore explained the meaning of the stealing and suggested that she should find a good moment in her relationship with the boy and make an interpretation to him. It appeared that she and John had a good relationship with each other for a few moments each evening after he had gone to bed; usually at such a time he would discuss the stars and the moon. This moment could be used.

I said: 'Why not tell him that you know that when he steals he is not wanting the things that he steals but he is looking for something that he has a right to; that he is making a claim on his mother and father because he feels deprived of their love.' I told her to use language which he could understand. I may say that I knew enough of this family, in which both the parents are musicians, to see how it was that this boy had become to some extent a deprived child, although he has a good home.

Some time later I had a letter telling me that she had done what I suggested. She wrote: 'I told him that what he really wanted when he stole money and food and things was his mum; and I must say I didn't really expect him to understand, but he did seem to. I asked him if he thought we didn't love him because he was so naughty sometimes, and he said right out that he didn't think we did, much. Poor little scrap! I felt so awful, I can't tell you. So I told him never, never to doubt it again and if he ever did feel doubtful to remind me to tell him again. But of course I shan't need reminding for a long time, it's been such a shock. One seems to need these shocks. So I'm being a lot more demonstrative to try and keep him from being doubtful any more. And up to now there's been absolutely no more stealing.'

The mother had had a talk with the form teacher and had explained to her that the boy was in need of love and appreciation, and had gained her co-operation although the boy gives a lot of trouble at school.

Now after eight months it is possible to report that there has been no return of stealing, and the relationship between the boy and his family has very much improved.

In considering this case it must be remembered that I had known the mother very well during her adolescence and to some extent had seen her through an antisocial phase of her own. She was the eldest in a large family. She had a very good home but very strong discipline was exerted by the father, especially at the time when she was a small child. What I did therefore had the effect of a double therapy, enabling this young woman to get insight into her own difficulties through the help that she was able to give to her son. When we are able to help parents to help their children we do in fact help them about themselves.

(In another paper I propose to give clinical examples illustrating the management of children with antisocial tendency; here I do no more than attempt a brief statement of the basis of my personal attitude to the clinical problem.)

NATURE OF ANTISOCIAL TENDENCY

The antisocial tendency *is not a diagnosis*. It does not compare directly with other diagnostic terms such as neurosis and psychosis. The antisocial tendency may be found in a normal individual, or in one that is neurotic or psychotic.

For the sake of simplicity I will refer only to children, but the antisocial tendency may be found at all ages. The various terms in use in Great Britain may be brought together in the following way:

A child becomes a *deprived child* when deprived of certain essential features of home life. Some degree of what might be called the 'deprived complex' becomes manifest. *Antisocial behaviour* will be manifest at home or in a wider sphere. On account of *the antisocial tendency* the child may eventually need to be *deemed maladjusted*, and to receive treatment in a *hostel for maladjusted children*, or may be brought before the courts as *beyond control*. The child, now *a delinquent*, may then become *a probationer* under a court order, or may be sent to *an approved school*. If the home ceases to function in an important respect the child may be taken over by the Children's Committee (under the Children Act, 1948) and be given 'care and protection'. If possible a foster home will be found. Should these measures fail the young adult may be said to have become a *psychopath* and may be sent by the courts to a *Borstal* or to prison. There may be an established tendency to repeat crimes for which we use the term *recidivism*.

All this makes no comment on the individual's psychiatric diagnosis.

The antisocial tendency is characterized by an *element in it which compels the environment to be important*. The patient through unconscious drives compels someone to attend to management. It is the task of the therapist to become involved in this the patient's unconscious drive, and the work is done by the therapist in terms of management, tolerance, and understanding.

The antisocial tendency implies hope. Lack of hope is the basic feature of the deprived child who, of course, is not all the time being antisocial. In the period of hope the child manifests an antisocial tendency. This may be awkward for society, and for you if it is your bicycle that is stolen, but those who are not personally involved can see the hope that underlies the compulsion to steal. Perhaps one of the reasons why we tend to leave the therapy of the delinquent to others is that we dislike being stolen from?

The understanding that the antisocial act is an expression of hope is vital in the treatment of children who show the antisocial tendency. Over and over again one sees the moment of hope wasted, or withered, because of mismanagement or intolerance. This is another way of saying that the treatment of the antisocial tendency is not psycho-analysis but management, a going to meet and match the moment of hope.

There is a direct relationship between the antisocial tendency and deprivation. This has long been known by specialists in the field, but it is largely due to John Bowlby that there is now a widespread recognition of the relationship that exists between the antisocial tendency in individuals and emotional deprivation, typically in the period of late infancy and the early toddler stage, round about the age of one and two years.

When there is an antisocial tendency *there has been a true deprivation* (not a simple privation); that is to say, there has been a loss of something good that has been positive in the child's experience up to a certain date,[1] and that has been withdrawn; the withdrawal has extended over a period of time longer than that over which the child can keep the memory of the experience alive. The comprehensive statement of deprivation, one that includes both the early and the late, both the pinpoint trauma and the sustained traumatic condition and also both the near normal and the clearly abnormal.

[1] This idea seems to be implied in Bowlby's *Maternal Care and Mental Health*, page 47, where he compares his observations with those of others and suggests that the different results are explained according to the age of a child at the time of deprivation.

Note

In a statement in my own language of Klein's depressive position (Chapter XXI) I have tried to make clear the intimate relationship that exists between Klein's concept and Bowlby's emphasis on deprivation. Bowlby's three stages of the clinical reaction of a child of two years who goes to hospital can be given a theoretical formulation in terms of the gradual loss of hope because of the death of the internal object or introjected version of the external object that is lost. What can be further discussed is the relative importance of death of the internal object through anger and contact of 'good objects' with hate products within the psyche, and ego maturity or immaturity in so far as this affects the capacity to keep alive a memory.

Bowlby needs Klein's intricate statement that is built round the understanding of melancholia, and that derives from Freud and Abraham; but it is also true that psycho-analysis needs Bowlby's emphasis on deprivation, if psycho-analysis is ever to come to terms with this special subject of the antisocial tendency.

There are always two trends in the antisocial tendency although the accent is sometimes more on one than on the other. One trend is represented typically in stealing, and the other in destructiveness. By *one* trend the child is looking for something, somewhere, and failing to find it seeks it elsewhere, when hopeful. By the *other* the child is seeking that amount of environmental stability which will stand the strain resulting from impulsive behaviour. This is a search for an environmental provision that has been lost, a human attitude, which, because it can be relied on, gives freedom to the individual to move and to act and to get excited.

It is particularly because of the second of these trends that the child provokes total environmental reactions, as if seeking an ever-widening frame, a circle which had as its first example the mother's arms or the mother's body. One can discern a series — the mother's body, the mother's arms, the parental relationship, the home, the family including cousins and near relations, the school, the locality with its police-stations, the country with its laws.

In examining the near-normal and (in terms of individual development) the early roots of the antisocial tendency I wish to keep in mind all the time these two trends: object-seeking and destruction.

STEALING

Stealing is at the centre of the antisocial tendency, with the associated lying.

The child who steals an object is not looking for *the object stolen but seeks the mother over whom he or she has rights.* These rights derive from the fact that (from the child's point of view) the mother was created by the child. The mother met the child's primary creativity, and so became the object that the child was ready to find. (The child could not have created the mother; also the mother's meaning for the child depends on the child's creativity.)

Is it possible to join up the two trends, the stealing and the destruction, the object-seeking and that which provokes, the libidinal and the aggressive compulsions? I suggest that the union of the two trends is in the child and that it represents *a tendency towards self-cure,* cure of a de-fusion of instincts.

When there is at the time of the original deprivation some fusion of aggressive (or motility) roots with the libidinal the child claims the mother by a mixture of stealing and hurting and messing, according to the specific details of that child's emotional developmental state. When there is less fusion the child's object-seeking and aggression are more separated off from each other, and there is a greater degree of dissociation in the child. This leads to the proposition that *the nuisance value of the antisocial child is an essential feature,* and is also, at its best, *a favourable feature* indicating again a potentiality for recovery of lost fusion of the libidinal and motility drives.

In ordinary infant care the mother is constantly dealing with the nuisance value of her infant. For instance, a baby commonly passes water on the mother's lap while feeding at the breast. At a later date this appears as a momentary regression in sleep or at the moment of waking and bed-wetting results. Any exaggeration of the nuisance value of an infant may indicate the existence of a degree of deprivation and antisocial tendency.

The manifestation of the antisocial tendency includes stealing and lying, incontinence and the making of a mess generally. Although each symptom has its specific meaning and value, the common factor for my purpose in my attempt to describe the antisocial tendency is *the nuisance value of the symptoms.* This nuisance value is exploited by the child, and is not a chance affair. Much of the motivation is unconscious, but not necessarily all.

FIRST SIGNS OF ANTISOCIAL TENDENCY

I suggest that the first signs of deprivation are so common that they pass for normal; take for example the imperious behaviour which most parents meet with a mixture of submission and reaction. *This is not infantile omnipotence,* which is a matter of psychic reality, not of behaviour.

A very common antisocial symptom is greediness, with the closely related inhibition of appetite. If we study greediness we shall find the deprived complex. In other words, if an infant is greedy there is some degree of deprivation and some compulsion towards seeking for a therapy in respect of this deprivation through the environment. The fact that the mother is herself willing to cater for the infant's greediness makes for therapeutic success in the vast majority of cases in which this compulsion can be observed. Greediness in an infant is not the same as greed. The word greed is used in the theoretical statement of the tremendous instinctual claims that an infant makes on the mother at the beginning, that is to say, at the time when the infant is only starting to allow the mother a separate existence, at the first acceptance of the reality principle.

In parenthesis, it is sometimes said that a mother must fail in her adaptation to her infant's needs. Is this not a mistaken idea based on a consideration of id needs and a neglect of the needs of the ego? A mother must fail in satisfying instinctual demands, but she may completely succeed in not 'letting the infant down', *in catering for ego needs*, until such a time as the infant may have an introjected ego-supportive mother, and may be old enough to maintain this introjection in spite of failures of ego support in the actual environment.

The (pre-ruth) primitive love impulse is not the same as ruthless greediness. In the process of the development of an infant the primitive love impulse and greediness are separated by the mother's adaptation. The mother necessarily fails to maintain a high degree of adaptation to id needs and to some extent therefore every infant may be deprived, but is able to get the mother to cure this sub-deprived state by her meeting the greediness and messiness, etc., these being symptoms of deprivation. The greediness is part of the infant's compulsion to seek for a cure from the mother who caused the deprivation. This greediness is antisocial; it is the precursor of stealing, and it can be met and cured by the mother's therapeutic adaptation, so easily mistaken for spoiling. It should be said, however, that whatever the mother does, this does not annul the fact that the mother first failed in her adaptation to her infant's ego needs. The mother is usually able to meet the compulsive claims of the infant, and so to do a successful *therapy* of the deprived complex which is near its point of origin. She gets near to a cure because she enables the infant's hate to be expressed while she, the therapist, is in fact the depriving mother.

It will be noted that whereas the infant is under no obligation to the mother in respect of her meeting the primitive love impulse, there is some feeling of obligation as the result of the mother's therapy, that is to say her willingness to meet the claims arising out of frustration, claims that begin to have a nuisance value. Therapy by the mother may cure, but this is not mother-love.

This way of looking at the mother's indulgence of her infant involves a more complex statement of mothering than is usually acceptable. Mother-love is often thought of in terms of this indulgence, which in fact is a *therapy in respect of a failure of mother-love*. It is a therapy, a second chance given to mothers who cannot always be expected to succeed in their initial most delicate task of primary love. If a mother does this therapy as a reaction formation arising out of her own complexes, then what she does is called spoiling. In so far as she is able to do it because she sees the necessity for the child's claims to be met, and for the child's compulsive greediness to be indulged, then it is a therapy that is usually successful. Not only the mother, but the father, and indeed the family, may be involved.

Clinically, there is an awkward borderline between the mother's therapy which is successful and that which is unsuccessful. Often we watch a mother spoiling an infant and yet this therapy will not be successful, the initial deprivation having been too severe for mending 'by first intention' (to borrow a term from the surgery of wounds).

Just as greediness may be a manifestation of the reaction to deprivation and of an antisocial tendency, so may messiness and wetting and compulsive destructiveness. All these manifestations are closely interrelated. In bedwetting, which is so common a complaint, the accent is on regression at the moment of the dream, or on the antisocial compulsion to claim the right to wet on mother's body.

In a more complete study of stealing I would need to refer to the compulsion to go out and buy something, which is a common manifestation of the antisocial tendency that we meet in our psycho-analytic patients. It is possible to do a long and interesting analysis of a patient without affecting this sort of symptom, which belongs not to the patient's neurotic or psychotic defences but which does belong to the antisocial tendency, that which is a reaction to deprivation of a special kind and that took place at a special time. From this it will be clear that birthday presents and pocket money absorb some of the antisocial tendency that is to be normally expected.

In the same category as the shopping expedition we find, clinically, a 'going out', without aim, *truancy*, a centrifugal tendency that replaces the centripetal gesture which is implicit in thieving.

THE ORIGINAL LOSS

There is one special point that I wish to make. At the basis of the antisocial tendency is a good early experience that has been lost. Surely, *it is an essential feature that the infant has reached to a capacity to perceive that the cause of the disaster lies in an environmental failure.* Correct knowledge that the cause of the depression or disintegration is an external one, and not an internal one, is responsible for the personality distortion and for the urge to seek for a cure by new environmental provision. The state of ego maturity enabling perception of this kind determines the development of an antisocial tendency instead of a psychotic illness. A great number of antisocial compulsions present and become successfully treated in the early stages by the parents.

313

Antisocial children, however, are constantly pressing for this cure by environmental provision (unconsciously, or by unconscious motivation) but are unable to make use of it.

It would appear that the time of the original deprivation is during the period when in the infant or small child the ego is in process of achieving fusion of the libidinal and aggressive (or motility) id roots. In the hopeful moment the child:

> Perceives a new setting that has some elements of reliability.
>
> Experiences a drive that could be called object-seeking.
>
> Recognizes the fact that ruthlessness is about to become a feature and so Stirs up the immediate environment in an effort to make it alert to danger, and organized to tolerate nuisance.
>
> If the situation holds, the environment must be tested and retested in its capacity to stand the aggression, to prevent or repair the destruction, to tolerate the nuisance, to recognize the positive element in the antisocial tendency, to provide and preserve the object that is to be sought and found.

In a favourable case, when there is not too much madness or unconscious compulsion or paranoid organization, etc., the favourable conditions may in the course of time enable the child to find and love a person, instead of continuing the search through laying claims on substitute objects that had lost their symbolic value.

In the next stage the child needs to be able to experience despair in a relationship, instead of hope alone. Beyond this is the real possibility of a life for the child. When the wardens and staff of a hostel carry a child through all the processes *they have done a therapy that is surely comparable to analytic work*.

Commonly, parents do this complete job with one of their own children. But many parents who are well able to bring up normal children are not able to succeed with one of their children who happens to manifest an antisocial tendency.

In this statement I have deliberately omitted references to the relationship of the antisocial tendency to:

> Acting out.
>
> Masturbation.
>
> Pathological super-ego, unconscious guilt.
>
> Stages of libidinal development.
>
> Repetition compulsion.
>
> Regression to pre-concern.
>
> Paranoid defence.
>
> Sex-linkage in respect of symptomatology.

TREATMENT

Briefly, the treatment of the antisocial tendency is not psycho-analysis. It is the provision of child care which can be rediscovered by the child, and into which the child can experiment again with the id impulses, and which can be tested. It is the stability of the new environmental provision which gives the therapeutics. Id impulses must be experienced, if they are to make sense, in a framework of ego relatedness, and when the patient is a deprived child ego relatedness must derive support from the therapist's side of the relationship. According to the theory put forward in this paper it is the environment that must give new opportunity for ego relatedness since the child has perceived that it was an environmental failure in ego support that originally led to the antisocial tendency.

If the child is in analysis, the analyst must either allow the weight of the transference to develop outside the analysis, or else must expect the antisocial tendency to develop full strength in the analytic situation, and must be prepared to bear the brunt.

Chapter XXVI

Pædiatrics and Childhood Neurosis[1]
[1956]

THE WORD neurosis has two connotations. In popular speech it covers the whole subject of psychological disease. It is difficult for me to know whether I am expected to deal with neurosis in a general way or whether those who planned this programme wished for a brief statement of neurosis in the more strict and restricted psychiatric sense of the term.

For the psychiatrist, neurosis refers rather specifically to the difficulties inherent in the personal life, and not on the whole to troubles arising out of faulty management. Moreover, neurosis does not include psychosis, or a latent psychosis, or a mood disorder, or a paranoid tendency, or an antisocial tendency.

Neurosis proper denotes *unconscious conflict*. It relates to *the instinctual life* of the child. Its main point of origin is at the toddler stage, before the age generally accepted for education at a school. At this stage the family setting is of maximal value.

It will be evident that the existence of true neurosis implies healthy emotional growth at the very important earlier stages in infancy, where dependence on the mother is near-absolute, and where failure of care produces psychiatric illness more serious than neurosis.

Neurotic illness takes its origin in the very severe *anxiety* that results from the instinctual drives of the child. By anxiety I mean the sort of affect that breaks through in the nightmare. These instinctual drives have biological backing.

Fantasy is the imaginative elaboration of physical function. In the play and in the conscious and unconscious fantasy of the small child we find all that is to be found in the lives of adults, except the full capacity for instinctual

[1] Paper read by invitation before the Eighth International Congress of Paediatrics, Copenhagen, Denmark, 25th July, 1956.

experience of genital kind. The arrival of this latter capacity presents the child with new problems at puberty.

At the root of neurosis is anxiety, especially that arising out of the violent conflicts in the unconscious fantasy, and in the child's personal inner reality.

When we get to this root of neurosis in the analysis of *adults* we regularly find the root is in this period of the *childhood* of the adult under analysis. As paediatricians, therefore, we may see (if we look) not only childhood neurosis, but also (and even more so) the latent tendency which may become manifest as neurosis at some time in adult life. (This is even more true if we consider psychosis. The prevention of mental hospital illness is in the hands of the paediatrician, did he but know it. It is safe to assert, however, that the paediatrician does not know it, and his life is thereby made sweeter.)

Unconscious conflicts of love and hate, of heterosexual and homosexual trends, and so on, lead to the organization of *patterns of defence*, and it is these patterns of defence that constitute *organized neurosis*.

The paediatrician, should he wish, and if he should have the technical skill for getting into touch with unconscious processes, can witness the battle while it is in progress at the toddler stage, after infancy and before the latency period; can watch the fight which is *for instinctual freedom* in relation to internal fears that paralyse. These fears are so great that external strictness can act as a relief.

In the latency period the child is relieved temporarily from the burden of changing and developing instinctual processes, but at puberty, because of the new biological drives, the battle restarts, the pattern of the defences having become already laid down.

I need hardly mention that a personal and steady environment helps and that a neurotic or unreliable environment hinders when the child is thus engaged — engaged in dealing with internal strains and stresses, strains and stresses of a very high order, inherent in life itself.

Health is not, at this stage, an absence of symptomatology. Normality is to be defined on a much broader basis, one which takes into account the essential conflicts, chiefly unconscious, that belong to health, that simply mean that the child is alive and lively.

It is important for me to convey the *degree of complexity* of neurosis rather than to attempt to concentrate the subject into a tabloid that can be taken without tax on the digestive system. Much work has now been done on the emotional development of the human infant, and much is generally accepted.

Neurosis being an organized defensive pattern, it is necessary for me to enumerate the main defences.

The main defences against the intolerable anxiety that belongs to conflict in the unconscious associated with the instinctual life are of several kinds.

317

First, instinct itself becomes inhibited, becomes unacceptable to the total self, or only acceptable under conditions that make instinctual satisfaction precarious.

Second, guilt roused on account of the conflict of love and hate is allayed by obsessional rituals, a kind of religion with a dead god.

Third, some of the emotional conflict becomes changed into conflict in terms of physical functioning, such as colic, or an hysterical paresis.

Fourth, by organized phobias the child becomes able to avoid certain situations that stimulate anxiety, or objects that symbolize the things which produce fear.

At times anxiety breaks through, and then a parent or nurse must be available to come to the rescue.

Further, the child gets a certain amount of relief by being able to regress, that is to say by being able to return to the instinctual patterns of infancy, where intake and output were the chief functions, and where the mother successfully met the infant's dependence. Or, regression takes place as a form of breakdown, apart altogether from the expectation of having dependence met.

In other words, the chief anxieties in *neurosis* (contrast psychosis and latent psychosis) belong to forward movement towards a genital and away from an alimentary type of instinct.

This forward movement leads to anxiety about the genital itself, and to essential differences in the fantasies, fears, and defences according to the sex of the child.

When we think of illness and health in terms of neurosis and the absence of neurosis we are taking it for granted that the child has reached a stage of development in which it makes sense to refer to *interpersonal relationships*. Whole children are related to whole people. This cannot be said in a description of the earlier stages where infants are related to part-objects, or are themselves far from being established as units.

At the root of neurosis proper is the triangular situation, the relationship between three people as this first appears in the child's life. Boys and girls develop differently at this stage, but there are always the two triangles, that based on the heterosexual position and that based on the homosexual position. It can readily be seen that there is room for great complexity here.

From all these possibilities Freud singled out for study the Oedipus complex and by this term we signify our recognition of the whole of the problem that arises out of the child's achievement of a capacity to be related as a human being to two other human beings, the mother and the father at one and the same time.

It is just here that the major anxieties arise because it is precisely here that the instincts are maximally roused, and in the child's dream, which is accompanied by bodily excitement, there is everything at stake. True neurosis is not necessarily an illness, and first we should think of it as a tribute to the fact that life is difficult. We diagnose illness and abnormality only if the degree of disturbance is crippling to the child, or boring for the parent, or inconvenient for the family.

In the *prevention* of neurosis we try to give what is needed in the earliest stages of infancy, where there is great dependence, and where the mother lays down the basis for the child's mental health by what she does through devotion to her own infant.

In *treatment* we have several methods available.

1. Sometimes we are able to modify the immediate environment by giving the parents such understanding as will enable them to carry on where they were failing; but this does not lead to a sudden cessation of symptoms. Indeed, an improved emotional environment may lead to an increase of symptoms, because the small child needs room for the acting out of samples of fantasy, and for the discovery of the self through play.

2. There is a great deal of relief to be given by the usual modifications — sending the child away for a holiday, finding a suitable school, getting relief for the over-worked mother, mobilizing the odd uncle or aunt, buying a dog, etc., etc. But I need not elaborate here; rather I would point to the tremendous complexity of every human situation and to the need for humility in planning for someone else's life.

3. Then there is the whole question of the giving of personal help to the child. I can only stress that *intuition is not good enough in psychological practice.*

If a paediatrician asks me how to proceed I must advise him to take the psycho-analytical training, and then to modify what he has learned to meet the special case.

There may be a place for personal work with children by those who have not been able to become analysts; but this can only be true if the doctor, by temperament, can maintain a non-moralistic attitude and can easily be reliable in the important respects, especially in not having a pressing emotional need of his own which will gradually supersede that of the child. I have paediatric colleagues who do psychotherapy and who intend to do more, and who do it well. In spite of this, I must state here, in my attempt to be simple and categorical, that personal psychotherapy of children and adults should be done by those who have trained as analysts. *This is what we must advise our younger colleagues, and it is to those who will have the double qualification that the ball will pass in the next decade.*

It is better for a paediatrician to work on equal terms with trained (perhaps non-medical) analysts than for him to attempt psychotherapy that he is not qualified to do.

I would rather see psycho-analysis held back for fifty years than witness a rapid extension of psychotherapy by those who have not studied the vast complexities of this subject and the human nature that it must go out to meet.

But this is all common knowledge. It is in the books. It has long come into the training of psychiatric social workers and indeed of all social workers who do casework.

For some reason or other in the last thirty years paediatrics has gone ahead in one direction but has lagged behind in another.

In these thirty years there has been an amazing advance in theory and practice in physical paediatrics, and it is this advance that has laid bare and made evident the existence and extent of emotional disorder. It is understandable that there has been no time for psychology, and those drawn into paediatrics were often attracted by the fact that the problems to be tackled would be of a physical nature.

Is it because paediatrics is still fully occupied on the physical side that at the Institute of Psycho-Analysis in London, where we are training thirty analysts to treat and to study children, it is not (with a few exceptions) paediatricians who are applying for such training? By the way, psychology is already being practised, and well practised, outside the medical profession, by psychiatric social workers, and child-care workers who deal with deprived children, by probation officers, and by the staffs of hostels for so-called maladjusted children and hosts of other groups of professional workers with organizations of their own. Many of these workers have seen the need for a personal analysis. The standard of casework is often high. It is paediatrics that has held back.

On the subject of neurosis you have heard my summary of well-known, well-accepted theory. I cannot leave it at this. My contribution must be to make an examination of the difficulty that paediatrics is in.

There is something wrong somewhere, and it can be assumed that if something is wrong we would all wish to put it right.

It is often said that paediatricians are necessarily good with children. This I believe to be true.

Here, however, it is my job to make the further observation that being good with children is not psychology. It is altogether a different subject.

In this Congress *physical* paediatrics is showing a warm-hearted attitude towards the other half of paediatrics, that which concerns *emotional* development, and yet the way seems blocked. Surely the explanation is that those who are physically-minded base their work on the physical sciences, anatomy and physiology and biochemistry, and they do not know what science to turn to and on which to base any excursion they may make into psychological territory. What is there in psychology corresponding to the physical sciences?

At this point I shall be dogmatic and personal. I have spent my professional life with one foot in paediatrics and the other in psycho-analysis. Treating many thousands of cases, I have also had the privilege of conducting about a hundred long personal analyses of adults and children. I have also played my part in the training of psycho-analysts.

I am making it my main point in this contribution that sooner or later it must be recognized that the science underlying psychological paediatrics *already exists* in dynamic psychology, or the psychology of conscious and unconscious processes that derives from Freud. Psycho-analysis, both as a science and because of the training it can offer, deserves co-existence with physiology. I do ask here and now for respect from the physical sciences for psycho-analysis, and I ask this especially *from those who dislike it*. Disliking it is no argument against it.

There *must* be those who dislike psycho-analysis, because of the fact that it studies human nature objectively; it invades the realms where previously belief, intuition, and empathy held sway. Moreover, psychology introduces a new element into clinical work: as psychiatrists we must expect to find *in ourselves* the same difficulties and neurotic defence organizations that we find in our patients.

There is a rich literature for those who wish to make a further examination of neurosis, and plenty of neurosis exists for clinical study. My main point has been a suggestion in regard to the *post*-postgraduate training of those young paediatricians who can look ahead and see themselves as practitioners in the psychological half of our common subject, paediatrics. They need to train in psycho-analysis.

Bibliography

ABRAHAM, K. (1916). 'The First Pregenital Stage of the Libido.' *Selected Papers on Psycho-Analysis.* London: Hogarth Press.

ABRAHAM, K. (1927). *Selected Papers on Psycho-Analysis.* London: Hogarth Press.

ABRAHAM, K. (1955). *Clinical Papers and Essays on Psycho-Analysis.* London: Hogarth Press.

AICHHORN, A. (1925). *Wayward Youth.* London: Imago.

BALINT, M. (1955). 'Friendly Expanses—Horrid Empty Spaces.' *Int. J. Psycho-Anal.,* Vol. XXXVI.

BENDER, L. (1947). 'Childhood Schizophrenia.' *Am. J. Orthopsychiat.,* Vol. XVII.

BOWLBY, J. (1951). *Maternal Care and Mental Health.* Geneva: World Health Organization.

BOWLBY, J., ROBERTSON, J., and ROSENBLUTH, D. (1952). 'A Two-Year-Old Goes to Hospital.' *Psychoanal. Study Child,* Vol. VII. London: Imago.

BRIERLEY, M. (1951). *Trends in Psycho-Analysis.* London: Hogarth Press.

BRITTON, C. (1955). 'Casework Techniques in the Child Care Services.' *Case Conference,* Vol I, No. 9.

BURLINGHAM, D., and FREUD, ANNA. (1942). *Young Children in Wartime: a Year's Work in a Residential War Nursery.* London: Allen & Unwin.

CASTERET, N. (1947). *My Caves.* London: Dent.

CREAK, M. (1951). 'Psychoses in Childhood.' *J. ment. Sci.,* Vol. XCVII.

CREAK, M. (1952). 'Psychoses in Childhood.' *Proc. R. Soc. Med.,* Vol. XLV.

FAIRBAIRN, W. R. D. (1952). *Psychoanalytic Studies of the Personality.* London: Tavistock Publications.

FREUD, ANNA. (1937). *The Ego and the Mechanisms of Defence.* London: Hogarth Press.

FREUD, ANNA. (1947). 'Aggression in Relation to Emotional Development; Normal and Pathological.' *Psychoanal. Study Child,* Vol. III–IV. London: Imago.

FREUD, ANNA. (1947). 'Emotional and Instinctive Development.' In *Child Health and Development.* Ed. by Prof. R. W. B. Ellis. London: John Churchill.

FREUD, ANNA. (1952). 'A Connection Between the States of Negativism and of Emotional Surrender (Hörigkeit).' *Int. J. Psycho-Anal.,* Vol. XXXIII.

FREUD, ANNA. (1952). 'The Role of Bodily Illness in the Mental Life of Children.' *Psychoanal. Study Child,* Vol. VII. London: Imago.

FREUD, ANNA. (1953). 'Some Remarks on Infant Observation.' *Psychoanal. Study Child,* Vol. VIII. London: Imago.

FREUD, ANNA. (1954). 'Problems of Infantile Neurosis: a Discussion.' *Psychoanal. Study Child,* Vol. IX. London: Imago.

FREUD, ANNA. (1954). 'The Widening Scope of Indications for Psycho-Analysis.' *J. Amer. Psychoanal. Assoc.,* Vol. II, No. 4.

FREUD, ANNA, and BURLINGHAM, D. (1942). *Young Children in Wartime: a Year's Work in a Residential War Nursery.* London: Allen & Unwin.

FREUD, SIGMUND. (1905). 'Fragment of an Analysis of a Case of Hysteria.' *Complete Psychological Works of Sigmund Freud.* Vol. VII, pp. 51–2. London: Hogarth Press.

FREUD, SIGMUND. (1905). 'Three Essays on the Theory of Sexuality.' *Complete Psychological Works of Sigmund Freud.* Vol. VII. London: Hogarth Press.

FREUD, SIGMUND. (1909). 'Notes upon a Case of Obsessional Neurosis.' *Complete Psychological Works of Sigmund Freud.* Vol. X. London: Hogarth Press.

FREUD, SIGMUND. (1914). 'On Narcissism: an Introduction.' *Collected Papers.* Vol. IV. London: Hogarth Press.

FREUD, SIGMUND. (1915) 'Instincts and their Vicissitudes.' *Collected Papers.* Vol. IV. London: Hogarth Press.

FREUD, SIGMUND. (1917). 'Mourning and Melancholia.' *Collected Papers.* Vol. IV. London: Hogarth Press.

FREUD, SIGMUND. (1920). 'Beyond the Pleasure Principle.' *Complete Psychological Works of Sigmund Freud.* Vol. XVIII. London: Hogarth Press.

FREUD, SIGMUND. (1921). 'Group Psychology and the Analysis of the Ego.' *Complete Psychological Works of Sigmund Freud.* Vol. XVIII. London: Hogarth Press.

FREUD, SIGMUND. (1923). *The Ego and the Id.* London: Hogarth Press.

FREUD, SIGMUND. (1926). *Inhibitions, Symptoms and Anxiety.* London: Hogarth Press.

FREUD, SIGMUND. *The Origins of Psycho-Analysis.* London: Imago. 1950 (1954).

FRIEDLANDER, K. (1947). *The Psychoanalytical Approach to Juvenile Delinquency.* London: Kegan Paul, Trench, Trubner.

GLOVER, E. (1932). 'A Psychoanalytic Approach to the Classification of Mental Disorders.' In *On the Early Development of Mind.* Chap. XI. London: Imago.

GLOVER, E. (1945). 'An Examination of the Klein System of Child Psychology.' *Psychoanal. Study Child,* Vol. I. London: Imago.

GLOVER, E. (1949). 'The Position of Psycho-Analysis in Great Britain.' In *On the Early Development of Mind.* Chap. XXIII. London: Imago.

GREENACRE, P. (1941). 'The Predisposition to Anxiety.' In *Trauma, Growth and Personality.* London: Hogarth Press.

GREENACRE, P. (1945). 'The Biological Economy of Birth.' In *Trauma, Growth and Personality.* London: Hogarth Press.

GREENACRE, P. (1954). 'Problems of Infantile Neurosis: a Discussion.' *Psychoanal. Study Child,* Vol. IX. London: Imago.

HARTMANN, H. (1952). 'Mutual Influences in the Development of Ego and Id.' *Psychoanal. Study Child*, Vol. VII. London: Imago.

HENOCH, E. (1889). 'Lectures on Children's Diseases.' Trans. by John Thomson. London: The New Sydenham Society.

HOFFER, W. (1949). 'Mouth, Hand, and Ego-Integration.' *Psychoanal. Study Child*, Vol. III–IV. London: Imago.

ILLINGWORTH, R. S. (1951). 'Sleep Disturbances in Young Children.' *Brit. med. J.*

JONES, E. (1946). 'A Valedictory Address.' *Int. J. Psycho-Anal.*, Vol. XXVII.

JUNG, C. G. *The Collected Works of C. G. Jung*. Ed. Herbert Read, Michael Fordham, *et al.* London: Routledge & Kegan Paul.

KANNER, L. (1943). 'Autistic Disturbances of Affective Contact.' *The Nervous Child*. Vol. II.

KLEIN, M., and RIVIERE, J. (1936). 'Love, Hate and Reparation.' *Psycho-Analytical Epitomes*. No. 2. London: Hogarth Press, 1937.

KLEIN, M. (1932). *Psycho-Analysis of Children*. London: Hogarth Press.

KLEIN, M. (1948). *Contributions to Psycho-Analysis, 1921–45*. London: Hogarth Press.

KLEIN, M., HEIMANN, P., and MONEY-KYRLE, R. (1952). *Developments in Psycho-Analysis*. London: Hogarth Press.

KLEIN, M., HEIMANN, P., ISAACS, S., and RIVIERE, J. (1955). *New Directions in Psycho-Analysis*. London: Tavistock Publications; New York: Basic Books.

LINDNER, S. (1879). 'Das Saugen an den Fingern, Lippen, bei den Kindern (Ludeln)'. *Jb. Kinderheilk*, N.F. 14.68. (179).

MACALPINE, I. (1952). 'Psychosomatic Symptom Formation.' *Lancet*, Feb. 9.

MAHLER, M. S. (1952). 'On Child Psychosis and Schizophrenia.' *Psychoanal. Study Child*, Vol. VII. London: Imago.

MAHLER, M. S. (1954). 'Problems of Infantile Neurosis: a Discussion.' *Psychoanal. Study Child*, Vol. IX. London: Imago.

MARTY, P. et FAIN, M. (1955). 'La Motricité dans la Relation d'objet.' *Rev. française Psychanal*. Tome XIX, Nos. 1–2. Presses Universitaires de France.

MIDDLEMORE, M. P. (1941). *The Nursing Couple*. London: Hamish Hamilton.

MILNER, M. (1952). 'Aspects of Symbolism in Comprehension of the Not-Self.' *Int. J. Psycho-Anal.*, Vol. XXXIII.

RANK, O. (1924). *The Trauma of Birth*. London: Kegan Paul.

READ, G. D. (1942). *Revelation of Childbirth*. London: Heinemann.

READ, G. D. (1950). *Introduction to Motherhood*. London: Whitefriars Press.

RICKMAN, J. (1928). 'The Development of the Psycho-Analytical Theory of the Psychoses.' *Supplement No. 2 Int. J. Psycho-Anal.* London: Baillière, Tindall and Cox.

RICKMAN, J. (1951). 'Methodology and Research in Psychopathology.' *Brit. J. med. Psychol.*, Vol. XXIV.

RIVIERE, J. (1936). 'On the Genesis of Psychical Conflict in Earliest Infancy.' *Int. J. Psycho-Anal.*, Vol. XVII.

RIVIERE, J., and KLEIN, M. (1936). 'Love, Hate and Reparation.' *Psycho-Analytical Epitomes*, No. 2. London: Hogarth Press, 1937.

ROBERTSON, J., BOWLBY, J., and ROSENBLUTH, DINA. (1952). 'A Two-Year-Old Goes to Hospital.' *Psychoanal. Study Child*, Vol. VII. London: Imago.

RYCROFT, C. F. (1953). 'Some Observations on a Case of Vertigo.' *Int. J. Psycho-Anal.*, Vol. XXXIV.

SCOTT, W. C. M. (1949). 'The Body Scheme in Psychotherapy.' *Brit. J. med. Psychol.*, Vol. XXII.

SCOTT, W. C. M. (1955). 'A Note on Blathering.' *Int. J. Psycho-Anal.*, Vol. XXXVI.

SEARL, N. (1929). 'The Flight to Reality.' *Int. J. Psycho-Anal.*, Vol. X.

SECHEHAYE, M. A. (1951). *Symbolic Realization*. New York: International Universities Press.

SPITZ, R. A. (1945). 'Hospitalism. An Inquiry into the Genesis of Psychiatric Conditions in Early Childhood.' *Psychoanal. Study Child*, Vol. I. London: Imago.

SPITZ, R. A., and WOLF, K. M. (1946). 'Anaclitic Depression: an inquiry into the genesis of psychiatric conditions in early childhood.' *Psychoanal. Study Child*, Vol. II. London: Imago.

SPITZ, R. A. (1950). 'Relevancy of Direct Infant Observation.' *Psychoanal. Study Child*, Vol. V. London: Imago.

STEVENSON, O. (1954). 'The First Treasured Possession.' *Psychoanal. Study Child*, Vol. IX. London: Imago.

WHITEHEAD, A. N. (1933). *Adventures of Ideas*. Harmondsworth, Pelican Books.

WINNICOTT, D. W. (1931). *Clinical Notes on Disorders of Childhood*. London: Heinemann.

WINNICOTT, D. W. (1945). *Getting to Know Your Baby*. London: Heinemann. Republished in *The Child and the Family*. London: Tavistock Publications, 1957; New York: Basic Books.

WINNICOTT, D. W. (1947). 'Physical Therapy of Mental Disorder.' *Brit. med. J.* correspondence. *Brit. med. J.*, May 17th, 1947, p. 688.

WINNICOTT, D. W. (1949). 'Leucotomy.' *Brit. Med. Students' J.* Spring 1949, 3, 2, 35.

WINNICOTT, D. W. (1949). *The Ordinary Devoted Mother and Her Baby*. Nine Broadcast Talks. Republished in *The Child and the Family*. London: Tavistock Publications, 1957; New York: Basic Books.

WINNICOTT, D. W. (1950). 'Some Thoughts on the Meaning of the Word Democracy.' *Human Relations*. Vol. III, No. 2, June 1950.

WINNICOTT, D. W. (1957a). *The Child and the Family*. London: Tavistock Publications; New York: Basic Books. (p. 141).

WINNICOTT, D. W. (1957b). *The Child and the Outside World*. London: Tavistock Publications; New York: Basic Books.

WOLF, K. M. and SPITZ, R. A. (1946). 'Anaclitic Depression: an inquiry into the genesis of psychiatric conditions in early childhood.' *Psychoanal. Study Child.*, Vol. II. London: Imago.

WULFF, M. (1946). 'Fetishism and Object Choice in Early Childhood.' *Psychoanal. Quart.*, Vol. XV.

Index

N.B. Italicized page numbers refer to case histories.

Abnormal behaviour
anxiety basis of, 7
ABRAHAM, KARL, 221, 234n
Absolute dependence (see also Dependence)
in infancy, 163
Absolute independence
in infancy, 163
Abstract thinking (see also Mind), 185
Acting out
recapturing of primitive experiences through, 249–50
role of, in regression, 288–90
Adaptation (see also Infant care; 'Primary Maternal Preoccupation'; Psyche-Soma; Regression)
active, by environment to infant's needs, 115, 189
infant's ways of dealing with failures of near-perfect adaptation by mother, 238
in infant care, 100
near-perfect, by mother, 189, 237–8
100 per cent, and illusion, 238–9
Addiction
and transitional phenomena, 242
Adolescents
need for special environment in analysis of, 168–9
Adoption, 9
Affect
true, behind hysterical acting, 180
Affectionateness
capacity for, v. sensual experiences, 271
Aggression (see also Behaviour; Birth Trauma; Psyche-Soma)

and instinctual experience, 205
and unconscious jealousy, 6
dependent on opposition, 214–16
development of healthy early, 214–16
independent of reaction to frustration in infancy, 215
in relation to emotional development, XVI
needs external objects for satisfaction, 215–7
primitive and early roots of, 210
problems in studying, 204, 214
socialization of, 207–9
variability of aggression potential, 216
AICHHORN, AUGUST, 306
Ambivalence
analysis of, 146–7
as hate in countertransference, XV
in childhood, 6
Anaclitic relationship (see also Dependence; Infant-Care; Regression), 268, 301
Anger
and frustration, 207
reactive and birth-experience, 188
Animals
nightmares about, 41
Annihilation
of object, through satisfaction, 153
threat of, from failures in infant care, 303–4
Antisocial Tendency (see also Delinquency), XXV
as a tendency towards self-cure, 311
as an attempt at cure of de-fusion of instincts, 311
basis of, in a lost good experience, 313

326

characterized by an element in it which compels environment to be important, 309

distinguished from delinquency, 306

dynamics of behaviour in, 314

first signs of, 311–2

implies hope, 309

importance of infant's perception of early loss in, 313

meaning of its nuisance value, 311

meaning of stealing and destructiveness in, 310

not a diagnosis, 308–9

result of early true deprivation, and not privation, 309

stage of ego-development at the start of, 313–14

treatment by management and not psycho-analysis, 309, 315

treatment by specialized environmental care, *307–8*, 315

v. psychotic illness, 313

Anxiety (*see also* Aggression; Birth Trauma; Depressive Position; Infant-care; Psyche-Soma; Regression), *7*

about infant's own inside, 268–9

about object of instinctual love, 268–9

and abnormal behaviour, 7

and appetite disorders, 34

and being held, 98

and greed, 33

and insecurity, VIII

and normality, I, 3

and physical ill-health, 7

and symptom formation in childhood, 3–5

as threat of annihilation, 303–4

birth memories, birth trauma and, XIV

cause of, in infant care, 98

depressive, 129–30

depressive, and doubt, 130

depressive, and manic defence, 131

depressive, and transitional objects, 232

depressive, defences against, 272–4

effect on fantasy, 17

experience of, presupposes minimal maturation, 181

fear of lack of, in regression, 100

infantile, and 'set situation', 69

in 'set situation', 59

masking physical disease, 20–1

normal in childhood, *6*

not directly related to traumatic birth, 189–90

physical symptoms of, case histories: I, II

physiology of, 62

prevention of, by good-enough infant care, 98

psychotic, in a girl, *121–2*

relief from testing capacity for, 100

root of neurosis, 316–17

three types of, from failure in infant care, 99

two types of, following instinctual experiences in infants 268–9

Anxiety hysteria, *11–3*

Anxious

meaning of the state, 181

Appetite

and emotional disorder, III, 33

and relation to greed, 33

disorder and depression, 34

disorders of, case histories, *37–51*

disorders, symptoms of, 33–4

disturbances, 40

disturbances and psychiatric illnesses, 33

inhibition of, and suspiciousness, 40–1

loss of, *3–4, 8*

Archetypes

and depressive position, 273

Armistice Day, 139–40

Art (*see also* Primary creativity; Transitional Object)

and inner world fantasy, 35

and madness, 224

Artist

and partial recognition of inner reality, 133

Artistic creation

and dreams, 152

basis in guilt-feeling, 270

resolution of objectivity v. subjectivity in, 172

Artistic expression

and primitive experiences, 150n

Asthma
  and anxiousness, 16
  and control of impulse, 59
  and fear of breast, 63
  and over-control, 63
  in an infant, *56–61*
Auto-erotic activities
  and transitional phenomena, 231–2
Auto-erotism, 238
  and flight to external reality (manic defence), 133

Baby
  'no such thing as a', 99
BALINT, ALICE, 98
BALINT, MICHAEL, 100
Behaviour
  aggressive, and return from introversion, 207–8
Belly
  place of inner world fantasy, *35*
Birth
  importance of infant's maturity at, 148
  memories, birth trauma and anxiety, XIV
  normal, experience of, 183, 211
Birth experience (*see also* Psyche-Soma; Psycho-analytic Set-up; Regression)
  and sleep in analysis, 178–9
  cataloguing of reactions to, 247–50
  normal, not apparent in analysis, 180
  relived in analysis of a defective boy, *177–8*
  relived through black-out, *179–80*
  setting up acute reaction patterns, 182–3
  v. birth trauma, 180–1
Birth trauma
  body-memories of, 186
  features of its reappearance in analytic set-up, 189
  leading to congenital paranoia, *185–6*
  leads not to anxiety but persecution, 189
  pattern of, repeated in analyses, 180
  psychotic delusions deriving from, 187
Black-outs (*see also* Birth trauma)

and physical unconsciousness, *179–80*
Blindness
  and guilt, 87
  fear of, 85
  hysterical, 87
Body
  children's relation to, 85
  memory of birth experience in children's play, 180
Body-Scheme
  and 'environment-individual set-up', 222n
  and psyche-soma development, 251
  concept of, 243
Body-surface
  interest in, and flight from inner reality, *140*
Borderline disorders
  and their relation to depressive position, 262
Bottle-feeding, 235n
BOWLBY, JOHN, 147, 221, 309–10
Breast (*see also* Depressive position; Infant care; Mother; Weaning)
  and spatula, 47
  as a whole person (mother), 264
  as whole technique of mothering, 239n
  created by infant, 163, 238–9
  -feeding, 165
  good internalized, 47
  mother's, and illusion, 152
  mother's, and primitive emotional development, 152
  mother's, and primitive integration, 152
  mother's, as primary external reality, 152
  play with, in infancy, 165
Breathing
  control of, in mystical practices, 188
  fantasy of, 63
  initiation of, non-significant in normal birth, 191
BRIERLEY, MARJORIE, 95, 135n
BRITTON, CLARE, 126
BURLINGHAM, DOROTHY, 221
Buying
  compulsion towards, and antisocial tendency, 313

Cases
  assessment of role of early environment in classification of, 279–80
  care of schizoid, and infant care, 171
  classification and choice of, for analysis, 278–9
CASTERET, NORBERT, 186
Cataloguing
  of reactions to impingements, 247–8, *248–51*
Chaos
  in child's fantasy world, *73*
Character-formation
  and fidgetiness, 23
  and inhibitions of greed, *39–40*
  in children in relation to mother's depression, 91–3
Chemotherapy
  result of advances in, 101
Chest
  experiences in birth trauma, 187–8
Child
  antisocial, and objective hate in the care-taker, 199–200
  antisocial, and 'primary maternal preoccupation', 303
Child analysis, 60
  and infant observation, 61
  and problem of management, *72*
  and provision for a home for cases, 74, 81, 306–7
  case histories, V
  contra indications for, V
  problems of impracticability of, 70–2
Child analysts, 84
Child care (*see also* Infant care)
  and prophylaxis, 4
  and psychoses, XVII
Childhood
  ocular psychoneurosis of, VI
  psychosis in, 219
Child psychiatry
  and case-management at home, 126
  and paediatrics, 102
  and value of symptoms, 102
Children
  problem of testing out in, from broken homes, *199–200*
Chorea, 26, *78*
  and emotional instability, 25

  and fidgetiness, 22
  and tics, *27*
  and trauma, *27*
  anxiety symptoms mistaken for, *12*
  diagnostic symptoms of, 24–6
Circle
  as diagram of self, 253
Clinic
  outpatient children's, and hypochondria in mothers, 92
Colds
  and excitedness, 16
  and over-stimulation, 16
Compliance
  as pathogenic developmental factor, 225
Concern (*see also* Depressive position; Primitive emotional development)
  and capacity for guilt, 206
  normal, and hypochondriacal worry, 87
  role of aggression in, 206–7
  stage of, and depressive position, XXI, 206–27
Conflict
  emotional, and physical illness, 4–5
  role of, in development, 3–6
Confusional states
  resulting from tantalizing early environment, 246–7
Consciousness
  transfer of, from individual to care-technique, 99
Consultations
  and case management, V
  and prospect of analytic treatment, 76
  and transference interpretation, *73*
  Child Department, V, 70
  failure of, with adolescents, 72
  value of therapeutic, V
Continuity
  conditions for establishment of, in earliest infancy, 189
  disruption of, through birth trauma, XIV
  effect of normal or traumatic birth experience on, 183
  provision of, by mother in infant care, 161

Control
   magical, and inner world, *41–3*
Couch
   meaning of analytic, in regression, 288
Countertransference
   and primitive object-needs in patients, 146–7
   and reassurance, 292–3
   hate in, XV
   met with in treatment of regressions, 280
   objective, 196
   phenomena, classification of, 196
CREAK, MILDRED, 219, 303
Creative activity
   and illusion and transitional objects, XVII, XVIII
   primary, XIX, 170, 230, 311
Crocodile
   as symbol of ruthless primitive self, 155n
Crucifixion and resurrection, 135
Culture
   and reparative potential of the individual, 94
Curiosity
   parental attitudes to sexual, *10*

DAVIES, W. H., 166
Day-dreams
   and external reality, 130
Death
   and fear of annihilation, 303
   denial of, and manic defence, 131
Defences (*see also* Anxiety; Dissociation; Manic defence; Psyche-Soma)
   against anxiety, 61, 272–4, 318
   organized ego, and false self, 281
Delinquency
   and antisocial tendency, 306
   and psycho-analysis, 306
   case histories, IX, *136–40*
   Regression to ruthlessness in, 154
   treatment of, 139
Denial
   of depression in children, 87
Dependence (*see also* Infant care; Mother; Regression: Transference)
   absolute, in infancy, *113*

denial of, by identification with environment, 247
   experience of, in regression, 297
   regression to, 284, 286–7, 290–1
Depersonalization (*see also* 'False self')
   and childhood imaginary companions, 151
   and regression to primitive emotional development, 151
   from failure in infant care, 99
Depression, 220–1
   and appetite disorders, 34
   and anxious restlessness, 87
   and ocular psychoneurosis, 86
   and transference, 146–7
   as a healing mechanism, 275
   child's, v. mother's, 92
   denial of, by false liveliness in children, 87
   distinguished from depressive position achievements, 265, 271–2, 275
   mother's, and mania in the boy, 77
   mother's defence against, and child's false reparation, 91
   reparation in respect of mother's organized defence against, VII
   suicidal elements of, in children, 88
'Depressive-ascensive', 134–5, *137*
Depressive position (*see also* Infant care; Primitive emotional development; Psyche-Soma; Regression; Transference)
   age of infant at, 263
   as factor in classification of cases, 279
   benign circle of, 269–72
   concept of, 91, 95
   developmental stages prior to, 274–5
   distinguished from depression, 265, 271–2
   effects of failures in, 271–2
   in treatments, 139–41
   its relation to manic defence, XI
   value of, to family life, 94
Deprivation
   and antisocial tendency, 309–10
   and depressive position, 310
Deprived child, 309
Destructive impulses
   and guilt, 65
   and inner reality, 61

Destructiveness
  and antisocial tendency, 310
  as testing of environment, 310
  fears of, 36
Devaluation
  in manic defence, 132
Development (*see also* Depressive position; Infant care; Primitive emotional development; Psyche-Soma)
  enrichment of, by unwellness, 4
  from conflict, 4
Devotion (*see* also 'Primary maternal preoccupation'; Psyche-Soma)
  mother's, in infant care, 220
Diagnostic interviews
  as miniature analytic treatments, 159
  failure of, through rigidity, *169*
  fruitful only as therapeutic interviews, *159*
Diarrhoea, 62
  v. 'hesitation phase' in 'set situation', 62
Diary-keeping
  as projection of mental apparatus, *252*
Direct access
  need for, in infancy and treatment, *167–9*
Disillusionment
  and weaning, 221, 240
Disintegration, 99
  and primary unintegration, 98, 149–50, 155
  as a defence, 98
  regressive, 149
Displacement
  of feeling from self to care-technique, 99
Dissociation (*see also* 'False self'; Infant care; Psyche-Soma; Regression), 152
  and unintegration, 151
  and waking life of infant, 152
Doctor
  and children's growth, 4
  attitude of, to psychological symptoms, 4–5, 102
  role of, and hypochondria in mothers, 88
Dreams, 96, *185–6*
  analyst's, *197–8*

and dissociation, 151
and magic, *110–11*
and reality-contact, 171–*172*
dealing with withdrawal states, *259–60*
manic defence in, *141*
Drug-addiction, 34

Earth
  and mother, 97
Eating
  and greed, 33
Education
  and childhood conflict, 4
Ego (*see also* 'False self'; Infant care; Mother; Psyche-Soma; Regression)
  assimilation into, of 'mother holding the situation', 271
  beginnings and primitive threats of annihilation, 304
  development at the start of antisocial tendency, 313–4
  development from analyst's adaptation in transference, 298
  development, role of aggressiveness at various stages of, 205–6
  disruption by prenatal reactions to traumata, *182–3*
  disturbances derived from birth trauma, 187
  early developments of, and role of environment, 283
  establishment and 'Primary maternal preoccupation', 303–4
  extremely immature, effects of acute environmental impingements on, 185, 303
  maturation, essential for the capacity to hate, 201
  maturity and immaturity, 305
  -needs and maternal care, 312
  -needs emerge from body-needs, 304
  observing, in regressions, 289
  organization enabling regression, 281
  organized-ego-defence mechanism in 'false self' and regression, 281
  primitive beginnings of, and good-enough environment, 213–4
  processes and instinctual experiences in infancy, 268n

-relatedness and 'Primary maternal preoccupation', 304

-relatedness provided by therapist in treatment of antisocial tendency, 315

role in transference-neurosis, 295

strengthened by normal birth experience, 181

surrender of true self to, through regression, 286–7

Ego-nuclei
primitive, and effect of birth experience, *184–5*, 186–8

Ego-split
and squint, *89–90*

Ego-spontaneity
role of aggression in, 217

Elation
and denial of inner reality, 133

Emotional development (*see also* Conflict; Primitive emotional development; Psyche-Soma; Regression)
aggression in relation to, XVI
and anxiety, 5
depressive position in, XXI

Emotional disorder
and appetite, III, 33

Encephalitis lethargica, 20

End of hour
and hate in the analyst, 197
and primitive emotional experience, 147
anxiety about, *142*

Enuresis, 5
and antisocial tendency, 313
and regression, *108ff*, 115–16
case history, Philip, IX, *103ff*

Environment
as adverse aetiological factor, *8–10*
assessment of role of, in analyses, 176
early, assessment of its role in classification of cases, 279
early, failure and regression, 281
effects of perfect v. bad, in infancy, 245
effects of tantalizing early, 246–7
its significance for antisocial tendency, 309, 311
necessity for perfect, in infancy, 162
perfect, and psyche-soma development, XIII, XXIV, 244

reactive to individual abnormality, *47*

role of, in early ego-development, 283

role of, in infancy, 300

'Environment-individual set-up' (*see also* Narcissism), XVII, 99
as matrix of primary narcissism, 266
beginnings of individual in, 221–2
diagrams of, 223
schizoid states and failures of, 222

Envy, 65

Epistaxis, 16

Equilibrium
disturbances of, and vertigo, 97
homeostatic, 300–1

Erotic experiences
and fusion with aggression, 214–18
conditions for satisfaction of early, 215
leading to sense of unreality, 213

Erotization
of aggression v. fusion of motility and erotic potential, 213

Excitement (*see also* Manic defence)
and eyes, 87
and organ changes, 17
anxiety about, *12*

Exhaustion (*see also* Psycho-analyst; Regression)
in treatment of delinquents, *138–40*, 214

Expectation
infant's, and external reality, 163, 169–70

External reality
advantages from acceptance of, 153
and fantasy, 129–30, 133
and illusion, 152
and illusion in infancy, 163
and primitive greed, 163
and psychoses, 152
as ballast to fantasy, 153
as part of self, 155
contact with, in quiet periods in infancy, 163
flight to, 133
primary relation to, and integration, 152
true relation to, and transference, 152
v. inner reality, 129, 133

External (not-me) objects
  aggressive component drives to first
    need for, 215, 217
External world
  in infant experiences, 98–100
Eye, VI
  and emotional conflict, 18
  and guilt, 18
  and hypochondria, 87
  and projection, 90
  and sadness, 87
  as substitute-organ, 87
  psychological illness and, 86
  rest of, in sleep, 89
  role in defence against depression, 88
  significance of, 85
  symbolic activities of, 90
  symptoms and guilt, 87
  tiredness of, 87
Eye-rubbing
  and depression, 86

Faecal retention
  absence of, 48
  enjoyment of, 48
'Failure situations'
  and fixation, 282
  'freezing' of, 281–2
  instinctual v. environmental, 282–3
  regression to, 282–3
FAIN, MICHEL, 204n, 211
Fainting (see also Unconscious—physical), 16
FAIRBAIRN, W. RONALD D., 229n, 269n
'False self'
  and compliance, 225
  and sense of futility, 286
  and transference, 296–9
  as care-taker self, 71–2, 281
  as ego-defence organization, 281, 292
  development through failure of in-
    fant care, 100
  early development of, 280
Fantasy
  and anxiety, 17
  and external reality, 129–30
  and frustration, 153
  and functional experience of body, 48
  and inner world experiences, 35
  and instinctual experiences, 146

and pain, 35
and psyche, 244
as imaginative elaboration of functions, 267–278, 316
flight from, to reality, 41
in early infancy, 60–1
more primary than reality, 153
of birth distinguished from memory
  of birth, 186–91
omnipotent, and denial of inner
  reality, 130
oral, placing of, inside body, 34
role in hypochondria, 146
role in psycho-analysis, 146
v. fantasying, 130n, 153
Father
  conflict about, 50
  importance of, in development, 113
  in inner reality, 131
  's role in consultation, 64, 77
Fear
  lack of, 41
Feeding (see also 'First feed') III, XVI
  experience, various implications of,
    268–9
Feeding disturbances, III, XVI
  paediatrics and infant care, 164–5
Feelings
  denial of expression of, in manic
    defence, 134
Fetishes
  and transitional objects, 236–7, 241–2
Fidgetiness (see also Manic Defence)
  II, 28
  and anxiety, 12, 15
  and anxious excitement, 22
  and character-formation, 23
  and chorea, 22
  and conflict over masturbation, 14
  and mastery of anxiety, 23
  and tics, 22
  causes of, 22–3
  from anxiety, 14
  symptoms accompanying, 23
'First feed'
  diagram, 223
Fits, 16
Fixation
  points and 'freezing of failure situa-
    tions', 282–3

Foetus
and experience of birth, 175
role of motility, aggression and life-
force in, 216–17
Folklore, 7
FREUD, ANNA, 50, 98, 147, 160, 209n,
221, 239n, 266, 269n, 296, 300, 301
FREUD, SIGMUND, 7, 54n, 58, 60–1, 64,
67–9, 157, 174–5, 180–2, 191,
200–1, 221, 231, 237, 237n, 247n,
263, 275, 278–9, 284, 284n, 285–6,
295, 306, 318, 321
FRIEDLANDER, KATE, 160
Frustration
and fantasy, 153
and infant's needs, 301
and splitting of objects into good and
bad, 207
experience of, in early infancy, 300,
304
need for, by reality, 4, 211
v. graduated failure, 216
Fusion
v. de-fusion, or erotic and aggressive
components, 214–7
Futility, 305
sense of, from loss of true self,
161–8, 212

Games (see also Spatula game; Squiggle
game)
manic-defence in, 136–9
Genital organs
and emotional development, 7–8
Giving
first, of infants, 269
Glasses
and need for punishment, 86
GLOVER, EDWARD, 95, 225
'Good breast'
examination of the concept, 276
'Good-enough environment'
experiences essential, 67
quality of, 67
role in primitive ego development,
213–4
wholeness of, 67
'Good mother'
compulsion to be, to others, 247

Grabbing
inhibition of, a symptom, 60
Grasping
inhibition of, and feeding difficulties,
50
in infancy, 147
Greed, III, XVI
and appetite, 33, 39–40
and destructive impulses, 65
and ego-experiences, 33
as symptom of anxiety, 33
case histories, 37–51
craving for medicines and, 34n
inhibition of, and its results, 34n, 38,
51
relation to love and hate, 33
symptoms of, 38
Greediness
and anxiety, 33
as symptom of antisocial tendency,
311–12
GREENACRE, PHYLLIS, 174n, 175–6, 180,
190, 301
Grief
and depressive position, 275
Group
individual's role in, based on capacity
for personal guilt, 96
-life v. individuality, 94–5
work with, 94
Guilt
and aggressive and destructive impulses, 91
and eye-symptoms, 87
and manic defence, 143–4
and physical illness, 21
and reparation, 91
and stage of concern, 206
and symptom-formation, 19
capacity for, 96
-feelings, roots of, in instinctual
attack on mother, 270
from projection of reactions to early
environmental impingements, 248
mother's unconscious, and child's
false reparation, 91
personal, and group-participation, 96
personal, and reparation to scientific
groups, 96
personal source of, 270

roots in early destructive impulses, 65
-sense and affectionateness, 271

Hallucination
and creative potential of first feed, 223
and external reality, 152–3
and illusion, 152–3
and mother's breast, 152–3
and regression, 97
as vehicle of instinct tension in infancy, 163
role in primitive emotional development, 154
Hands
and breast-play in infancy, 165–6
HARTMANN, HEINZ, 211
HASKELL, ARNOLD, 93
Hate
capacity to, based on ego maturation, 201
child's need to be hated, *199–200*, 202
coincident love and hate in psychotics, 195–6
in the countertransference, XV
justified, in analytic setting, 196
mother's initial, of infant, 201–2
non-existent in very primitive ego experience, 210
unconscious v. objective hate, 196–7
Head
as remembered in birth experience, 186–7
significance of placing mind in, 247, *250*, 252
Headache, 15, 247
cause of, in birth trauma, 186
in analysis, *260*
Helplessness
and aggression, 207
experience of, in traumatic birth, 184–6
HERMANN, IRME, 98
Heterosexuality
compulsive and manic defence, 133
History-taking, III, 45
paediatric, 158
HOFFER, WILLI, 231
'Homeostatic equilibrium', 300–1

Homosexuality
father's unconscious, and child's reaction, *79*
Hope
implied in antisocial tendency, 309, 314
role of, in regression, 283
Hopelessness
about attaining personal life, 184
Hostels
the value of, 314
Hostility
unconscious, and hysterical symptoms, 18–9
Humour
and acknowledgement of inner world fantasies, *35*
Humpty Dumpty, 226
Hunger
in infancy and object-expectancy, 163
Hyperaemia, 17
Hyperaesthesia, 17
Hypnotism, 16
Hypochondria, 34
and denial of fantasy, 133
and fantasy of internal objects, 146
and manic defence, 133
mother's v. child's, 88
of the mother, and outpatient children's clinic, 92
Hypochondriacal
pains and inner anxieties, 62
worry and normal concern, 87
Hypomanic patient, 195
Hysteria
masking madness, 100

Id experience (*see also* Depressive position; Instinctual experience)
and motility, 211–12
pre-history of aggression in earliest, 211–12
Id impulse
and concern about love object, 270–1
Id satisfaction
and fear of annihilation, 153
frustration of, and reactive aggression, 210
Idealization
pathological, of good breast, 276

Ideals
  achievement of, and early development, 8
Identification
  in false reparation, 91
  male, in a girl, *121*
  male, in mother interferes with 'Primary maternal preoccupation', 302
  of mother with infant, 300–1
  with environment and denial of dependence, 247
  with the aggressor, 209n
Identity
  loss of, through reactions, 184
  personal, and role of failure, 93
ILLINGWORTH, RONALD S., 232
Illness (*see also* Conflict; Unwellness)
Illusion (*see also* Psyche-Soma; Transitional object)
  and transitional objects and phenomena, XVIII
  and transitional object, diagram, 239–40
  as link between psyche and environment, diagram, 223–4
  in infancy, art and religion, 230–1
  merging of external reality and hallucination in, 154
  mother's role in establishing, in infancy, 163
  provided by mother's 100 per cent adaptation, 238–9
  requirements for provision of, 154
  results from infant-expectation being met by external reality, 169–70
  role and experience of, in early infancy, XIII
  role in primitive emotional development, 152
Imaginary companions
  childhood, and depersonalization, 151
Imagination
  impoverishment from inhibition of greed, *49*
Impingements
  early, leading to pathological reactions, diagrams, 222–4
  from birth trauma, 183–4
  leading to set reaction patterns, 183–4

reaction to, and loss of true self, 211–13
Impulsiveness
  and motility, 204–5, 211, 213–14
  and ruthless love, 265
  inability to attain, *255*
Incontinence
  as dissociation, 152
Incorporation
  psychic and physical, of objects, 46–8
Indebtedness
  unawareness v. acknowledgement of, 230
Individual differentiation
  beginnings of, 99
Indulgence
  and mother love, 312–13
Infancy
  development in early, 162
  pre-object-relationship stage in, 163
Infants
  basis of health or ill-health in emotional development of, 159
  development of, before six months, 147–8
  development of, at 5–6 months, 148–9
  symptoms of psychiatrically ill, 170–1
  their need of hate in mother, 202
  their ways of dealing with graduated maternal failure, 238
Infant care, XIII, XIX
  and 'Primary maternal preoccupation,' XXIV, 303
  and psychiatry, *166–8*
  as agent of personality integration, 150
  disruptions of, relived in analysis, *166–70*
  essentials of, 160–1
  failure in, and three types of anxiety, 98–9
  failures of, result in splitting, 170
  graduated failure of perfect adaptation v. frustration in, 215–16, 301
  importance of own mother in, 153
  link with care of mentally sick, 158
  mother's handling of quiet and excited states in, 266–8

role of good-enough, in neutralizing earliest anxieties, 99
techniques of, 98
understanding of, and transference, 286–7, 295–9
Infant-mother relationship, 98
and 'Primary maternal preoccupation', XXIV
earliest, 154
Infant observation, III, *45*
and spatula game, III, 45–8, 51
and transitional objects and phenomena, XVIII
descriptions of clinic setting, 52–4
in a 'set situation', IV, 52
Inhibitions
of instinct from failure of depressive position, 271
Inner reality, 230
and depressive anxiety, 129
and fantasy, 130
and transference, 132
denial of, and manic defence, 129, 131–3
good and bad, 61
partial recognition of, 133
v. external reality, 61, 129
Inner world (*see also* Depressive position; Manic defence; Primitive emotional development; Psyche-Soma)
and anxiety, 35
and magical control, *42*
and oral fantasy, 34
and spatula game, 47
development of, 269–72
fantasies of, and physical disease, 35
good and bad objects in, *37*
growth of, 207–8
harm from clinical exposure of fantasies of, 36
impoverishment of, from inhibition of oral fantasy, *48*
over-control of, 35
role of aggression in growth of, 207
Insane
emotional burden in the care of the, 194–5
Insecurity
and anxiety, VIII

Inside
anxiety about, following instinctual experiences, 268–9
significance of, 130
Instinct
and depressive position, XXI
and ego-development in infancy, 305
cure of de-fusion of, element in anti-social tendency, 311
-development and regression, 282–3
genital, and neurosis, 318
interplay of, primary environment and self, 154–5, 155n
mastery of, and symptom-formation, 5
Instinctual experience (*see also* Illusion; Psyche-Soma; Regression)
acute, and integration of personality, 150
aggressive v. erotic roots of, and the analyst, 214
and aggression, 205
annihilation of object from satisfaction in, 153
its effect on infant's relation to mother, 268–70
Instinctual needs
and maternal care, XVIII, XXI, XXIV
mother's failure about, 312
Institute of Psycho-Analysis, 96, 320
its role as consultation clinic, 83
Integration (*see also* Depressive position; Illusion; Infant care)
from infant care and instinctual experiences, 150
in child of the split between care-taking and exciting environment made by good-enough mothering, 267–8
in earliest infancy, diagram, 226
in primitive emotional development, XVIII, XIX, XXI, XXII, *149*, 150, 152–3
Intellect (*see also* Mental activity; Mind; Psyche-Soma; Regression)
as enemy of psyche, 225
defensive exploitation of, 225
dissociated from psyche by birth trauma, 191–2
function of, to memorize primitive experiences of impingements, 191–2

role of, in making not-good-enough environmental adaptation good-enough, 225

Intellectual development
  precocious or retarded, related to false integration, 185

Internalization
  as defence mechanism, 208–9

Internal object, III, XXI, 130–1
  and manic defence, 131
  and transitional objects, 237
  denial of good, 133
  omnipotent control of, *136–44*

Interpersonal relationships, 230, 279

Interpretation
  and greed, 67
  discretion about, *114*
  in consultation, *73*
  of analyst's hate to the patient, 202–3
  of birth trauma, 180–1
  v. importance of setting in treatment, 297

Intra-uterine
  experiences, 98
  state, psyche in, 191
  state, regression to, relived in analysis, 191

Introjection
  of ego-supportive mother, 312
  leading to one-body relationship, 99

Introspection
  and manic defence, 132

Introversion, 155
  and paranoid states, 227
  and squint, 90
  return from, and aggression, 207–8

Isolation
  meaning of, in psychotic distortions, 222–3

Jealousy, *3, 4, 6, 65*
Jokes
  and denial of depressive position, *140*
JONES, ERNEST, 139, 139n, 243
JUNG, CARL G., 96, 155n, 273

KANNER, LEO, 303
King
  role of, in inner reality, 131

KLEIN, MELANIE, 33–4, 60–1, 68, 95, 129, 132n, 139n, 146n, 190, 206, 209n, 221, 226n, 237, 239n, 240, 262, 265–6, 270, 275, 301

Labour
  infant's experience during, 184

Laughter
  and depressive anxiety, *142*
  in analysis, *142*

Leucotomy, 194, 253–4, 287

Life-force
  in the foetus, 216–17

Light-headedness, 135

Lilith
  mythological figure of, 154n

LINDNER, S., 234

LITTLE, MARGARET, 192

Liveliness
  false, and denial of depression, 87

Loneliness, *80–1*

Looking
  as giving life, *142*

Loss
  reaction to, and depressive position, 275

Love (*see also* Primitive love)
  and food fads, 40
  aggression as part of primitive expression of, 205–6
  coincident love and hate from early environmental failure, 195–6
  doubt about, 40
  impoverishment of capacity for, from avoidance of guilt, 207
  mother's, of infant, 161
  ruthless, in infancy, 200–1

Love-object
  anxiety about, following instinctual experience, 268–70

MACALPINE, IDA, 244

Madness
  and infant care, 98
  fear of, 100
  in infancy, 224

Magic (*see also* Omnipotent control)
  and dreams, *110–11*
  and persecution, 227

MAHLER, MARGARET S., 300, 303

Management, XXII, XXIII, XXV
    as inherent necessity of analytic work
        with psychotics, 195–6
    in treatment of antisocial tendency,
        309
    its role in analytic treatments, 279–80
    of regression at home: case histories,
        IX, X
    v. psychotherapy, *119*
Mania
    and inner world deadness, 209
    and pneumonia, 20
    differences from manic defence, 209
    in boy, reactive to mother's depres-
        sion, *77*
Manic defence (*see also* Fidgetiness), II,
    XI
    and denial of inner reality, 129
    and depressive anxiety, 130–1
    and life, 131
    and symbolism, *135–43*
    characteristics of, 132ff
    denial of depressive position in, 272
    distinguished from mania, 209
Marital
    difficulties and inhibition of greed,
        44–5
MARTY, PIERRE, 204n, 211
Masochism
    and disturbances of fusion of early
        motility and id impulses, 213, 217
Masturbation
    and anxiety, 17
    and fidgetiness, 14
    and regression to pregenital stages, 17
    masked by flight to external reality, 133
Maternal failure
    graduated, infant's ways of dealing
        with, 238
Me and Not-me, XVIII, XXI
    role of aggression in differentiation
        of, 215–17
Medicines
    and inhibition of greed, 34n
    craving for, 34n
Melancholia, 34
Memorizing
    as a defensive function of intellect
        against persecutions, 191–2
    of birth experience, *248–50*

Memory
    true birth, 184
Mental activity
    as a thing in itself, 246–7
    as cataloguing reactions to impinge-
        ments, *246–50*
    as substitute care-taking of psyche-
        soma, 246
    excessive, based on erratic maternal
        behaviour, 246
    turns good-enough into perfect
        mothering, 245
Mental defect
    and psychosis, 225
    as result of tantalizing early environ-
        ment, 246
    case history of boy, *177–8*
    from disruption of infant care, 170
Mental disorders
    psychological basis of, 158
Mental health
    basis in mother's devotion and infant
        care, 7, 150, 219–20, 227–8
Mental structure
    complexity of, in infants, 34n
Mental v. physical
    a false distinction, 244, 254
Metapsychology
    delay in its direct application in
        treatments, 295
Micturition
    and fidgetiness, 23
    increased frequency and anxiety, *6, 8*
MIDDLEMORE, MERELL P., 158, 164
MILNER, MARION, 237n
Mimicry
    defence against derision, *106*
Mind (*see also* Mental activity)
    and its relation to psyche-soma, XIX
    in pathology usurping care-taking
        function of environment, 246
    localized in head, 247, *250*, 252
    -psyche, development of, 246–7
    theory of, 244–6
Mother (*see also* Infant care; Psyche-
        Soma; Transitional object)
    and paediatricians, 161–2
    as internal possession, 68
    as providing the setting for illusion in
        infancy, 163

as therapist in infancy, 312
as total environment of infancy, 150
as transitional object, *236*
dependence on, and vertigo, 97
false reparation and identification with, 91
fantasy of re-entry into, derived from birth trauma, *187*
importance of care by own, 153
loss of, 68
management of regression by, case histories, IX, X
meaning of actual, to infant, 160
pre- and post-natal experiences of depressed, *182-3*
reparation in respect of mother's organized defence against depression, VII
sought in the stolen object, 311
Mother's
    body and oral fantasy, 34
    depression, 140n
    depression and specific character formation in children, 91-3
    devotion, 163-4
    function to provide graduated failure of adaptation, 245-6
    hate of baby, 200-1
    hypochondria and outpatient children's clinic, 92
    hypochondria v. concern in child care, 92
    job in infant care, 160-1
    mood providing a task for the child, *93-4*
    need of moral support to enjoy infant care, 165
    task of holding a situation for infant, 263-71
    two functions in relation to excited or quiet states, 266-8
Motility   (*see   also*   Psyche-Soma; Regression)
    and aggression, 204-5
    experienced as reaction to impingements, 212-13
    failures of early fusion of, and erotic potential, basis of masochism, 213
    fusion of, with erotic potential in health, 213

role of, in id experience, 211-12
summation of motility experiences and ego-beginnings, 213-14
Mourning, 275
    and manic defence, 131
Mouth
    hallucinations of, *178*

Nail-biting, 155-6
Narcissism (*see also* Primary narcissism) 142-3
Nasal congestion
    and destructive wishes, 18
    and excitement, 15
    and rage, 15
    from prolonged excitement, 17
Needs
    distinguished from wishes in analysis, 288
    in infancy, 301
    met by analyst's active adaptation, 298-9
Negative transference
    v. objective anger about analyst's failures, 299
Nervousness
    cause of, in erotism and hostility, 20
    physical causes of, 20
Neurosis (*see* Psychoneurosis)
Neurotic people
    intolerance of triangular relationships in, 65, 288
Normality
    and anxiety, I, 3
    and unwellness, 5
Nose-picking, 18
Not-me possession
    first, XVIII
Nuisance value
    significance of, of antisocial child, 311
Nursing couple, 99, 164

Objectivity (*see also* Subjectivity)
    early roots of, 153
    in analyst's hate of the patient, *196*
    leading to loss of capacity for illusion, 171
Object relationship (*see also* Depressive position; Internal object; Primitive emotional development)

primitive, 146ff
prior to first, 99
v. object-expectancy in primitive instinct tension, 163
Objects
splitting into good and bad, 207, 207n
Object-seeking
in antisocial tendency, 310
Obsessional neurosis
and cataloguing of reactions to impingements, 247–8, 247n
Ocular psychoneurosis (*see also* Psychoneurosis)
and depression, 86
and personality structure, 86
of childhood, VI, 85
Oedipus complex, 262, 277
and fixation points, 282–3
and neurosis, 7, 318
Omnipotence (*see also* Manic defence)
infantile and antisocial tendency, 311
Omnipotent control
and magic, 227
and manipulation in manic defence, 132
One-body relationship
capacity for, 99
Ophthalmologists
and psychology, *85*
Opposition
need for, in aggression, 214–16
Oral erotism
and aggression, 205
intermediate area between true object relationship and, 230
Oral fantasy, 34
and 'inner world', 34
inhibition and impoverishment of 'inner world', *48*
in 'set situation', 60
of good and bad, *37*
Oral function, 34
Oral gratification, 34
role of, in development, 17
Oral instinct, 34
and infant care, 98
conflict over, in spatula play, 49
Oral sadism
analysis of, and lessening of inner persecution, 273

Organ changes
from excitement, 17
Orgasm, 17

Paediatrics
and childhood neurosis, XXVI
and exploitation of 'false self', 225
and mental health, 219–20
and psychiatry, XIII
and psycho-analysis, 319–21
and 'support-without-interference' for mothers, 161–2
clinical, and emotional conflicts, 5
prophylaxis against psychosis responsibility of, 228
symptom tolerance in, case history, IX
Paranoia
congenital (not inherited) resulting from severe birth trauma, *185–6*, 190
problem of analytic handling of pre-oral factors in, 190
Paranoid defensive organization
case history, X
Paranoid position (Klein), 226n
and birth trauma, 190
Paranoid state
and first integration of self, 99, diagram, 226–7
and introversion, 227
Parents
on helping, 308
Patient's
fantasies of analyst, 195
need of object hate in the analyst, 199
wishes as needs, 202–3
Penis envy
and stealing, *75*
Perception
objective and subjective, and transitional objects, 241
objective v. subjective sight, 88
Persecution
and depression, 275
and depressive position, 275
derived from de-fusion of primitive aggressive and erotic components, 215–18
patterns of, set by birth trauma, 189–90

Persecutory anxiety, IV, VI, XI, XVI, XXI, *136–8*

Person
start of being a, 98–9

Personality-development
divisible into three parts, 217
normal, and reparation, 91

Personality-structure
and ocular psychoneurosis, 86
wholeness of, as factor in classification of cases, 279–80

Personalization, XII
in primitive emotional development, *149*, 151

Perversions (*see also* Fetishes; Masochism; Transitional object)
possible cause in chest memories of birth trauma, 187–8

Physical changes
from emotional causes and conflicts, 13–14, *15*, 16–17

Physical disease
and emotional disturbances, 5, *12*

Physical health
and emotional strain, 3
and unconscious conflicts, 5

Physical illness
as criterion of emotional ill-health, 5
from emotional conflict, 13
its use for emotional growth, 103–4
relation to 'inner world' fantasies, 35

Placement
v. psycho-analysis of delinquents, *306–7*

Play
and giving (depressive position), 271
and transitional phenomena, 241
body-memories of birth experiences in children's, *177–8*, 180
schizoid child's, 227
with breast in infancy, 165–6
working through of defences against depressive anxiety in, 69, 274–5

Pleasure
and injury to love-object, 155

Pleasure-principle, 237

Possession (*see also* Transitional objects)
capacity for, of object, XVIII, 68

Potency, 270–1

Pre-concern stage
in primitive emotional development, III, XII, XVI, XVIII, XXI, XXIV, 154–5
of ego-development and aggression, 206

Pregnancy
fantasies, their defensive function, 36
mother's, child's reaction to, *3, 73*

Prenatal (*see also* Psyche-Soma; Regression)
emotional development and later ego-strength, 182
experiences in regression in analysis, *248–50*

Pressure
its meaning as love, *250*

Primal scene
in spatula play, 50

Primary creativity (*see also* Transitional objects)
and antisocial tendency, 311

Primary identification
and transference, 295

'Primary maternal preoccupation', XXIV, 184n
and ego-relatedness in infants, 304
and society's role with antisocial children, 303
definition of, 302
disturbances of, 302–3

Primary narcissism (*see also* 'Environment-individual set-up')
and absolute dependence, XVII, 262
and motility, 211–12
and reactions to impingements, 212
and regression in analysis, 286
as the earliest 'environment-individual set-up', XVII, 266

Primary process (*see also* Process), 295
following of, in transference, 297–8

Primitive emotional development, III, XII, XIV, XV, XVIII, XIX, XXIV, XXV
diagrams of, 223–6
effects of perfect or bad environment on, 245
possibilities for observation of, in analysis, 221
three processes of, 149

Primitive love
 and pre-ruth stage, 210
 as greed, 163
 roots of the destructive elements in, 211
 ruthless, in infancy, 200–1
Process
 following patient's, in analysis, 278
 respect for, by active adaptation in therapy, 222–3
Projection
 and eyes, 90
 of early environmental impingements as source of guilt, 248
Prophylaxis, XXVI, 228, 319
 in child care, 4
Pseudologia fantastica
 and transitional phenomena, 242
Pseudo-maturity
 and 'false self', 225, 296
Psyche
 definition of, 244
 dissociation of, from intellect, 191–2
 in intra-uterine state, 191
 intellect as enemy of, 225
 lodging of, in body, 226
 seduction of, into mind-psyche, 247
Psyche-Soma, XIV, XVI, XVII, XVIII, XXII
 early development of (diagrams), 222–6
 mind and its relation to, XIX
 perfect environment an absolute need of early development of, 245
 split in, from infant-care failures, 99
Psychiatric illness
 roots in early infancy, 51
Psychiatry
 and countertransference, 195
 and infant care, 166–70
 and psycho-analysis, 194–5
 and study of mental illnesses, 171
 and treatment of psychotics, 194–5
 paediatrics and, XIII
Psychic reality, 129n
Psycho-analysis, 7
 and infant observation, 37–8
 and delinquency, 306
 and paediatrics, 102–3, 164, 319–21, XXVI

and placement problems of delinquents, 306–7
and research in psychoses, 145, 221
and the unconscious, 61
and treatment of psychoses, 287
assessment of various environmental factors in, 176
cf. 'set situation', 67
classification and choice of cases for, 278–9
contra-indications for, V, 309, 315
features of birth material in, 189, 192
idea of, as art v. study of regressions, 291
its help to psychiatry, 194–5
management of primitive infant-care aspects in, 167–70
not indicated for treatment of anti-social tendency, 309, 315
of adolescents, 169
of artists, 133
of neurotics v. that of psychotics, 196–7
of normal adults: research value, 159
of religious patients, 133
patient's feverish pleasure in, 140
problems of 'false self' met with in, 213
provision of special environment in, 166–70
reliving of birth-experience in, of a psychotic boy, 177–8
role of mother's mood in, 93
three types of, 146
treatment v. technique in, 278
Psycho-analyst
 actively presenting good mothering, 281–2
 and mother's hypochondriacal anxiety, 92
 as parent-substitute in therapy, 93–4
 as patient's 'creation', 169
 attitude of, to depressive position, 264
 attitudes of various analysts to regression, 290–1
 behaviour of, in analytic setting, 284–6
 coincident love and hate of, in psychotics, 195–6

comparative strain on, whether meeting aggressive or erotic roots of patients' impulses, 138–40, 214

fantasies about, in various illnesses, 146–7

handling of patient's primary process by, 297–8

hate of, of psychotic patient compared to mother's hate of baby, 201–2

healing dreams of, *197–8*

importance of infant-care aspects for, 295–6

incorporating the, *73*

patient's compliance with analyst's unconscious demand, 95–6

patient's fantasies of, *73*, 195

patient's use of failures of, 298

role of, in handling a parent's mood in patients, 94

strain on, in handling regressions, 298–9

subjectivity and objectivity in, 95

success of, with treatment through displacing depressed parent, 94

survival of, as dynamic factor in treatments, 279

Psycho-analytic setting (*see also* Birth trauma; Transference)

as a medium, *256–60*

examination of Freud's, 284–6

in regression, XXII, 297

in regression, represents mother with her technique, 286–94

more important than interpretation in regression, XXII, 297

recapitulation of birth trauma in, XIV, 181

regression within, XXII

role of, in withdrawal states, XX, XXII, XXIII

role of management in, 279, *280–*

Psychoneurosis, 284

aetiology in childhood, 7, 101–2, 157, 316–17

and anxiety, 317

and Oedipus complex, 318

and patterns of defence, 317

childhood, and paediatrics, XXVI

ocular, of childhood, VI

prevention of, 319

treatment of, 319

Psychosis (*see also* Psychotic patient)

aetiology of, in infancy development, 157

an environmental deficiency disease, 246

analysis of, 145

and child care, XVII

and environmental failure, 286

and infancy emotional development, 149

closely related to health, 284

in childhood, *81–2*, 219

organized v. chaotic illness in, 287

prophylaxis of, responsibility of paediatricians, 228

spontaneous recovery from, 283

Psychosomatic

disorders, 244, 254

disorders and birth trauma, 186–8, 191

Psychotherapy

through case-management, 85

through management at home, *115ff*

v. tolerance of symptoms, 86

Psychotic behaviour

in a girl, 121–2

Psychotic patient

analyst's dream about, *197–8*

analyst's hate in treatment of, XV

concreteness of analyst's behaviour for, 198–9

management of coincident love and hate in, 195–6

objective countertransference in the analysis of, 196

psychiatric treatments of, 194–5

Punishment

denial of, *42–3*

Rage, 15

RANK, OTTO, 185

Reaction (*see also* Psyche-Soma; Regression), XIV, XV, XIX, XXI, XXII

accumulation of, instead of real self experiences, 216–17

and loss of identity, 184

mental cataloguing of, to impingements, *247–50*

patterns and birth-experience, 182–3
to impingements as pathogenic factor
in primitive emotional development, *182–3*, 184–5
READ, GRANTLY DICK, 176
Reading
and emotional use of eyes, 88–9
compulsive, and thumb-sucking,
156
Real
feeling of the, roots in infancy, 171,
304–5
Reality (*see also* External reality; Inner
reality, XVIII, XXI
flight to, 130
shared, need for, from infancy to
adult life, *163–70*
Reality-testing, 230, 240
Realization, XII
in primitive emotional development,
149
Reassurance
and countertransference, 292–3
and regression, 292–3
children's reaction to, 88
use of opposites, 134
Regression, XX, XXII
advantages from, in analysis, 261
and enuresis, 115–16, case history, IX,
X
and reassurance contrasted, 292–3
and value of acting out, 288–90
as a healing mechanism, 293
as organized return to early dependence, 284, 286–7, 290–1
breakdown of identifications with
analyst in, 202
dealt with by management at home,
case history, IX
difference between *wishes* and *needs*
in, 288
distinguished from withdrawal and
split states, 283
distinguished from withdrawal states
in analysis, XX
from anxiety in infancy, 148
in analysis, *248–52*
in analytic setting, *255–61*
in analytic setting, of mother's technique in infant care, 285–6

in respect of instinct development v.
early environment failures, 282–3
in search of the true self, *280*
lack of anxiety at, and madness, 100
meaning of, 280–1, 283
not infantile behaviour, 281
organization in the individual to
enable, 281
to dependence and importance of
analytic setting, 297
to dependence, importance of, in
analytic treatment, 192–3
to dependence v. regression in respect
of erotogenic zones, 255
to fixation (id) points, *282*
'unfreezing' of 'failure situations' in,
281–2, 287
vicissitudes of observing ego in, 289
within psycho-analytic set-up, XXII
Religion, 135
and illusion, 224
in analytic treatment, 133
Reparation (*see also* Depressive position), XII, XVIII, XXI, 61
and creativeness, 91
and guilt, 91
and mother's organized defence
against depression, VII, 91
capacity for, in healthy personality, 91
false, 91
false, and failure among students,
92–3
false, and identification with mother,
91
false v. personal guilt, 96
in relation to a group, 96
in relation to instinctual experiences,
269–70
v. magical re-creation, 264
Repression
and instinctual development, 317–18
and manic defence, 130
and psychoneurosis, 157
of male identification in a girl, *121–3*
Research
in analysis and self-analysis, 196
into emotional development: various
approaches, 158–9
Resistances
existence of, good prognosis, 213

Responsibility
impoverishment of personal, 95
Restlessness (see also Fidgetiness;
Manic defence)
and anxiety, 22, 36–8
anxious, and depression, 87
manic, different from persecutory, 272
symptoms of anxiety, 12
Restitution, XXI
false, through escape into mother's
depression, 92
Retaliation
role in primitive object relationship,
155
Rheumatic aches
from anxiety, 12–14
Rheumatic fever, 20
RICKMAN, JOHN, 99, 221
RIVIERE, JOAN, 33, 141, 211, 240
ROBERTSON, JAMES, 231
Ruthlessness, XII, XV, XVI, XXI
as stage in infancy development, 265
change from, to ruth, in depressive
position, 265–6
in primitive infant-mother relationship, 154–5
RYCROFT, CHARLES, 97–8, 100

Sadism, 213, 217
Sadness, 111
and eyes, 87
Sanity
defensive, 150, 150n
flight to, 287
Satisfaction, XXI, XXIV
and annihilation of object, 153–4
as being fobbed off, 154n, 268
SCHILDER, PAUL, 98
SCHMIDEBERG, MELITTA, 139
Schizoid
-character, without depressive position achievement, 264
-personality and thumb-sucking, 156
-personality cases, 171
-states, roots of, in disturbances of
earliest infancy, 222–3
-states, definition and diagram of,
226–7
-types and set interviews, 169

Schizophrenia (see also Psyche-Soma;
Psychosis, Regression; Schizoid)
analysis of, in experimental stage, 159
and feeding-disturbances of infancy,
165
an environmental deficiency disease,
162
case histories, 168–9
SCOTT, W. CLIFFORD M., 222n, 232n,
243, 251
Screaming
and anxiety in childhood, 4, 7
SEARL, NINA, 130
SECHEHAYE, M. A., 205n, 297
Seduction
of psyche into mind, 246–7, 254
Self (see also Depressive position;
'False self'; Psyche-Soma; Regression), XIII, XVII, XVIII, XIX,
XXI
-analysis, and countertransference in
treatment of regressions, 280, 284
and instinct: Jungian v. Freudian
hypothesis, 155n
conditions for beginning of true,
182–3
imaginative, development of, 244
localization of, in own body, 149
operating from kernel or shell, 98–9
true, hidden through reaction to environmental impingements, 212
Self-criticism
lack of, and manic defence, 132
Sensitivity
heightened, in mothers, XXIV, 302
Sensuality
and denial of inner deadness, 131
exploitation of, in anxiety, 48
Sentimentality, 202
Separation anxiety
and spatula play, 57–8, 68
'Set situation'
and analytic situation, 55
and relation to both parents, 66, 66n
and relation to internalized mother,
68–9
anxiety in, 59
asthmatic attack in an infant in, 58
behaviour in, 64
case histories, 52–, 58–60, 62

complexity of, 64
infant observations in, IV, 52
'moment of hesitation' in, 53–4, 56
role of primary oral fantasy in, 60
therapeutic possibilities of, 55
therapeutic role of, 66–7
Sex obsession
in a boy, *138–40*
Sexual enlightenment, *10–11*
Sexual intercourse
aggressive and erotic elements in, 218
Sibling rivalry
value of, *3*
Sight
value of, 85
Sleep
and intra-uterine existence, 175
as withdrawal state in analysis, *255–60*
deep, and depersonalization, 151
dissociation between, and waking in infancy, 151
disturbance and fidgetiness, 23
disturbance of, from anxiety, *5–7*
in analysis, and birth experience, 178–9
Social activity
based on personal guilt, 207
Society
danger to, from repressed personal aggressiveness, 204
Somnambulism
as dissociation, 152
Soul
conception of, and illusion, 154
Spatula game (*see also* 'Set situation')
III, IV, *45*, 63–4
and mastery of separation anxiety, 68
and observation of infants in a 'set situation', IV
and primal scene, 50
and relation to internalized mother, 68
and super-ego, 59–60
breast-significance of spatula in, 63–4
case histories, III, IV
cf. Freud's description of cotton-reel play in a child, 68
deviations from normal in, 56
importance of father-role in, 50

meaning of spatula in, 63–4
normal stages of, IV, 53–4
SPENCE, PROFESSOR SIR JAMES, 164
SPITZ, RENÉ, 221, 265
Splitting
basic, in personality development, diagram, 224–5
defence against guilt, 207
into good and bad objects, 207, 207n
relived in transference, 170
resulting from failure of infant care, 170
Spontaneity
and aggression, 217
and ego experience, 217
and motility, 204–5
Spontaneous recovery
in psychosis v. neurosis, 283–4
'Squiggle game'
in interview technique, *108ff*
Squint, 88–9
and acute introversion, 90
and split in ego, *89–90*
and unintegration in personality, 90
as dissociation, 152
cf. thumb-sucking, 88–9
Stealing
and antisocial tendency, *36–8*, 310
and regression, case history, IX
and search for mother in stolen object, 311
and transitional objects, 242
STEVENSON, OLIVE, 236
Students
failure among, and false reparation, 92–3
suitability of child cases for analytic, 74, 82–3
Success
breakdown after, and dependence on parents, 93
fear of mother stealing, 93
Suffocation
wish for, suicide and murder, 188
Suicide, 34, 188
and accident-proneness, 209
Super-ego (*see also* Depressive position; Primitive emotional development)
XII, XXI, 59–60
Surrealism, 35n

Suspended animation
as manic defence, 133
Suspicion, 72
and inhibition of greed, *40-1*
and spatula-play, *49*
Symbiosis, 301
Symbolism
and illusion, XVIII
and manic defence, *135-43*
and transitional object, 233-4
Symbols
examples of, 136
their role in neurotic v. psychotic patients, 199
Symptom-formation
and anxiety, *4-5*
and developmental conflicts, 5
as a defence against guilt, 19
due to environmental changes, *8*
Symptoms
as an SOS, 102
in mammals v. human beings, 5
multiplicity of, *11-13*
positive evaluation of, in child psychiatry, IX, 102
value of, and their role in psychotherapy, 86
violent, normal in childhood, 71
Symptom tolerance
in paediatrics, *IX*

TAYLOR, JAMES M., 134
Technique (*see also* Psycho-analysis; Psycho-analytic setting; Regression; Transference)
developments in, XII, XIV, XV, XX, XXII, XXIII, XXV, 146
Termination of analysis
and working through of depressive position, 143
Testing out (*see also* Antisocial tendency; Hate)
of love and hate in environment by children and psychotics, *199-200*
Thinness
result of anxiety, 13-14
Throat
hysterical symptoms of, 18-19
Thumb-sucking
and auto-erotism, 155-6

and hate, 155
and loss of object, 156
and primitive object-love, 155-6
and transitional phenomena, 231-2
Tics, 23-4
and fidgetiness, 22
Time
and the regressed patient, 288
importance of, factor in depressive position, 262-3
-sense in infancy and psychosis, 149
Toys
small, significance of, 139n
Transference (*see also* Countertransference; Psycho-analytic setting; Regression) VIII, XI, XII, XIV, XV, XVII, XX, XXII, XXIII, XXV
allowing past to *be* present in, 297-8
analyst's cashing in on good early relationships of the patient in, 198-9
and ambivalence, 146-7
and analysis of pre-depressive relationships, 147
and depression, 146-7
and depressive position, 273
and failure of early fusion of erotic and aggressive elements, 214-15
and inner reality, 132
and primary identification, 296
and primary relation to reality, 152
and problem of mother's mood in patient, 93
and psychosis, 150
and unintegration states, 150
as narcissistic state, *142-3*
clinical varieties of, XXIII
effects of good-enough adaptation by analyst in, 298
experience of depressive position in, 271
mother-role in, 141
need for direct access in, *167-70*
negative v. objective anger in patients, 299
-neurosis, and role of ego, 296
-neurosis, and Oedipus complex and fixations, *282*
primitive splitting relived in, 170

problem of 'age of patient' in, 181–2
recapitulation of primitive infant-care experiences in, 166–70
regression as withdrawal states in, *255–61*
repetition of parental depression in, 95–6
significance of infant care in, 295
Transitional objects
and illusion, 154; diagram, 223
and transitional phenomena, XVIII
as early stages of the use of illusion, 239
description of, 231–2
importance of the actuality of, 233
main function of, diagram, 239–40
metapsychological observations on, 236–7
relationship to internal object, 237
special qualities in relationship to, 233
typical, and distorted use of, *234–6*
Trauma (*see also* Psyche-Soma; Regression) XVII, XIX, XXII
actual, ill-effects of, *8–9*, 27–8
birth, birth memories and anxiety, XIV
link with fantasies, *9*
retrospective use of, 9
Treatment
management as part of, in analysis, 279, *280*
v. technique in analysis, 278
Truancy, 313
Tuberculosis, 6
Two-body relationships, 99

Unconscious (*see also* Conflict; Emotional development; Symptom-formation), 7
belief in, 10
conflict, 316
fear of, 62
following the patient's, 297–8
hostility and symptoms, 19
Unconsciousness—physical
and birth trauma, 184
as 'not-knowing', *250*
regressive meaning of, *249–52*

Unintegration, XII, XIV, XVII, XIX, XXII, XXIV, 99
in personality and squint, 90
phenomena in clinical work, 150
primary, 149
states of and infant care, 98
Unit-status
and external persecution, 18
Unreality
feeling of, and manic defence, *142*
feelings and craving for the new, 173
Unwellness
and developmental enrichment, 4
and normality, 5
Urticaria, 17

VAN GOGH, VINCENT, 172
Vasomotor skin changes, 17
Vertigo, 98
and dependence on mother, 97
and insecurity, VIII
defence against madness, 100
Vomiting
cyclic, and anxiety, I, 5, *15*, *43*

Waking
-life as dissociation, 152
Weaning (*see also* Depressive position; Transitional objects) III, XI, XVIII, XXI
and depressive position, 263, 275
and disillusionment, 163, 221
and illusion-disillusionment, 240
WHITEHEAD, A. N., 95
'Wish to be eaten'
mother's and analyst's, 276
Wishes
distinguished from *needs* in regression, 288
Withdrawal states (*see also* Introversion; Schizoid)
and regression, XX
handling of, in analysis, 255–60
meaning of, in analysis, 261
person's need for simplified setting in psychiatric care, 173
Wizard
in Philip's interview, *112–13*

Woman
    fear of, in men and women, 304
Womb
    not the inside, 36

WULFF, M., 234n, 237, 241

Zest
    and feed-experiences, 268